Methods of Group Exercise Instruction

THIRD EDITION

Carol Kennedy-Armbruster, PhD

Indiana University, Bloomington

Mary M. Yoke, MA, MM

Indiana University, Bloomington

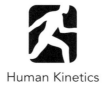

Human Kinetics

Library of Congress Cataloging-in-Publication Data

Kennedy, Carol A., 1958- author.
  Methods of group exercise instruction / Carol Kennedy-Armbruster and Mary M. Yoke. -- Third edition.
      p. ; cm.
  Includes bibliographical references and index.
  I. Yoke, Mary M., 1953- author. II. Title.
  [DNLM: 1. Physical Education and Training--methods. 2. Exercise Movement Techniques--methods. 3. Exercise. 4. Physical Fitness. QT 255]
  GV481
  613.7'107--dc23
                                        2013031977

ISBN-10: 1-4504-2189-X (print)
ISBN-13: 978-1-4504-2189-8 (print)

The web addresses cited in this text were current as of August 2013, unless otherwise noted.

Acquisitions Editor: Amy N. Tocco; **Developmental Editor:** Katherine Maurer; **Assistant Editor:** Susan Huls; **Copyeditor:** Ann Prisland; **Indexer:** Susan Hernandez; **Permissions Manager:** Dalene Reeder; **Graphic Designer:** Nancy Rasmus; **Graphic Artist:** Denise Lowry; **Cover Designer:** Keith Blomberg; **Photographer (cover):** Neil Bernstein © Human Kinetics; **Photographs (interior):** Neil Bernstein and Tom Roberts © Human Kinetics, figure 12.1 courtesy of the authors; **Photo Asset Manager:** Laura Fitch; **Visual Production Assistant:** Joyce Brumfield; **Photo Production Manager:** Jason Allen; **Art Manager:** Kelly Hendren; **Associate Art Manager:** Alan L. Wilborn; **Illustrations:** © Human Kinetics; **Printer:** Sheridan Books

We thank Indiana University in Bloomington, Indiana, for assistance in providing the location for the photo and video shoot for this book.

The video contents of this product are licensed for private home use and traditional, face-to-face classroom instruction only. For public performance licensing, please contact a sales representative at **www.HumanKinetics.com/SalesRepresentatives**.

Printed in the United States of America   10   9   8   7   6   5   4   3

The paper in this book is certified under a sustainable forestry program.

Human Kinetics
Web site: www.HumanKinetics.com

United States: Human Kinetics, P.O. Box 5076, Champaign, IL 61825-5076
800-747-4457
email: humank@hkusa.com

Canada: Human Kinetics, 475 Devonshire Road Unit 100, Windsor, ON N8Y 2L5
800-465-7301 (in Canada only)
email: info@hkcanada.com

Europe: Human Kinetics, 107 Bradford Road, Stanningley, Leeds LS28 6 AT, United Kingdom
+44 (0) 113 255 5665
email: hk@hkeurope.com

Australia: Human Kinetics, 57A Price Avenue, Lower Mitcham, South Australia 5062
08 8372 0999
e-mail: info@hkaustralia.com

New Zealand: Human Kinetics, P.O. Box 80, Mitcham Shopping Centre, South Australia 5062
0800 222 062
e-mail: info@hknewzealand.com

Contents

Part I   Fundamentals of Group Exercise Instruction

① Best Practices   3

② Social Aspects of Group Exercise   23

③ Foundational Components   35

④ Traditional Concepts   59

Part II   Primary Components of Group Exercise

Part III Group Exercise Modalities

Preface

Welcome to *Methods of Group Exercise Instruction*, 3rd Edition. The new view of group exercise is that it is more than just exercise; it is about connecting with others who want to enjoy movement experiences that enhance their health and well-being. Group exercise started over 50 years ago as *aerobics*, with an instructor leading participants. It has since evolved into a wide variety of formats that may not even contain an aerobics segment. In fact, the reason many people gravitate toward a group exercise experience is that it helps them adhere to regular movement, an increasingly important concept in light of what is called, "sitting disease," where we sit too much in our lives and at work. As our society continues to move toward sedentary life and work practices, group exercise will be even more important for improving quality of life; it is no longer just about how we look and move.

The many ways to exercise in a group include programs such as stationary indoor cycling, boot camp or sport conditioning, water exercise, kickboxing, Pilates, yoga, dance formats such as Zumba, or outdoor adventure experiences. Each decade there is another addition to the group exercise family of modalities. Group exercise programs can be found in a variety of settings, including fitness centers; workplaces; schools; universities; and community, church, and medical centers.

We anticipate that the demand for competent group fitness instructors who have the knowledge and skills to lead dynamic, safe, and effective movement experiences will only increase throughout the 21st century. Further, there is a demand for instructors who can lead more than one type of format and who can relate well to participants. Thus, group exercise instructors can enhance their marketability by becoming expert leaders in a variety of class formats and also by learning more about group dynamics in general. This book will introduce you to several common group exercise modalities and will spark your interest in creating new formats; this is essential in order for group exercise to grow and thrive. Learning the ins and outs of group movement experiences is beneficial for physical education, recreation, fitness, and dance professionals, as well as anyone passionate about helping others to lead healthy lives. Even if you are not planning to instruct group exercise, you may become a program director responsible for hiring, training, and evaluating group instructors; knowledge of class format, teaching progressions, and safety considerations will enhance your skills whether you lead experiences yourself or evaluate those who are instructors.

We believe that this book fills an important gap in the group exercise educational experience because it presents research-based information on a variety of group exercise modalities while maintaining a strong how-to, applied focus. Movement samples embedded in the book will also fire up your creativity and give you new ideas for your next class if you are already teaching group exercise. We are extremely pleased that Human Kinetics developed the accompanying online video resource to make it even easier for you to learn the practical skills necessary for leading effective group instruction. It is nearly impossible to become a competent instructor simply by reading a book; you must practice and experience the leadership and movement skills with your body as well. To that end, we have incorporated numerous devices to help you apply the information learned in our book, including practice drills and online videos. In many cases, these drills are shown in the online video as well as described in the text, so you can practice right along with the applicable video clip.

A major distinguishing feature of our book is that the information presented is based on research and best practices identified by many certifying organizations within the fitness industry. Since the early 1980s, a plethora of research has been conducted on group exercise, primarily regarding energy expenditure but also focusing on biomechanics, injury incidence, exercise adherence, and effectiveness of specific exercise programs. New research validates the importance of group dynamics for improving adherence to healthy movement. Our goal is to present scientific principles and relevant research whenever they are available; however, we are interested in making the scientific evidence come to life through our experience with the fun and fellowship of the group experience. Our first edition contained more than 250 research articles; we added another 200 + articles and citations to the second edition; and we have continued the trend with this edition, making this the most referenced group exercise book on the market.

We have divided our third edition into three parts. Part 1 focuses on the fundamentals of group exercise instruction. Part 2 focuses on movement science with a discussion of the primary components of group exercise. Finally, part 3 includes eight modalities that are common in many group exercise settings. New to this edition are a focus on the social aspects of group exercise, coaching-based approaches for classes such as boot camp and group personal training, and an enhanced emphasis on neuromotor and functional fitness training, which is part of the 2014 American College of Sports Medicine (ACSM) guidelines for exercise.

The purpose of this book is to provide you with the practical skills necessary for instructing group exercise. Numerous other texts on exercise instruction cover exercise physiology, kinesiology, nutrition, special populations, injury prevention, business matters, behavior modification, and more. Our book focuses on the nuts and bolts of instruction: the specific exercises you'll use and the techniques you'll need for moving to music, designing movement patterns in a systematic way, and cueing your participants. We'll introduce you to the most popular methods of group fitness and provide you with the basic skills required to lead.

How This Book Is Organized

The third edition of this book is divided into three parts. Part I (Fundamentals of Group Exercise Instruction) continues to provide a general overview of group exercise: the evolution and advantages of group exercise; the strategies for creating group cohesion within a class; the core concepts in class design; and the use of music, choreography, and cueing methods in designing a class. New to this section is a focus on the social aspects of group exercise, helping you understand that group exercise is more than about movement. It's also about camaraderie, friendship, and the fun of engaging in a group experience. We introduce a revised evaluation form that will be used throughout the book to evaluate group instruction, providing a template for gauging the effectiveness of the various modalities covered. Additionally, in part I we introduce communication skills, best practices, and traditional and coaching concepts.

Part II (Primary Components of Group Exercise) offers updated scientific guidelines for leading the four major segments of a group exercise: warm-up, cardiorespiratory training, muscular and neuromotor conditioning, and flexibility training. The basic concepts covered here pertain to all types of group exercise modalities. These concepts include intensity, safety, posture and alignment, anatomy, and joint actions. In chapter 8, the muscular conditioning and flexibility training chapter, we provide many specific exercises and cueing examples. This chapter covers all the major muscle groups and also includes important modifications for each exercise introduced.

Part III (Group Exercise Modalities) focuses on the practical teaching skills required for the most common modalities: kickboxing, step, stationary indoor cycling, sport conditioning, boot camp, water exercise, yoga, and Pilates. Basic moves, choreography (when applicable), and training systems are covered for each type of class. Part III is where we become modality specific; the drills, routines, and teaching skills covered are addressed on the accompanying online video as well as in the text. Many of the drills are demonstrated by an experienced instructor in the video clips, so you can practice skills such as anticipatory cueing and teaching to a 32-count phrase, as well as how to regress and progress a given movement. Also in part III, you'll find a chapter (chapter 17) on using alternative modalities. This final chapter presents practical application ideas that help you tie all the elements of group exercise together, so you can create any new format you would like, along with key points from the Group Exercise Class Evaluation Form (see appendix A), which is flexible enough to be adapted to any new format. Group exercise is ever evolving, and formats we currently have may be retired and replaced by newer and more popular ones. Having the skills to create and customize new formats is important for the future of group exercise.

Online Video and Instructor Resources

One change you'll notice in this edition is that the video content previously delivered on a DVD is now an online video resource. This new method for delivering the content allows you to more easily find and play the clips you want to view, and it gives you the flexibility to use your Human Kinetics web site login to view them from multiple locations and devices. If you have purchased a print book, visit www.Human Kinetics.com/MethodsOfGroupExercise Instruction to access the online video resource. If you have purchased a used book or an e-book that does not already include the video clips, you may also purchase access to the online video resource separately from the Human Kinetics site.

Instructors using this text to teach courses in group exercise instruction will find a wealth of useful ancillary materials available at www.Human Kinetics.com/MethodsOfGroupExercise Instruction. These resources are free to instructors who have adopted this text for their courses and include an instructor guide, test package, and, new to this edition, an image bank that provides all the figures, tables, and photos from the book for use in custom presentations.

About Us

We have each taught group exercise for 30+ years, and in that time we have seen it evolve from traditional aerobics to the broad spectrum of modalities available today. In addition to our graduate degrees in exercise science, we have accumulated several certifications in group exercise and attended countless continuing education conferences and workshops for coaching all the modalities covered in this text, and more. We have presented at numerous national and international fitness and wellness conferences, and we continue to teach group exercise to the general public, constantly improving our own practical teaching skills. We have each been involved in several research studies, Carol primarily in the area of water exercise and functional movement, and Mary in the areas of high- and low-impact step exercise, slide energy expenditures, and the efficacy of exercise on Pilates apparatus—in fact, we first met while speaking about our research at an IDEA research symposium back in 1989! We served together for 6 years on the credentialing committee of the American College of Sports Medicine (ACSM), working primarily in the area of group exercise. This book is used in health and fitness curricula around the world. Additionally, we have authored books individually, and we have coauthored another book together. We believe we bring a unique perspective to this text because we are both committed to a hands-on approach yet are thoroughly familiar with the demands of academia and the requirements of science.

As with all formal teaching, skill comes with practice. Teaching group exercise takes courage, perseverance, and energy. It requires continual learning, rehearsal, and discipline. However, the work is worth it because helping others live more healthful lives by having fun while exercising feels great! There's no better way to help other people than by improving their quality of life. Making a difference by educating, caring for, and motivating your participants is a gift both to them and to yourself. We hope this book helps you become an agent of change for people wanting to embrace healthy lifestyles. We can't think of a better gift you can give to yourself and others.

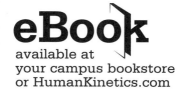

eBook available at your campus bookstore or HumanKinetics.com

Accessing the Online Video

New to this third edition is online streaming video, including over 100 minutes of content demonstrating key principles and exercises from the book. You can access the online video by visiting www.HumanKinetics.com/Methods OfGroupExerciseInstruction. If you purchased a new print book, follow the instructions on the orange-framed page at the front of your book. That page includes access steps and the unique key code that you'll need the first time you visit the *Methods of Group Exercise Instruction* website. If you purchased an e-book from HumanKinetics. com, follow the access instructions that were e-mailed to you after your purchase. If you have purchased a used book, you can purchase access to the online video separately by following the links at www.HumanKinetics.com/MethodsOf GroupExerciseInstruction.

Once at the *Methods of Group Exercise Instruction* website, select Online Video in the ancillary items box in the upper-left corner of the screen. You'll then see an Online Video page with information about the video. Select the link to open the online video web page.

On the online video page, you will see a set of buttons that correspond to the chapters in the text that have accompanying video. Select the button for the chapter's videos you want to watch. Once you select a chapter, a player will appear. In the player, the clips for that chapter will appear vertically along the right side, numbered as they are in the text. Select the video you would like to watch and view it in the main player window. You can use the buttons at the bottom of the main player window to view the video full screen and to pause, fast-forward, or reverse.

The online video replaces and expands the DVD content from the previous edition. Following is a list of the clips in the online video.

Video 3.1 Creating a positive atmosphere

Video 3.2 Training opposing muscle groups

Video 3.3 Using the progressive functional training continuum

Video 4.1 Counting out the beat practice drill

Video 4.2 Basic 2-count and 4-count moves

Video 4.3 High-low arm patterns

Video 4.4 Elements of variation practice drill

Video 4.5 Smooth transitions

Video 4.6 Changing the lead foot

Video 4.7 Building a basic combination

Video 4.8 Sample combination with high- and low-impact moves

Video 4.9 A combination at three intensity levels

Video 4.10 Freestyle choreography practice drill

Video 4.11 Anticipatory cueing practice drill

Video 4.12 Correcting alignment for a stationary lunge

Video 6.1 Warm-up for a high-low impact class

Video 6.2 Warm-up for a step class

Video 6.3 Warm-up for a sport conditioning or boot camp class

Video 7.1 Using intensity options and effective cueing

Video 7.2 Monitoring intensity in a group exercise class

Video 7.3 Cool-down after a cardio segment

Video 8.1 Cueing and progression for some basic muscle conditioning exercises

Video 8.2 Flexibility training segment

Video 8.3 Muscle conditioning exercises for the biceps

Video 8.4 Muscle conditioning exercises for the triceps

Video 8.5 Muscle conditioning exercises for the hamstrings

Video 9.1 Exercises for balance and neuromotor training

Video 9.2 Sample functional training exercises

Acknowledgments

We are very grateful to the many people who have influenced the writing of this book. This book is a tribute to those who have made a difference in our lives. Our parents inspired us to follow our passion and to work hard to make our passion a reality. Thanks to Joan and Bob Caster (Carol's parents) and James and Margaret Yoke (Mary's parents) for their belief in us and for their continuous support over the years. To our adult children, Tony and Jessica Kennedy, Nathaniel Yoke, and Zachary Ripka, thank you for keeping us fascinated with your growth into adulthood. Being empty nesters certainly created time for edition #3! To Marty Armbruster, Carol's husband, thanks for your encouragement and for driving the older adults in Ch. 9 to Bloomington for our photo shoot. We also acknowledge and thank all the people we have encountered through the years who have influenced our perception of group exercise.

Thanks to the following people and organizations for their inspiration and input: ACSM, ACE, AFAA, AEA, Ken Alan, Elisabeth Andrews, Chris Arterberry, Susan Bane, Kim Beetham-Maxwell, Lawrence Biscontinni, Teri Bladen, Jay Blahnik, Penny Black-Steen, Andy Blome, Sharon Bogen, Jane Bradley, Peggy Buchanan, Donna Burch, Can-Fit-Pro, Sharon Cheng, Denise Contessa, Robyn Deterding, Julie Downing, April Durrett, Dr. Jane Ellery, Dr. Ellen Evans, Melinda Flegel, Tere Filer, Dr. Bud Getchell, Nancy Gillette, Laura Gladwin, Maureen Hagan, Lisa Hamlin, Cher Harris, Sara Hillard, Lisa Hoffman, Shayla Holtkamp, IDEA Health and Fitness Association, Janet Johnson, Gail Johnston, Graham Melstand, Mindy King, Dr. Dave Koceja, Dr. Len Kravitz, Susan Kundrat, Alison Kyle, , Karen Leatherman, Deb Legel, Deena Luft-Ellin, Graham Melstrand, Dr. John Shea, Dr. Larry Golding, Pat Maloney, Patti Mantia, Patti McCord, Colleen Curry, Michelle Miller, Margaret Moore, Ghada Muasher, NASM, Maria Nardini, NSCA, Kris Neely, Greg Niederlander, Charlotte Norton, Tony Ordas, Dr. Bob Otto, Karen Pierce, Jacque Pedgrift, Dr. Bob Perez, Dr. Jim Peterson, Linda Pfeffer, Debi Ban-Pillarella, Bill Ramos, Lauri Reimer, Mark Robertson, Pat Ryan, Dr. Mary Sanders, Pearlas Sanborn, Holly Schell, Lisa Sexauer, Dr. Marty Siegel, Robert Sherman, Linda Shelton, Sarah Shore-Beck, Siri Sitton, Mike Spezzano, Dr. Dixie Stanforth, Kathy Stevens, Lisa Stuppy, Steve Tharrett, Dr. Walt Thompson, Kelly Walker-Haley, John Wygand, and Mandy Zulkoski.

Special thanks to the Indiana University School of Public Health for their assistance with the video clips. The use of their facilities and equipment made the video and still photos possible. The video and still photo instructors include Lori Adams, David Auman, Joan Armbruster, Marty Armbruster, Yulia Azriel, Andrew Baer, Allison Berger, Bridget Black, Teri Bladen, Erin Brace, Jackie Braspenninx, Sarah Bruno, Allison Chopra, Katie Collins, Chad Coplen, Theresa Collison, Lisandra Cuadrado, Joe Denk, Ceceila Fortune, Abby Gray, Katie Grove, Malvika Gulati, Alyssa Hinnefeld, Lisa Hoffman, Leigh Ann Hoy, Bryan Hurst, Ann Houtoon, Brittany Ignas, April and Michael Jackson, Jennifer Jeffers, Jake Jones, Jessica Kennedy, Mindy King, Margie Kobow, Tatiana Kolovou, Walter Kyles, Guo Lei, Kayla Little, Evangeline Magno, Gerry and Diana McAfee, Colleen McCracken, Evan McDowell, Cara McGowan, Jessica Mcintire, Devin Mcguire, Cherry Merritt-Darriau, Kellin Miller, Samia Mooney, Tammy Nichols, Patrick O'Brien, Tricia Oxford, Tiffany Owen, Bobby Papariella, Matt Prewitt, Branden Price, Kelly Baute, Jill Rensick, Wendi Robinson, Camilla Saulsbury, Misty Schneider, Meagan Shipley, Earl Sims, Naima Solomon, Andrew Souder, Jennifer Starr, Will Thornton, Cameron Troxell, Mai Tran, Brock Waller, Jacki Watson, Zhangfan Xu, Margaret Yoke, Katie Zukerman and IU Summer One P218 class.

Finally, great big thanks to the staff at Human Kinetics, especially Judy Patterson Wright, who convinced us to write this book; Amy Tocco for her continued encouragement and support of the need to write another edition; and Kate Maurer, our faithful developmental editor who possesses the patience of a saint along with detailed organizational skills to keep us all on track. Thanks also to Neil Bernstein for his professionalism and high-quality photos. Special thanks to Doug Fink, Gregg Henness, and Roger Francisco who produced all three editions of the video clips. We've had a blast working with you guys over the years. Many thanks!

Part I

Fundamentals of Group Exercise Instruction

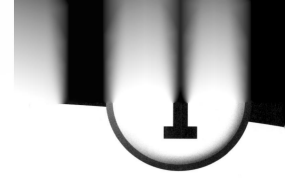

Best Practices

Chapter Objectives

By the end of this chapter, you will be able to

- review the evolution of group exercise;
- understand the important role of group exercise in the fitness industry;
- create healthy marketing tactics for group exercise;
- become familiar with current trends in group exercise formats and focus;
- review branded, extreme conditioning, and commercial off-the-shelf programs;
- understand basic business practices for group exercise programming; and
- understand the major professional certifications and educational organizations in group fitness instruction.

Group exercise is an exciting field; although it originated in aerobic dance, its current devotees participate in a wide range of activities such as stationary indoor cycling and group TRX classes. Given the great variety and complexity of group activities, we might ask, what are best practices for group exercise? How do we create healthy marketing tactics for group exercise that include all levels of group exercise participants and promote proper exercise progressions and regressions? What about branded programs, extreme conditioning programs, and commercial off-the-shelf programs? How do these products affect and encourage or discourage healthy group exercise participation? Finally, with all the various credentials available to health and fitness professionals, there is a need to understand basic business practices for group exercise programming and how an instructor's qualifications can make a difference. Therefore, a thorough understanding of the major professional certifications and educational organizations in group fitness instruction is essential. As the need for preventive health practices becomes even greater in our society, professional group exercise instruction will take on an even more important role. If you

are reading this book, you are most likely striving to be a professional who is seeking knowledge and experience on how to be a better group exercise instructor. We encourage you to take the information in this book and help change the lives of your participants who seek a better quality of life through participation in group movement experiences.

Evolution of Group Exercise

What is the origin of group exercise? A great deal of credit belongs to Jacki Sorensen, who was directly involved with Dr. Kenneth Cooper's early work on aerobic capacity (Schuster 1979). Aerobic dance was born in 1969 when Sorenson was asked to launch an exercise program on closed-circuit TV for the wives of the U.S. Air Force men stationed in Puerto Rico. While preparing for the show, she studied the famed Air Force aerobics program, which was developed by Dr. Cooper. Sorensen took Dr. Cooper's 12-minute running test, which evaluates a person's cardiorespiratory fitness based on how far a person can jog or run in 12 minutes. When she scored well on the test even though

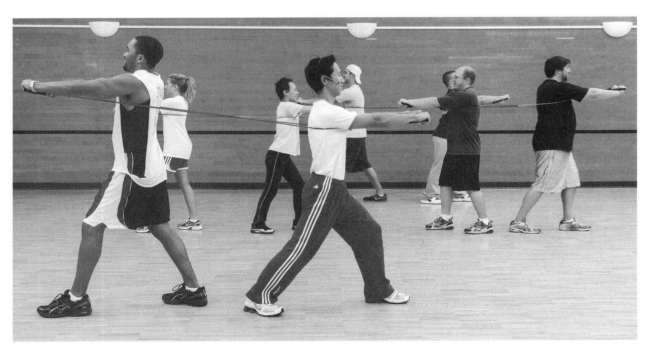

Group exercise classes provide structured and interactive movement experiences that help increase adherence in beginning to advanced participants.

she had never run before, Sorensen figured that her lifetime of dancing had not only kept her figure trim but had also kept her heart and lungs in shape. This realization gave her the idea of combining dance with aerobic exercise (Sorenson and Bruns 1983). With this inspiration, she devised specific dance movements to music that others could copy and teach. The intent of the routines was to elevate the heart rate and keep people moving to music to enhance their fitness for both health and aesthetic purposes.

In that same year (1969), Judi Sheppard Missett founded the Jazzercise program and turned her love of jazz dance into a worldwide dance exercise phenomenon. Jazzercise has expanded to offer a fusion of jazz dance, resistance training, Pilates, yoga, and kickboxing and has improved the health of millions of people worldwide. According to Tharrett, O'Rourke, and Peterson (2011). Jazzercise has evolved into the largest fitness franchise in the world with over 32,000 classes held annually in more than three dozen countries. The program is still going strong and is often offered in churches and community centers, where it can reach the average participant (Jazzercise 2008). Currently, the perception of group exercise is that it is offered within fitness facilities when, in fact, its beginnings with Sorenson and Missett occurred in community centers.

In the 1980s aerobic dance provided an outlet for many people, especially women, to exercise in a group. The aerobic dance movement brought intentional exercise to the forefront; before this time, intentional exercise was not in the mainstream. The Aerobics and Fitness Association of America (AFAA) created the first standards and guidelines for group exercise in 1983. It also started the first nationally recognized certification for group exercise fitness (which was the first certification both authors of this book took in the industry). In 1984 the IDEA Health and Fitness Association (then called the International Dance Exercise Association) held its first international convention. Also during this time the National Sporting Goods Association reported that 24.4 million Americans participated in aerobics (IDEA 2007). Aerobic dance became a pop culture phenomenon—in 1982, *Jane Fonda's Workout Book* (Fonda 1981)

topped the best sellers and was followed by her successful high-impact workout video.

However, enthusiasm for this new exercise diminished when its injury rates began increasing. Injuries to the shins, feet, and knees were particularly common in high-impact aerobics (Mutoh et al. 1988; Richie et al. 1985). DuToit and Smith (2001) also noted the high injury rate in instructors. Their survey of instructors in 18 fitness centers in Australia determined that 77% of instructors were experiencing lower-extremity injuries. Clearly, the activity of aerobic dance was fun but potentially not sustainable over time if instructors were experiencing such a high injury rate. Garrick, Gillien, and Whiteside (1986), however, noted that injuries were most common with those participants who lacked prior involvement in other fitness activities. The injury rate may, in fact, have been due to many beginning exercisers (particularly female exercises) gravitating toward aerobic dance as their first fitness experience.

Many variations of aerobic dance, such as low-impact aerobics, were developed to provide more variety and promote a safer way of exercising to music. One study (Brown and O'Neill 1990) found that 66% of participants in high-impact aerobics experienced injuries compared with only 9% of people in low-impact aerobics. Low-impact aerobics became the craze of the late 1980s, and some experts believed it to be a better option than traditional aerobic dance (Koszuta 1986). Less impact produced less jarring on the joints, and thus low-impact aerobics still provided fitness benefits while reducing the risk of injury to the musculoskeletal system. In the late 1980s aerobics participants started to overcome the no pain, no gain experiences that were so prevalent in the early 1980s (Francis and Francis 1988).

Kernodle (1992) believes that step aerobics was invented to cope with a lack of space for activities engaging large-muscle groups. He wrote that aerobic dance exercisers became "pioneers in moving in small spaces" (1992, p. 68). In 1990 Gin Miller, the developer of step aerobics, presented step to a large group of instructors at AFAA's APEX convention. She stated her reason for inventing step was to have fun while rehabilitating her knee. In a gym, 20 to 30 people can move effectively in an aerobic dance class. By adding steps that make vertical movement possible, almost twice as many people can participate within the same space. Step was also developed to maximize space and prevent injury (Francis 1990). Step uses gravity to overload the body. It reduces the injury risk because it allows the whole body to work against gravity without subjecting the lower body to the impact forces of high- or low-impact aerobics. Step instructors have figured out ways to add impact into the activity by having participants run on or jump onto the step. This activity is mostly low impact, but it can become high impact if participants prefer, and the instructor gives choices for impact movements.

The step movement of the 1990s led to the development of many other forms of group exercise. Water exercise, stationary indoor cycling, trekking, and many other kinds of group activities surfaced. Many of the group classes developed in the 1990s did not require dance skills or even rhythm. Therefore, the term *aerobic dance* was replaced by *group exercise* to better describe the broad scope of activities that had emerged. In 1996 Eller noticed that many clubs had dropped the word *dance* from their schedules. He believed that the dance choreography had become too difficult and was keeping participants from enjoying the activity, and so people were looking for other class options. The activity of aerobic dance had originated as a predominantly female activity, at least in the United States. As different formats of the activity arose over time, the range of participants broadened. Many males attended stationary indoor cycling, boot camp, and core-strengthening formats. Hence, the name aerobic dance did not fit the activity as well as it had as a fitness choice in the 1980s.

Since the 1990s, group exercise has grown into a diverse offering, providing options for almost every ability and preference (see table 1.1). For example, Zumba is a dance format that blends dance and fitness. Many formats are no longer limited to one type of movement option. Fusion classes are more the norm, with combination cardio–strength designs such as cycle–strength or cardio–core class formats. These formats offer split time between cardio options and muscular strength and conditioning. Most fitness businesses have strength and conditioning areas, but group exercise participation also includes an element of entertainment and socialization for exercisers. As a result, instructors have been motivated and encouraged to develop innovative movement experiences. Zumba, for example, can introduce dance movements to copy in social dance situations. Stationary indoor cycling classes have brought more cyclists onto the road as they learn the skill of cycling and take it outdoors. Another popular group exercise option is group personal training. According to Thompson (2012), the ACSM 2013 trends reveal that group personal training and functional training are in the top 10 trends for fitness programming. These trends may influence the depth and breadth of future group exercise offerings. One thing is for sure: Having a skill in group exercise instruction will provide a lot of opportunities for future employment.

Role of Group Exercise

Group exercise classes are the lifelines of many fitness programs. They generate enthusiasm and create the connectedness needed to keep people coming back. When group exercise first

TABLE 1.1   Possible Group Exercise Class Choices

Category	Examples
Choreographed to music	Step, kickboxing, hip-hop, Zumba
Stretch and strengthen	Stretching, stability or BOSU ball, circuit strength, boot camp
Mind and body	Yoga, Pilates, tai chi, qigong
Coaching and non-beat driven	Water exercise, stationary cycling, group strength using machines, equipment-based instruction on treadmills, rowers, etc.
Combination or fusion	Cardio core, cycle strength, dance fusion, yogilates

emerged, many people considered it to be a fad, but by now it has become clear that group exercise is here to stay. The U.S. Healthy People 2020 (2012) objectives as well as public health goals in many countries emphasize increasing the proportion of the population that is at a healthy weight, increasing physical activity, and reducing the number of people who have functional limitations. Individuals may engage in the U.S. Centers for Disease Control and Prevention (CDC)–recommended 150 minutes of physical activity for adults per week (2012); however, what happens in the remaining 6,500 minutes of the waking week is also important for health. While traditional fitness (wellness) programming delivery methods for group exercise instruction may be a productive option for individuals who can afford a fitness membership and who are intrinsically motivated to exercise, the issue arises concerning capturing the large portion of the population not engaged in fitness (wellness) experiences.

In addition to the need for regular physical activity, total time spent sitting is a health concern that has recently attracted more attention in the literature and one that is important for group fitness instructors to be aware of. Katzmarzky and colleagues (2009), Patel and colleagues (2010), and van der Ploeg and colleagues (2012) demonstrated a dose-response association between sitting time and mortality from all causes and between sitting time and cardiovascular disease, independent of leisure-time physical activity. In other words, a single leisure-time physical activity (such as attending a group exercise class) was not enough movement to compensate for too much sitting time in terms of improving health and mortality risk. Pate, O'Neill, and Lobelo (2008) define sedentary activities as those incurring no more than 1.6 metabolic equivalents (METS); this includes the specific behaviors of sitting and lying down. These behaviors are generally considered distinct from inactivity, which refers to a lack of moderate or vigorous physical activity. Taylor (2011) reviewed scientific research on sitting time from 2005-2010 and concluded that prolonged sitting is positively associated with an increase in mortality; although the conclusion was based on survey information.

Taylor (2011) recommends the inclusion of sitting time reduction as a part of future physical activity and fitness guidelines. Brown, Bauman, and Owen (2009) point out the need to focus on movement experiences beyond traditional fitness opportunities as our work becomes more sedentary in nature. No longer can we assume that participants who come to a group exercise class are active and ready to exercise. Using group time to remind participants of the importance of movement outside of class, finding out their movement histories in general conversation before and after class—these are essential components of building professional respect and group cohesion, and they can help create a class specific to the needs of your participants. We may have to rethink group exercise delivery methods and consider small-group training for those who need more instruction before participating in a large-group exercise session. We may also need to consider that future participants are less active and spend more time sitting outside of their intentional exercise experiences. Incorporating general movement-tracking programs (with pedometers or movement-tracking devices) and offering classes that are shorter in length are ways to help attract and involve the large percentage of the population who are not active and sit a lot in their daily activities.

According to Tharrett and Peterson (2012), within the last 8 to 10 years traditional health and fitness club memberships have held steady at 14% to 17% of the U.S. population with the international population having less market penetration than the U.S. For example, Asia has penetrated less than 1% of the eligible population; Europe 5%, South Korea 7.2%, and Japan 3.2%. There is a lot of growth potential in the international fitness market. However, evidence suggests that traditional facility-based fitness (wellness) programming may not be as inclusive as once thought. While traditional fitness (wellness) programming delivery methods may be a productive option for individuals who can afford a health club membership and who are intrinsically motivated to exercise, the issue arises concerning capturing the other 75% to 80% of the population not engaged in fitness (wellness) experiences. According to the U.S. Census Bureau, the population of the United

States was estimated at 308 million people in 2010. The International Health and Racquet Sportsclub Association (IHRSA) reported that in 2010, 50.2 million Americans held health club or fitness memberships at facilities. This accounts for approximately 16% of the U.S. population. Internationally, 8% to 10% of the population chooses to join a fitness facility. If we were to concede that every person holding a health club or fitness facility membership got the recommended amount of physical activity, that leaves over 250 million Americans plus millions of participants around the world to be served. Also, the rapid increase in the obesity pandemic over the last decade is a concern that is impacting the health and wellness of many nations. It might be time to rethink the delivery of fitness programming that will naturally move more participants toward a small-group experience, particularly participants who are beginners and are inactive in their daily living activities. Currently, personal training is popular, but in the same hour a personal trainer spends with one client, a group fitness instructor may reach 40 to 50 participants. Personal trainers who are also group exercise instructors may have many more opportunities to find clients due to their visibility as group instructors. The recent trends in personal training focus on group sessions versus one-on-one training as being beneficial to the clients and trainers.

According to the IDEA 2013 fitness programs and trends report (Schroeder & Donlin, 2013), 79% of responders stated that the most popular class duration was 60 minutes. Note that this survey is sent to business owners and instructors. It would be interesting to survey participants about preferred length of class time. Business managers and instructors often cater to the population that is intrinsically motivated and chooses to be in a fitness facility.

There continues to be an increase in the advanced exerciser demographic in fitness facilities. Could this mean we are catering to the fit to get them more fit? As obesity continues to increase, and fewer people participate in physical activity, a person might question why the number of advanced participants at fitness facilities is increasing when fewer members of the general public are exercising regularly

(Jakicic and Otto 2005). Church and colleagues (2011) showed that during the last 50 years in the United States, there has been a progressive decrease in the percentage of individuals employed in occupations that require moderately intense physical activity. Their review of changes in the labor force since 1960 suggests that a large portion of the national weight gain may be explained by declining physical activity patterns during the work day. As group exercise instructors, we might ask if we are remaining in touch with the general public. Might we be more successful going out into the community and reaching the population that may not come into a health and fitness facility? We need to start thinking of group exercise as an option in less traditional venues such as church facilities, workplaces, outdoors, or simply as a part of our leisure experience. Principles of exercise progression would warrant the need to have class sessions start at 30 minutes and progress in duration. It is important that fitness professionals remain in touch with the general public and tailor programming to improve the overall health and wellness of the population at large rather than cater to a population that is already moving and would continue to move even if there were not any fitness facilities available. Reaching out to all participants is an important goal of the group exercise programmer.

The most recent ACSM recommendations are presented in the "Summary of the 2014 ACSM Evidence-Based Recommendations for Exercise for Healthy Adults" in this chapter. These recommendations will be outlined in more detail in successive chapters. The recommended duration for cardiorespiratory exercise is 30 to 60 minutes of purposeful moderate exercise or 20 to 60 minutes of vigorous exercise, or a combination of moderate and vigorous exercise with a note that 20 minutes of exercise per day can be beneficial, especially in previously sedentary individuals. Including 30-minute group classes in facility programming is a good way to attract participants who may be new to group exercise and help them meet the guidelines for exercise participation. Many facilities are finding success with 30-minute or shorter classes; Lofshult (2002) suggested that the most popular class length is 30 minutes because it accommodates the busy lives

Summary of the 2014 ACSM Evidence-Based Recommendations for Exercise for Healthy Adults

Cardiorespiratory: > 5 days per week of moderate exercise, or > 3 days per week of vigorous exercise, or a combination of moderate and vigorous exercise on 3-5 days. 30-60 minutes of purposeful moderate exercise or 20-60 minutes of vigorous exercise, or a combination of moderate and vigorous exercise per day in either one continuous session or in multiple sessions of > 10 minutes to accumulate the desired duration.

Resistance Training: On 2-3 days/wk, adults should also perform resistance exercises for each of the major muscle groups, 8-20 repetitions of 1-4 sets depending on what training outcomes are desired.

Flexibility: Crucial to maintaining joint range of movement, completing a series of flexibility exercises for each of the major muscle–tendon groups on > 2-3 days/wk and performing 60 seconds of total stretching time for each flexibility exercise.

Neuromotor: Involves balance, agility, coordination, and gait and are recommended on > 2-3 days per week for 20-30 min for a total of 60 minutes of neuromotor exercise per week.

Adapted from ACSM 2014.

of today's participants. Yet our fitness trends and contemporary sitting time health research demonstrate that many fitness programs cater to the advanced participant. It is important that our scientific principles match our business and marketing practices if we are going to be seen as group exercise professionals that deliver our services to all types of participants.

Trends in Group Exercise

The IDEA survey (Schroeder & Donlin 2013) lists small equipment as the most frequently used by respondents. Of that equipment, 92 % utilize resistance tubing or bands, 91 % stability balls, 89 % barbells and dumbbells, 84 % foam rollers and small balls, 83 % balance equipment, and

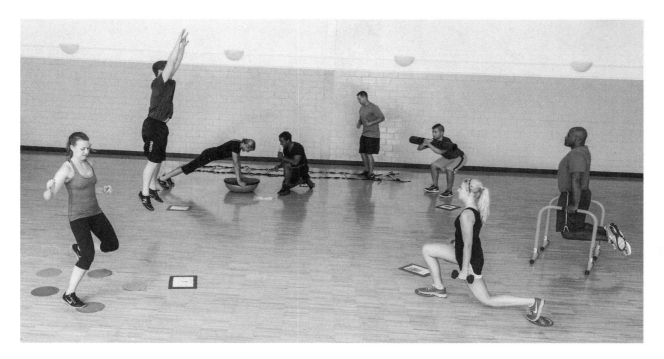

Boot camp and sport conditioning classes have grown in popularity in recent years.

82% medicine balls. All these pieces of equipment are often used in a group exercise setting. In terms of program offerings related to group instruction, the top five group exercise trends were ranked in the following order; body weight leverage training, core-conditioning classes, boot camp classes, strength training, and dance. It's also interesting to note that group exercise is venturing out of the four walls of a gym setting and working around the entire fitness facility as well as outdoors.

The 2013 survey also found that 98% of instructors and directors surveyed described clients as apparently healthy. Yet, they also identified that 90% were older adults, with 87% stating they had special medical needs. Other findings from the IDEA 2013 Fitness Programs and Equipment Trends report identified the top five mind-body program trends as yoga, mind-

body fusion, pilates and yoga fusion, pilates, meditation, and group reformer. Zumba, which is a branded, choreographed program, appears to be popular because the moves tend to be simpler with large amounts of repetition, and participants generally feel it is less important to be in sync with everyone than it is to simply have fun.

The American College of Sports Medicine (ACSM) published its observations on fitness trends (Thompson 2012) in its *Health and Fitness Journal*. The ACSM is attempting to understand and define a trend versus a fad in the fitness industry. Health fitness professionals who filled out this survey often have college degrees in kinesiology or other health-related fields. The worldwide 2012 survey was sent to over 26,000 fitness professionals certified by the ACSM. Figure 1.1 identifies the trends from 2007 through 2011, which show that since 2007

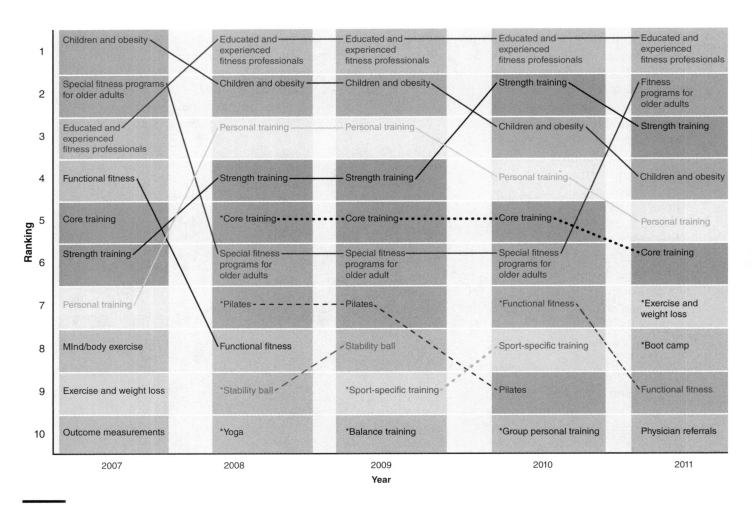

FIGURE 1.1   Trends in the fitness industry.

the number one fitness trend, as identified by fitness professionals having ACSM certifications, is that more clients are looking for educated and experienced fitness professionals. The potential bias of this survey is that the respondents were ACSM certified and thus were themselves educated and experienced fitness professionals. The order of trends might be different if the survey was sent to participants. Other interesting findings from this survey are that 10 of the top 20 trends involved fitness instruction in a group setting. Group exercise is not a fad, as many said it was when it first began. It has become a staple that will be part of the fitness industry for a long time. Thus, as group exercise instructors, we must realize who we are programming for, and how we direct that programming, will be important in making a difference in the overall health and wellness of the population. Let's also not forget that in many facilities, group exercise sessions generate a profit (Nogawa-Wasman 2002) on top of providing health benefits for participants.

It is interesting to note that the current ACSM evidence-based guidelines (2014) validate a typical group exercise class format dating back to the inception of group exercise in the 1970s. The guidelines include cardiorespiratory, muscular strength and endurance, neuromotor movement, and flexibility training, all of which have been a part of the group exercise experience for a long time. A contemporary focus on incorporating neuromotor (specifically balance) and flexibility exercises into group exercise experiences is relatively new to the ACSM evidence-based guidelines; this emphasis reflects trends toward a focus on functional fitness and concerns about the fitness of an aging population. Recommendations for volume, pattern, and progression of these neuromotor exercises and progression of flexibility exercise are not known, but the importance of these exercises is being recognized. Balance and agility exercises are recommended in the ACSM guidelines for older adults (Nelson et al. 2007). The 2014 ACSM guidelines for the general population refer to balance exercises as "functional training and neuromotor exercises." Incorporating balance exercises into the group experience not only helps prevent falls in older adults, but also enhances the neuromuscular

system in order to prevent the deterioration of balance that occurs with age. As the baby boomers age, they continue to influence group exercise programming.

From a business and marketing perspective improved movement and function also saves health care dollars (see "Creating Healthy Marketing Tactics for Group Exercise"). In a meta-analysis of the literature on costs and savings associated with workplace chronic disease prevention and wellness programs, Harvard researchers (Baicker, Cutler, and Song 2010) reported that for every dollar spent on wellness programs, US medical costs are reduced by $3.27 and absenteeism costs are reduced by $2.73. Regarding productivity or reduction of "presenteeism," Pronk and colleagues (2004) concluded that lifestyle-related modifiable health risk factors significantly affect employee work performance. As health care costs continue to rise, conscientious action must be taken to combat the deteriorating health of American workers (Eriksson et al. 2010). The economics of physical inactivity and obesity are at the forefront in the United States, with approximately 17% of the U.S. Gross National Product being dedicated to health care costs (Johnson 2012). Over the last 50 years the number of Americans in the labor force has increased from approximately 40% to 50% due in part to the increase of women in the workplace (Lee and Mather 2012). The IDEA 2013 fitness programs and trends survey had a 69% response rate from females. As women become busy in both their work and home life the trends in group fitness program offerings may need to change. We may observe group movement experiences showing up in the workplace environment as a regular part of the work day to augment some of these issues related to increasing health care costs and efficient use of time for working mothers and fathers.

Demographics

The shift from aesthetics to health is not necessarily occurring with younger populations, but it is more likely a result of baby boomers experiencing a lack of function in their later years. A 70-year-old client signed up for personal training because he could no longer open jars. Another

Creating Healthy Marketing Tactics for Group Exercise

The gluteus medius muscle abducts the hip, but why does a participant need to strengthen this muscle, and what exercises work the muscle effectively? During the aesthetic movement of the 1970s through the 2000s, the main purpose for exercising was to lose weight and look better, and many of us still select exercises based on cultural influences that dictate what our bodies should look like. You can't turn on a screen device without seeing an advertisement about how some exercise program helped Susie or Joe look "like this." Looks will always be important to us, but we also need more out of fitness: We want to feel and move better. We want to have more energy to enjoy life regardless of our age, and we want to maintain our independence as long as possible by performing daily tasks with vigor. It is estimated that the average person loses 13 to 15 years to dysfunction: While we may live a long life, we typically spend the last few years of that life unable to function independently. Thus, each of us will be fighting to maintain our independence in our later years.

As formats of group exercise continue to be created and studied, the ACSM evidence-based guidelines on the quantity and quality of fitness for healthy adults continue to evolve (ACSM 2014). It is important that our marketing practices for fitness follow the science as well as the trends. Too many times a program will resort to aesthetic marketing practices by putting up a sign that reads "sign up now for Zumba to lose weight by New Years!" A better marketing tactic based on the science of exercise might read "sign up now for Zumba so you will feel better and enjoy your holiday." A business manager will tell you this is not what works in the long run, but combining science with marketing is what a fitness professional does. You would not see a lawyer post a sign that says "get a divorce by the holidays; I'll help you." That would be unprofessional. Until our profession begins to present ourselves in a professional way by how we market our programs, it will be difficult to receive respect and support from other professionals. According to a recent National Business Group health survey (2011), 80% of U.S. companies plan to offer financial rewards as a part of worksite wellness programs in order to reduce health care costs and thus create a more thriving economy. Marketing to business groups is a good idea. They need our help right now, but they must perceive us as professionals who can help them.

client could not pick up a bar of soap dropped in the shower and so sought help to improve his ability to perform adult daily living (ADL) tasks. The inability to perform ADL tasks often leads people into an exercise setting. In the United States, according to Sipes and Ritchie (2012), every day for the next 17 years 10,000 baby boomers will turn 65. The U.S. senior population will double by the year 2040 as compared to the year 2010. According to the 2012 U.S. Census Bureau report, the worldwide population of persons aged 65 years or older was an estimated 420 million, a 9.5 million increase from 1999. During 2000 to 2030, the worldwide population aged 65 years or older is projected to increase by approximately 550 million to 973 million, increasing from 6.9% to 12.0% worldwide, from 15.5% to 24.3% in Europe, from 12.6% to 20.3% in North America, from 6.0% to 12.0% in Asia, and from 5.5% to 11.6% in Latin America and the Caribbean. The needs of this age group are largely responsible for the term *functional training*. This segment is growing, and we will need to adapt our group exercise experiences to their needs. On the other hand, the echo boomers (children of baby boomers) have grown up in a different era. They like experiences and tend to appreciate outdoor, real-life fitness opportunities—hence, the stationary indoor cycling, boot camp era that began in the late 1990s. According to Tharrett, O'Rourke, and Peterson (2011), current facility demographics include the following: 10% are under 18 years of age, 31% are 18 to 34 years old, 37% are 35 to 54 years old, and 23% are 55 and over. The future of group exercise needs to be changed both in format and offerings in order to cater to such a vast age spectrum and diverse interests within the participant age groups.

The baby boomers started the fitness movement, and they still dominate the demographics.

Table 1.2 outlines the effects the baby boomers have had on group exercise instruction and how the functional training movement has developed. Astrand's (1992) article titled "Why Exercise?" contained the first hints of the functional training movement. In this article Dr. Astrand describes a connection between exercise physiology, human performance, and the functional requirements of living. Wolf (2001) suggested that "training movements and not muscles may be the paradigm shift needed for today's functional conditioning." Santana (2002) defined functional training as "exercising for a specific duty or purpose of a person or thing." Functional training develops the muscles and movement patterns that make the performance of everyday activities easier, smoother, safer, and more efficient. Functional exercises improve a person's ability to function independently or perform a sport more effectively. This focus underlies what is perhaps the most important benefit of attaining fitness: Everyday activities become easier, and quality of life improves. Other research (Flegal et al. 2005) looking at the estimated number of deaths in the United States associated with being underweight, overweight, and obese found that being overweight alone is not associated with excess mortality. Overweight individuals can improve their health by attending group exercise in the same way leaner individuals can. According to Blair (2009) physical inactivity could be the biggest risk factor for preventing early death for all disease causes. Segar, Eccles, and Richardson (2012) found that exercise goals related to quality of life enhancement significantly improved exercise adherence.

As our population ages and the cost of health care continues to escalate, we will move further away from a fitness-related focus on aesthetics to one that emphasizes purposeful movement and enhanced quality of life. For example, Whitmer et al. (2005) inserted linked obesity to an increased risk for dementia. This study indicated that obesity in middle age is an independent risk factor for future dementia. Thus, staying active and maintaining a normal weight may not just be important for overall increased length of life; it may also be important for being free from other diseases that limit functional capacity.

Branded and Off-the-Shelf Programs

According to Tharrett, O'Rourke, and Peterson (2011), Phil Mills is the founder of Les Mills International, which was one of the first international branded group exercise programs brought into the fitness market in the 1990s. Les Mills International was founded in 1997, seven years after its creators had developed their first exercise program, Body Pump, which was initially introduced in Australia in 1995. By 1998 Les Mills had created four new programs (Body Combat, Body Balance, Body Step, and RPM). At the present time, Les Mills programs are offered in over 13,000 facilities around the world. The Les Mills–branded programs are a lot like the Sorensen and Missett early group exercise programs—prepackaged choreographed programs and the music to go along with them sold as a package. As new prepackaged routines are developed by Mills and his associates, they are passed on to the organizations that buy the rights to use them. The instructors are trained as Les Mills certified, and they are the only ones who can teach a Les Mills–branded class. Our opinion of these programs is that they are good

TABLE 1.2 Baby Boomers' Influence on Fitness Trends

Decade	Baby boomers' age	Trend
1970s	20s	High-impact aerobics, running 10K races
1980s	30s	Low-impact aerobics, walking, running 5K races
1990s	40s	Step, slide, water exercise, stationary indoor cycling, yoga
2000s	50s	Functional fitness, stability balls, balance devices
2010s	60s	Core strength, neuromuscular and proprioceptive emphasis, preventing falls
2020s	70s	Chair exercise, walking, corrective exercise, foam rollers

if a facility does not have a trained, certified group exercise program director. However, we believe that having a trained, certified group exercise professional on site is essential. Each population is different, and every participant is different. To think that we can prechoreograph a workout and not have to modify a routine for participants is unrealistic. If we are there for the health and wellness of our participants, then on-the-spot modifications will need to be made. Branded programs such as Les Mills assume that all individuals can move the same and at the same intensity and speed. This can be dangerous for the participant and the instructor if modifications are necessary and not appropriately provided.

Other types of branded programs that are more often on the Internet or television in contrast to being offered within a fitness facility are P90X, CrossFit, Insanity, and Gym Jones; we are quite certain there will eventually be many more. These are commercial off-the shelf (COTS) products also known as extreme conditioning programs (ECPs). Often these programs are presented with words such as "extreme," "elite," or "high intensity" to help sell them as one of the best ways to get in shape quickly. These programs may be good for the individual who is on the run and needs to get a workout in a hotel room or basement, or a participant who lacks structure and wants to have a program that can be purchased to get started on a fitness path. There is increasing acceptance of these programs because they are marketed largely through anecdotal reports of major gains in physical fitness and performance (Bergeron et al. 2011).

One of the limitations to these types of programs is that the instruction is not specific to the group or individual. How can an individual on a screen know how to modify the activity for your needs and also adjust for your specific movement patterns if he or she cannot see you? These programs are often presented as quick fixes. For example, the name P90X relates to the idea that the program is 90 days long, and after that you will be fit. The program does not emphasize how difficult it is to sustain fitness once you have reached the level you want. Jones, Christensen, and Young (2000) reported a 35% increase in weight-training injuries since 1978 from the misuse or abuse of weight-training equipment. A more recent study on weight-training injuries (Kerr, Collings, and Comstock 2010) reported in U.S. hospital emergency rooms found that the proportion of overexertion injuries increased significantly with age. We attribute some of this increase in weight-training injuries to programs like COTS or ECPs that are often not supervised or vetted for scientific principles and that often can be dangerous for the older adult who begins a weight-training regimen later in life. Our opinion of unsupervised extreme conditioning programs is that you may learn some effective motivational techniques and some good movement ideas for your class. However, be careful and do not assume that everyone can do all the exercises that are portrayed. In many ECP programs the participants are often young and fit. Such programs may be good for the participant who wants to take fitness to another level, but they certainly are not appropriate for anyone with special needs or for the average participant just beginning an exercise program.

Another type of branded program on the rise which is often offered through a commercial facility chain is CrossFit. At this time there are actual CrossFit competitions published in many screen venues from the Internet to television. Much of the CrossFit instruction and many of the competitions are in small groups and use weights or challenging body-weight exercises. Group cohesiveness and interaction are encouraged and promoted in CrossFit facilities. Olympic lifts like the snatch or the clean and jerk movement are excellent for total body conditioning when instruction is specific to the individual and there is a progression leading to the proper performance of these exercises. Many CrossFit exercises are touted as functional training, yet they are specific to military maneuvers even though they are given to the general exerciser. At this time there is no evidence that these practices are in fact functional. Extreme conditioning programs may be appropriate for the very fit exerciser. However, encouraging these types of movements for the general public without extensive exercise progressive training can be troublesome.

An ACSM consortium (Bergeron et al. 2011) published a paper on extreme conditioning programs such as CrossFit, P90X, and Insanity. The authors of this paper included representatives from the military as well as exercise researchers. The pros and cons of extreme conditioning programs were analyzed and reported. Physicians and primary care providers have apparently identified the potential emerging problem of disproportionate musculoskeletal injury risk from ECPs, particularly for novice participants (Hadeed, Juehl, and Elliot 2011).

As Seidman (2007) so eloquently states in his book *How: Why How We Do Anything Means Everything*, we need to learn how to create a "wave" (much like a fan wave that cascades around a football stadium) in our group exercise program marketing practices. We need to get beyond selling fitness practices to the 14% to 17% of the population who are already fit, while also marketing body image changes to those who lack fitness. Seidman believes that sustainable values (integrity, honesty, truth, hope) are those that connect us deeply as humans. Seligman (2011, p. 60) states in his book *Flourish* that "good science requires the interplay of analysis and synthesis." Therefore, our hope is that you look deeper at why marketing extreme group exercise options and focusing on weight loss are potentially unsustainable premises for the general population. We hope you will think about the true purpose of exercise and physical activity and not confuse it with the notion that fitness must be quick, easy, tough, or extremely intense. Acquiring and sustaining a healthy lifestyle is a lifelong process of preserving and protecting our bodies so we can enjoy life and leisure to the fullest for all our remaining years.

Business Basics for Group Exercise

The role of the group exercise instructor is far reaching. As business operators begin to embrace the importance of developing relationships with clients, the importance of the group exercise instructor will continue to increase. Most group exercise instructors work part-time, and many teach for several organizations and facilities. A group exercise employee can make or break a member's experience based on his or her attitudes and organizational skills. Instructors need to arrive early, perform class setup duties, and greet participants and interact before their classes. Many instructors are paid for their preparation time as well as their actual teaching time. This preparation time is arguably the most important for developing good relationships with participants. Outstanding group exercise instructors will help retain clients for facilities and, because of their relational skills, will help sustain participant fitness. We cannot underestimate the importance of the group exercise instructor in the business practices of group fitness instruction.

Teaching group exercise requires a unique set of skills. Instructors must be able to entertain, educate, role model, and think on their feet. In his bestselling book *Blink: The Power of Thinking Without Thinking*, Gladwell (2005) suggests that falling back on involuntary subconscious processes can be more effective than using higher-level cognitive functions when completing certain tasks. In many ways his book describes and appreciates the skill set needed to teach group exercise. An instructor has little time to process all that needs to be processed. Decisions must be made within the blink of an eye. A qualified leader is essential for a high-quality group exercise program, and hiring appropriate instructors can save time and money often spent on initial training.

According to the international American Council on Exercise (ACE) (2010) fitness compensation survey, part-time group fitness instructors make an average of US$24.50 per hour, specialty instructors make an average of US$27.50 per hour, and yoga or Pilates instructors make an average of US$29.50 per hour. Since a program that offers group exercise has a large financial investment, let's review practices that will enhance both the instructor's and the supervisor's knowledge of the business of group exercise.

Fostering Teamwork

Excellence begins with teamwork. Instructors who are part of an excellent group exercise staff cooperate by doing their jobs and covering their classes; everyone feels as if he or she is part of a team and works to support the team. Griffith (2005) made some notable suggestions for team-building activities that foster fun and enthusiasm within a group exercise staff:

- Divide your staff members into teams based on their specialty areas and assign them tasks.
- Create a choreography notebook of types of moves (e.g., step, boot camp, high- and low-impact, etc.) developed by all the group exercise instructors on staff.
- Create an overall schedule for group strength classes so instructors and participants know which muscles will be worked in which class.
- Have the mind–body class instructors develop a flier that describes the differences between yoga and Pilates.

Tharrett and Peterson (2012) suggest the following four Es for building a successful fitness team:

- Identify *expectations* to set the course for the team.
- *Equip* the team through education and opportunities for professional growth.
- *Encourage* the team—encouragement is the fuel of champions.
- *Evaluate* whether goals and expectations are met.

Whenever possible, have the instructors work together to solve problems. This creates a sense of ownership for instructors, and their loyalty to the program will skyrocket. Instructors who do not feel a part of the team often seek employment at another facility, so keeping group exercise instructors happy is important. Remember that group exercise is often the heart of the facility. If the heart of the facility is happy, then so are the facility members. Fostering teamwork is good business practice.

Recruiting and Retaining Group Exercise Instructors

Gregor (2006) suggests that all prospective instructors be put through a detailed hiring and auditioning process before being offered a job. A personal interview, an audition, shadow teaching, and a final evaluation make up the standard process for hiring and preparing an instructor to teach. Several examples of how to recruit and train instructors are available (Brathwaite et al. 2006; Davidson et al. 2006). Tharrett and Peterson's *Fitness Management* (2012) contains many interview questions specific to fitness interviewing and recruiting. If you are a fitness manager or director of group exercise instructors, we encourage you to read business books for information on how to retain and recruit staff.

As an instructor, you are a consumer of the industry. Strive to find a position in a facility or program that will create the best experience for you. A good workplace experience often occurs because of sound business practices. Check the facility group exercise schedule. Is the program diverse? Are 30-minute classes offered so you know health and wellness are a priority for the owners? If the class schedule contains mostly hour to hour-and-a-half classes, the facility may not be one that caters to the average population and thus may have fewer participants overall in the program. The management's priority is often the bottom line. It can become the job of the staff and instructors to keep the health and wellness of club members at the forefront. Hagan (2005) suggests that facility schedules should have start and finish dates for classes, offer multilevel classes, offer fusion classes, and highlight a new specialty class in order to enhance the adherence of participants. If you find such a schedule, then you will have most likely found a good club or facility that you will want to check into further. Look at the mission statement of the organization you are considering. If the mission focuses on enhancing the health and wellness of participants, and the organization demonstrates sound business practices, you will enjoy being a group exercise instructor at that facility. Always check into a company's business practices before auditioning to be an instructor for that organization.

Education, Credentialing, and Certification

A group exercise class must be built on the foundation of participant safety. An important aspect of learning about safety is becoming certified by a national organization. You do not necessarily have to be certified in order to teach group exercise, but certification proves that you have content knowledge and are serious about your role as a professional fitness instructor. Malek and colleagues (2002) confirmed the value of formal education when they found that a bachelor's degree in exercise science and an ACSM or National Strength and Conditioning Association (NSCA) certification, as opposed to other certifications, were strong predictors of a personal trainer's knowledge. We suggest that similar credentials might be strong predictors of a group exercise instructor's knowledge. An ACSM article on credentialing (Whaley 2003) discussed the importance of formal academic education for the creation of knowledgeable and skilled fitness professionals. Many universities now offer degree programs for those wishing to pursue careers in the fitness Industry. The ACE website (see "Group Fitness Certification and Continuing Education Organizations" later in this chapter) endorses university partners. This list of universities might be a good place for you to start researching if you're serious about a career as a fitness professional.

When the fitness profession was just starting, it was difficult to find a university that had a degree program in fitness leadership. However, many programs are now available. We encourage you to continue your formal education, especially if you want to manage a fitness center and enhance healthy living for your participants. Fitness instructors who desire to place their participants' health and well-being at the forefront of group exercise need to gain as much knowledge about how the body works as possible. IHRSA recommends that club owners hire fitness instructors with certifications from agencies accredited through the National Commission for Certifying Agencies (NCCA). IHRSA believes that doing so will help fitness professionals take a legitimate place on the health care continuum because accreditation of a credentialing organization by NCCA is the standard for many other allied health professionals (nurses, athletic trainers, and so on). The Distance Education and Training Council (DETC) is another credentialing organization. DETC does not extend accreditation to certification programs but only to distance learning

courses and programs that prepare individuals to sit for independently administered certification examinations. Several fitness certifications are accredited through DETC. According to the American Council on Exercise (2005), certification is the hardware of the fitness business, and education is the software. We recommend getting certified and attending continuing education offerings so that you can be the best fitness professional you can be.

Many national certifications involve written and practical exams for which an instructor must demonstrate basic skills in exercise leadership and its related components (e.g., anatomy and physiology, intensity monitoring, injury prevention). We recommend taking nationally recognized certifications because these tests are designed by many professionals who agree on pertinent knowledge in the field of exercise instruction. Local or club certifications or training programs are always a good place to start getting the education you need to take a national certification exam. Most nationally recognized certifications require you to have cardiopulmonary resuscitation (CPR) and automated external defibrillator (AED) certifications before sitting for the exam. At the end of this section is a list of organizations that provide fitness training and certification. We have been involved with many of these organizations and know they all have good training programs for group exercise instructors.

Many organizations and universities train group exercise leaders, and it is good to experience different kinds of training; however, when it comes to certification, make sure the organizations you choose are credible, and that their tests are professional. Many fitness professionals have more than one certification depending on what skills they need and use. Usually, it's good to have both a group-focused certification and a one-on-one certification. We recommend taking more than one certification exam because completing each is a learning experience. It is our hope that more universities will offer exercise leadership classes so that certification will become simply a verification of knowledge. We also hope that this book will prompt faculty and staff within universities to provide academic training for group leadership. Currently, many academic institutions offer degrees in kinesiology (the study of movement) or exercise physiology, but often these degrees do not include a group exercise leadership component. Since ACSM added knowledge and skills of group leadership to the ACSM guidelines (2014) in both their 2010 and 2014 editions, we hope that scientists in the fitness field are acknowledging the importance of this activity. There is a difference between a fitness professional and an instructor who works part-time leading fitness classes. The fitness professional often has had formal training and education in exercise prescription and fitness assessment. However, we know few fitness professionals who do not instruct group exercise.

This book is written for the fitness professional who instructs group exercise. We will not be covering just one format but rather principles of science that are to be included in any group exercise class format. What is included in this book is information derived from the training manuals of many widely recognized certification organizations.

Continuing Education

An excellent group exercise program requires and provides continuing education that keeps its instructors stimulated and updated. Often, facilities bring in speakers or pay stipends for instructors to attend conferences. An excellent organization not only retains instructors via incentives to perform continuing education but also regularly evaluates its instructors. Feedback

---

Group Fitness Certification and Continuing Education Organizations

Aerobics and Fitness Association of America (AFAA)

15250 Ventura Blvd., Ste. 200
Sherman Oaks, CA 91403
877-968-7263
www.afaa.com

Aerobics and Fitness Association of America—AFAA does not require a four-year degree to take its Primary Group Exercise exam. The exam includes both a written and a practical component and is accredited by the DETC. AFAA offers additional certifications for group instructors, including step, kickboxing, and emergency response. AFAA also offers many continuing education one-day workshops such as Practical Teaching Skills and Choreography; Perinatal Fitness, Older Adult Fitness, Floor, Core, and More for Personal Trainers; Practical Pilates; Practical Yoga Instructor Training; Midlife Fitness for Women; and Mechanics of Injury Prevention. Most of these workshops are available online as well as in person, delivered by master trainers.

Alberta Fitness Leadership Certification Association (AFLCA)

c/o Provincial Fitness Unit
University of Alberta
Edmonton, Alberta T6G 2H9
780-492-4435
www.provincialfitnessunit.ca

Alberta Fitness Leadership Certification Association—AFLCA is a nonprofit organization dedicated to creating, promoting, and implementing national standards for the training and certification of group exercise leaders. AFLCA provides a minimum of 44 hours of training involving a written theory exam, specialty training courses, and assessment of practical skills. AFLCA-approved trainers currently offer a wide variety of certification and accreditation training programs, including the following subject areas: exercise theory, group exercise fundamentals, resistance training, aquatic exercise, fitness for the older adult, choreography, cycle, step, portable exercise equipment, and mind–body group exercise training.

American College of Sports Medicine (ACSM)

401 W. Michigan St.
Indianapolis, IN 46202-3233
317-637-9200
www.acsm.org

ACSM certification is recommended for the professional with a degree in a health-related field who supervises a program in a facility. A bachelor's degree from a four-year university is required to take most ACSM exams. The exam is administered online and requires knowledge of exercise science, fitness assessment skills, and leadership principles.

American Council on Exercise (ACE)

4851 Paramount Dr.
San Diego, CA 92123
800-825-3636
www.acefitness.org

A four-year degree is not necessary to take the ACE Group Fitness Instructor written-only certification exam. ACE has other certifications for personal trainers and wellness coaches and has developed an Advanced Health and Fitness Specialist Certification exam for the fitness professional who has a four-year degree in a health-related field. ACE and IDEA have a long-standing business relationship and together offer continuing education workshops and publish a monthly health and fitness journal.

Can-Fit-Pro

110-225 Consumers Road
Toronto, ON M2J 1RA
800-667-5622
www.canfitpro.com

Can-Fit-Pro offers a variety of certifications in group exercise, personal training, nutrition, pre- and postnatal exercise, older adult exercise, mind–body exercise, and sport conditioning. Program courses are delivered in person and range from 16 to 25 hours in length. Most certification exams consist of a written theory exam and an assessment of practical skills. Can-Fit-Pro courses and exams are delivered nationally by a team of trainers and master trainers.

SCW Fitness Education

1618 Orrington Ave., Ste. 202
Evanston, IL 60201
877-SCW-FITT
www.scwfitness.com

SCW Fitness Education—SCW certification blends practical, theoretical, and physiological knowledge of successful teaching techniques for group exercise. The emphasis is on class sequencing, warming up, proper progressions, creative delivery, musical phrasing, proper cueing, and choreography development. This certification focuses on leading in front of others and demonstrating proper teaching skills.

World Instructor Training Schools (WITS)

206 76th St.
Virginia Beach, VA 23451-1915
888-330-9487
www.witseducation.com

World Instructor Training Schools—WITS has schools nationwide in colleges and universities to meet the needs of serious students entering the fitness field. WITS provides a 6-week course that is

> continued

> continued

36 hours long and includes a final written and practical skills exam. Half of the course is theoretical and the other half is hands-on and practical. Students must develop actual group exercise routines, which they then lead in the final exam.

IDEA Health and Fitness Association

> 10455 Pacific Center Ct.
> San Diego, CA 92121-4339
> 800-999-4332
> www.ideafit.com

IDEA Health and Fitness Association—IDEA holds several conferences for fitness instructor education throughout the year, including an international conference, a personal training conference, a mind–body conference, and several others that are filled with group exercise ideas and education on fitness and health concepts. IDEA also publishes the *IDEA Fitness Journal*, which is an excellent resource for group exercise instructors as every edition has a section devoted to improving group exercise instruction.

YMCA of the USA

> 101 N. Wacker Dr.
> Chicago, IL 60606
> 800-872-9622
> www.ymca.net

YMCA of the USA—Each YMCA operates independently and therefore requires specific certifications and training procedures. Overall, the various YMCAs offer certifications both in group exercise and in personal training. Their trainings involve hands-on, practical skills for teaching group exercise.

is the breakfast of champions (Tharrett and Peterson 2012) and the way to grow as a professional. When applying to work for an organization, it is important to find out if you will be evaluated as a group exercise instructor. Ask for an evaluation of your class or videotape it yourself and watch yourself teaching. This is a wonderful way to learn about your abilities as a group exercise instructor. There are many tools that help evaluate the effectiveness of a class. One tool is our Group Exercise Class Evaluation Form, discussed in chapter 3 and provided in appendix A. There are others that have been introduced in the professional literature as well (Eickhoff-Shemek and Selde 2006).

Learning and growing as a professional is an important aspect of teaching group exercise. Always check to make sure the organization you are working for has sound business practices that

you are proud to represent. Many companies, recreation departments, and health clubs insist that their instructors be nationally certified. Others set up their own training or coursework that must be completed. Either method is a step toward elevating exercise instruction and ensuring a certain level of knowledge and expertise. But having a certification does not automatically mean that you will be a wonderful instructor. It just means that you are serious and are willing to increase your knowledge and experience. We have attended many workshops, lectures, and seminars from the organizations mentioned in this chapter. We keep our national certifications current but also continually update and improve our teaching skills through continuing education events held by many of these same organizations. Certification is very important; continuing education is equally important.

Chapter Wrap-Up

Group exercise can be powerful if participants feel welcome, learn new things, get to know others, are taught safely, and believe that their time is being well spent. The experience cannot only make a positive change in their emotional outlook but also improve their health and quality of living. Understanding the business practices of group exercise will help you choose to work for an organization that has both good fitness programs and business practices. Understanding what professional fitness organizations offer in terms of certification and continuing education is a step toward becoming a fitness professional. Once we move beyond emphasizing quantized fitness gains and aesthetics, we can understand that the real power of exercise lies in the experience itself. Group exercise can definitely be a terrific, life-enhancing experience, and the skills and knowledge of the instructor are key to making the experience as powerful as possible.

ASSIGNMENT

Write a 1- to 2-page, double-spaced paper on a current branded, extreme conditioning, or commercial off-the-shelf group exercise program. Research the program online in order to discover the company's marketing tactics, business practices, and requirements (if any) for instructor certification; include this information in your report. Either attend one of these classes live or perform a workout offered online by the company. Write about your experience and the quality of the instruction offered.

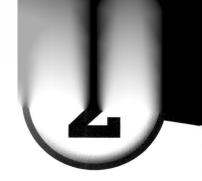

Social Aspects of Group Exercise

Chapter Objectives

By the end of this chapter, you will be able to

- implement behavioral strategies in a group exercise setting,
- understand group cohesion research as it applies to group exercise,
- understand the importance of role modeling for group exercise instructors,
- apply healthy emotional environment principles in group exercise, and
- understand the difference between student-centered and teacher-centered instruction.

As instructors, our overarching purpose for offering group classes is to help people live happier and healthier lives through exercise. We want our classes to enhance the quality of life of all our participants. Kravitz (2007) believes that the future of fitness professionals involves developing and endorsing programs that are directed toward the enhancement of health for clients. Francis (2012) cites a growing role for fitness professionals in public health education. We help educate participants by incorporating health-related fitness components into our program design. This book revolves around the health-related components of fitness. In fact, in chapters 6 through 9 within the Primary Components of Group Exercise section of this text, we review these fitness components and discuss how to accomplish them through group exercise program design. The health-related fitness components include cardiorespiratory endurance, muscular strength and endurance, flexibility, neuromotor fitness, and body composition. While focusing on the health-related components of fitness improves physiology, we also know that group dynamics can improve social dynamics, which also improves health (Seligman 2011).

Therefore, another important aspect of group exercise is the socialization and connectedness its participants experience. Research confirms that a low level of social support is associated with a two- to threefold increase in risk of cardiovascular disease and mortality (Mookadam and Arthur 2004). A lack of social support is also linked with an increased risk of death from cancer and infectious disease (Uchino 2006). Dr. Dean Ornish (1998), a preventive medicine physician, is known for saying, "Illness begins with 'I' and Wellness begins with 'we.'" in his many presentations based on his book *Love and Survival*. Many of the new forms of group exercise, such as stroller babies or organized outdoor walk or run and boot camp groups, increase not only physical activity but also social connectedness (McGonigal 2007). According to Estabrooks (2000), the presence of a highly task-cohesive group has the greatest influence on exercise adherence. For example, many group exercise classes offered at nine o'clock in the morning attract stay-at-home mothers or fathers who enjoy exercise and sharing stories about their children. Often, retirees find that their group exercise class is their social outlet. Some exercise classes celebrate birthdays together, go to lunch together, and form their own social networks.

This chapter will cover ways to integrate health-related components of fitness into practice and focus on the integration of healthy group dynamics in combination to promote safe and effective instruction with an emphasis on social connection principles that also improve health. Having a group exercise instructor who can affect a participant's health both in and outside the class is necessary from a public health perspective. With obesity on the rise in our society, it is imperative that instructors look beyond the mechanics of class instruction and appreciate the health practices they are imparting to their participants, both physically and socially.

Creating Group Cohesion

An excellent group exercise instructor encourages group cohesion while teaching. In fact, Bray and colleagues (2001) found that the fitness instructor's ability to connect with participants was an important predictor of exercise attendance. Popowych (2005) emphasized the importance of group connectedness and suggested that a specific focus on integrating this concept into a group format was warranted. Burke and colleagues (2006) performed a meta-analysis on types of group exercise. Their research showed that a group exercise class where group dynamics principles were used to increase adherence was superior to a standard group exercise class where the instructor showed up and taught the class with little interaction. Group cohesion can be accomplished only in a group setting. In strength and conditioning rooms, where the participants are using their own machines and performing their own routines (often while wearing iPods and headphones), group cohesion is less likely. Group exercise encourages interaction and can enhance emotional as well as physical wellness—especially if the instructor fosters an interactive environment.

The major emphasis in training programs for group exercise instructors has been on class content. What has been lacking is guidance on

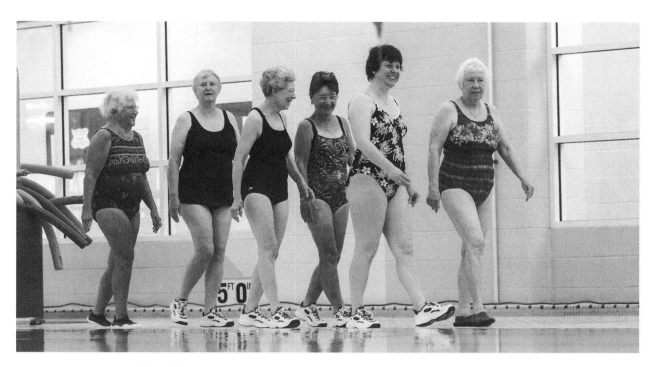

A focus on healthy lifestyle brings many seniors to group exercise classes, where they enjoy socialization benefits as well.

connecting the participants so that a sense of community develops within the group class, which has many benefits. Alan (2003) believes that this connection is often what brings older adults to a group exercise experience. Floyd and Moyer (2009) found that breast cancer survivors experienced greater improvements in their quality of life through group exercise instruction as compared to individually based exercise programs. Teaching group classes from a student-centered perspective with an emphasis on developing group cohesion can enhance adherence. According to Carron, Widmeyer, and Brawley (1988), group cohesiveness is related to individual adherence behavior. For example, when participants meet and socialize with others in the class, they are more likely to keep coming and therefore keep exercising. Carron and colleagues suggest that we all should examine how to keep groups of participants coming back to class so that we can enhance the health and wellness of the overall population. Therefore, investing resources in improving group exercise classes and creating a sense of community within a fitness facility is a logical step in improving national health.

Heinzelmann and Bagley (1970) reported that 90% of adult participants in an exercise program prefer to exercise in group settings. Similarly, Stephens and Craig (1990) reported that 65% of participants prefer to exercise in groups rather than alone. Group exercise programs also appear to produce higher rates of exercise maintenance than individual-based programs (Massie and Sheperd 1971). Spink and Carron (1992) found that group cohesion in female exercise participants played a role in adherence behaviors. Finally, Carron, Widmeyer, and Brawley (1988) had class participants, both those who dropped out and those who stayed with the program, assess the cohesiveness of their classes. Participants who stayed with the program held higher perceptions of cohesiveness.

Spink and Carron (1994) stated that while the university setting provides greater perceptions of task cohesion, the health club setting relies more on social factors for adherence. For example, when students are graded on attendance, their attendance improves. In clubs, creating social opportunities allows fitness classes to build cohesion and improve attendance. The current model within fitness or health clubs is not designed to foster group cohesion except in organized group exercise classes. Instructors can make or break the opportunity for group cohesion with how they teach. For example, compare and contrast the following scenarios: Jill comes in to teach her stationary indoor cycling class and reminds participants that she has a "no talking" rule during class so participants can focus on the workout. Contrast that with John who teaches another stationary indoor cycling class and asks participants to say hello to their neighbors before the class begins and ask them where they are from. These instructors have selected different methods to start their classes. John's method will foster more group cohesion than Jill's approach.

Older adults tend to have a better exercise experience when the experience includes social activities outside of the exercise class. Estabrooks and Carron (1999) found that elderly exercisers who have stronger beliefs in the social cohesiveness of their exercise class have more positive attitudes about exercise. In a study by Spink and Carron (1993), an exercise class that participated in a team-building intervention program had significantly fewer dropouts than a similar class that did not undergo the team-building program. Finally, Carron, Hausenblas, and Mack (1996) have shown that developing a highly cohesive group that is focused on the exercise task and its possible outcomes is likely to have a strong effect on compliance.

Research and participant stories tell us that as group exercise instructors, we need to do more than stand in front of a class and lead exercises. We need to engage in exercise together. By focusing on being student-centered teachers, we can make a difference in the cohesiveness of our classes, and ultimately this difference will improve the health and wellness of our participants. The following suggestions are practical ways for facilitating cohesion in a group exercise class:

- Learn your participants' names and have them learn one another's names.
- Schedule social outings.
- Create a Facebook page for your class and use it to share information and social gatherings.

- Create an e-mail list of participants and share it with everyone.
- Update your website with participant success stories for all to read.
- Share personal stories—be human with your participants!
- Use partner exercises and have participants introduce themselves while doing exercises.
- Discuss current health topics with participants.
- Have participants count down or up with you when performing exercises.
- Name movements after participants.
- Keep track of attendance and connect with participants who are not coming to class.
- Celebrate birthdays, anniversaries, and any other important dates with your groups.
- Have holiday themes or props, such as tying jingle bells on participants' shoes.
- Schedule a picture-sharing circuit class and have participants guess whose picture is at each station.

Instructors as Role Models

By looking back at the history of Reebok advertisements which promoted specific shoes for group exercise, we can witness the aesthetic movement in action. Many of the ads from athletic shoe companies in the 1970s, 1980s, and 1990s showed a small picture of the shoe and a large picture of a fit body (usually a female body). These ads contained two messages. The first was that if you bought the shoes, you would get the body in the picture. The second was that participating in group exercise would help you get the body in the picture. Several studies on exercise and weight loss conducted during the 1990s (Gaesser 1999; Miller 1999) encouraged people to place a greater emphasis on lifestyle change and pay less attention to aesthetics. Nike was one of the first companies to change its focus from aesthetics to promoting healthy lifestyles. According to Bednarski

(1993), who was a marketing executive for Nike at the time, it was difficult to convince male managers that the company needed a different marketing strategy for women, but eventually Nike created an empowering campaign geared toward women that featured shoe ads with testimonials about how it felt to be fit through sports and exercise. The focus was more on all the things people could do with this newfound energy than on what they looked like. Many of the ads did not feature any people; instead, they touted the health benefits of exercise. Enhancing self-esteem was seen as more important than changing body shape. Health clubs and workout videos also used body image to market programs and products. The *Buns of Steel* video campaign is one example. Naming group exercise sessions by body parts is another example. Classes such as Ultimate Abs, Butts and Guts, and Absolute Arms all played on the aesthetics message.

One way to move your program into the new functional fitness for health era is by naming your classes in a positive, educational way. One fitness center uses time to describe its classes. For example, it calls a class *Step 45* instead of *Ultimate Step* so that participants will know that the class lasts 45 minutes. The more hard core the class name sounds, the fewer beginners the class will attract (Kennedy 2004).

Aesthetics Versus Health

Much of the exercise equipment in the 1970s was designed to enhance aesthetics with little reference to improving functional abilities for health. For example, a seated biceps curl variable resistance machine improves the strength of the biceps, but if users lift with the arms and the low back gets injured while lifting, they have not trained the whole system but instead have trained the individual parts. Recently, researchers have begun to acknowledge that the body works as a system, and so it needs to be trained as a system for strength training to enhance our lives. De Vreede, Samson, and VanMeeteren (2005) studied 98 healthy women aged 70 years and older. One group was assigned to an exercise program based on functional tasks (e.g., performing sit-to-stand exercises), and another group was assigned a traditional resistance exercise program (using variable resistance machines in a circuit). Both groups exercised 3 times per week for 12 weeks. The results showed that the functional exercises were more effective than the resistance exercises when it came to improving functional task performance for older adults. Ginis, Jung, and Gauvin (2003) found that regardless of concern about body image, women who worked out in front of mirrors felt worse after exercising than women who exercised without mirrors. A study on body image among women who were strength training confirmed that the training improved not only strength but also body image (Ahmed, Wiltonm, and Pituch 2002).

Fitness is becoming a prominent part of people's lives as they find a sense of purpose in working out that goes deeper than how they look. The fitness movement may have initially been based on appearance, but this focus is certainly changing into the functional training era of movement for healthy living. Some people believe that soon we will no longer be discussing *exercise* and *fitness*. We will remove the *E* and *F* words for good and instead begin discussing the importance of physical activity in our lives. Use of the terms *exercise* and *fitness* has turned away some potential participants from enjoying movement experiences. Group exercise is more than a movement experience—it also has a social and educational component. We need to emphasize physical activity outcomes as well as promote the fun and social atmosphere of group exercise in order to bring back past participants who have had a bad experience with exercise and fitness. See Selected Obesity and Inactivity Research Findings later in this chapter.

The interconnectedness of systems is a pattern that has become evident in many disciplines. Capra (1982) drew on quantum physics, economics, and ecology to argue that the world should not be analyzed as made up of independent, isolated elements—the system should be considered as a whole. For example, a person may develop arteriosclerosis, a narrowing and hardening of the arteries, as the result of an unhealthy lifestyle that involves improper diet, lack of exercise, and excessive smoking. Surgical treatment for a blocked artery may temporarily alleviate the resulting chest pain, but it does not make the person well. The surgical intervention merely treats a local effect of a systemic disorder that will continue until the underlying problems are identified and resolved. An analogous scenario in the fitness setting is training individual muscle groups without training the core that houses those muscle groups. We cannot use the strength we gain by doing a bench press unless we also work on total-body strengthening. This concept is the essence of the new movement for healthy philosophy. Pilates, yoga, and tai chi are types of group exercise classes that have gained popularity because of the increasingly recognized importance of a systems approach to training the body.

Although we have come a long way in changing the message from aesthetics to function, we still have a long way to go. In an article on triathlon training, Kahlkoetter (2002) stated that "women often begin training for the purpose of losing weight and looking better, rather than for inner satisfaction and health" (p. 48). Hollywood, television, magazines, and movies are often to blame for the unrealistic images put before us. However, one example of an attempt to set things straight is that of Jamie Lee Curtis. After being featured in the fitness movie *Perfect,* she admitted to engaging in many unhealthy practices in an effort to keep her perfect body. In a *More* magazine article (Wallace 2002), Curtis posed for a picture with no makeup or body touch-ups so that people could see her true self. Ideally, her example will lead others to unveil the Hollywood myth of the perfect body. Men are not immune to the body image issue. According to Beals (2003), muscle dysmorphia (a form of body image disturbance found among male weightlifters) is on the rise; half of those with this disorder have tried anabolic steroids. Psychiatrists have connected the symptoms of muscle dysmorphia in males as being similar to those of anorexia nervosa in females, with the main difference being that muscle dysmorphia focuses on the acquisition of muscle mass and anorexia nervosa focuses on the shedding of body mass (Murray and Touyz 2012).

Fitness Instructors and Body Image

According to Westcott (1991), participants rate knowledge as the most important characteristic of their fitness instructor. Most participants also look up to their fitness instructor as a role model. This puts a lot of pressure on instructors: What kind of role models are we? In an article by Evans and Kennedy (1993), results of an informal research study of female fitness instructors showed that while their average body fat was 20% (which is quite low; the average in the United States is 32%), 46% of the fitness instructors believed they were very or somewhat overweight. A study (Nardini, Raglin, and Kennedy 1999) of 148 female fitness instructors found that 64% perceived an ideal body as one that was thinner than their current bodies. Olson and colleagues (1996) studied female aerobics instructors and found that 40% of the instructors indicated a previous experience with eating disorders. The aerobic dance instructors in this study had Eating Disorder Inventory scores that suggested behaviors and attitudes consistent with those of female athletes whose sports emphasize leanness and of women who have eating disorders such as anorexia and bulimia. A survey conducted at a large national conference on water fitness (Evans and Connor 1995) revealed that 48% of water fitness instructors agreed that they constantly worry about being or becoming fat. Another study (Krane et al. 2001), which looked at female athletes and regular exercisers, suggested that concern about excessive exercise in these women was warranted.

Fitness professionals experience a myriad of intrinsic and external pressures to achieve the coveted lean and toned appearance. These pressures may lead us to engage in dangerous exercise behaviors and weight-loss techniques. We must take care of ourselves as well as take care of our participants who may have body-image problems (see "Resources for Disordered Eating and Body Image" in this chapter). Yager and Jennifer (2005) identified the important role that educators play in preventing eating disorders. In order to screen potential instructors and create healthy environments, we must be healthy ourselves. If you are teaching group exercise classes but do not have a good body image, consider talking to a counselor or stepping down as a fitness instructor until you resolve your personal issues. You cannot be an effective role model if you cannot walk the talk. The good news is that several of the new group exercise formats are improving body image self-acceptance through increased body awareness. Impett, Daubenmier, and Hirschman (2006) found that frequent yoga practice is associated with greater body awareness, positive affect, and satisfaction with life as well as decreased negative affect.

Davis (1994) studied physical activity in the development and maintenance of eating disorders and found that, for a number of anorexic women, sport or exercise is an integral part of the progression toward self-starvation. She suggests that overactivity be viewed as a primary and not a secondary symptom of eating disorders. As instructors, we should not teach several classes in one day; by doing so we will be telling participants that overexercising is healthy. We also ought to role model healthy behaviors, such as taking the stairs instead of the elevator or parking the car farther away from the building so that we have a longer walk in. Modeling daily activities to participants is as important as modeling healthy intentional exercise patterns.

Freeman (1988) reminds us that body image is independent of physical characteristics. An attractive person can feel plain or unattractive. Because body image and self-esteem are perceptions, changing our bodies will not improve our image or self-esteem unless the physical changes are accompanied by changed perceptions. Improving body image involves changing how we think about our bodies. Taking charge of our own body image and educating participants about body image are important if we are to be positive role models.

Resources for Disordered Eating and Body Image

National Eating Disorders Organization
www.nationaleatingdisorders.org

American Dietetic Association
www.eatright.org

National Women's Health Information Center
www.womenshealth.gov

Creating a Healthy Emotional Environment

In addition to being positive role models, group exercise instructors need to establish a comfortable emotional environment for their participants. Education, motivation, and creative class content are not the only factors that keep participants coming back to group exercise. Tapping into participants' feelings is necessary to affect adherence. Bain, Wilson, and Chaikind (1989) performed a research study on overweight women taking part in an organized exercise program. The authors found that 35% of the participants who were overweight dropped out, while only 7% of the participants who were at their recommended weight quit the program. Although factors such as safety, comfort, and quality of instruction affected the women's exercise behaviors, the most powerful influences seemed to be the social circumstances of the exercise setting, especially concerns about visibility, embarrassment, and judgment by others. As the instructor, you should acknowledge all the participants—from the ones you know to the ones who always hide at the back of the room. What you do and say can affect class atmosphere, and a simple hello can make all the difference to a newcomer in group exercise. Ornish (1998) believes that interpersonal interaction might be the single most important ingredient for creating an accepting environment in a group exercise experience. Seligman (2011) created a Positive Psychology Center in 2005 based on his belief that schools need to teach skills of well-being as well as achievement. Apply Seligman's ideas to group exercise and we see that teaching movement patterns will improve health, but teaching and modeling a healthy emotional environment while instructing may also teach happiness life skills.

Goleman (2006) suggests that having social and emotional intelligence in any group setting dictates the success of the group experience. Goleman believes that "the emotional economy is the sum total of the exchanges of feeling among us. In subtle (or not so subtle) ways, we all make each other feel a bit better (or a lot worse) as part of any contact we have; every encounter can be weighted along a scale from emotionally toxic to nourishing" (1998, p. 165). A specific example of supporting others within a group exercise setting is to announce before class how great it feels to be there, improving overall health and well-being. Contrast this with telling the class how you ate two desserts the night before that you intend to work off during the session. The first statement leaves participants with a health-related sense of purpose for the workout. The second statement can send a message that punishment through exercise is recommended after overindulging. Seidman (2007) believes the most powerful form of human influence to be inspiration. The first syllable of inspiration is "in," signifying that the conduct is internal and intrinsic. Coercion and motivation happen to you; inspiration happens *in* you. Learn how to inspire your participants, and you will help create a healthy emotional environment.

A study on group dynamics in physical activity by Fox, Rejeski, and Gauvin (2000) found that enjoyment during physical activity is optimized when a positive and supportive leadership style is coupled with an enriched and supportive group environment. Instructors affect adherence and may be an important predictor of exercise behavior. We help create a sense of community that can often be what brings adults to our group exercise experience. Using social intelligence (Goleman 2006) as well as emotional intelligence in any group setting dictates the success of the group experience. A specific example of failing to apply social intelligence in a group exercise setting would be if you stayed in the front of the room and talked only to participants in the front row. The participants in the middle and back rows might feel unacknowledged. If instead you knew the names of everyone, greeted all the participants when they came into class, and moved around the room to encourage them throughout the workout, you would be creating a healthier emotional and social atmosphere. Social intelligence is a key ingredient for being a positive role model.

An environment where an instructor presents and flaunts a body beautiful can also intimidate participants. Eklund and Crawford (1994) compared two similar video exercise routines in which the instructor's apparel was different—in one, the instructor wore a thong-style exercise leotard, while in the other the same instructor wore shorts and a T-shirt. Physique-anxious participants rated the thong leotard video more unfavorably than the shorts and T-shirt video.

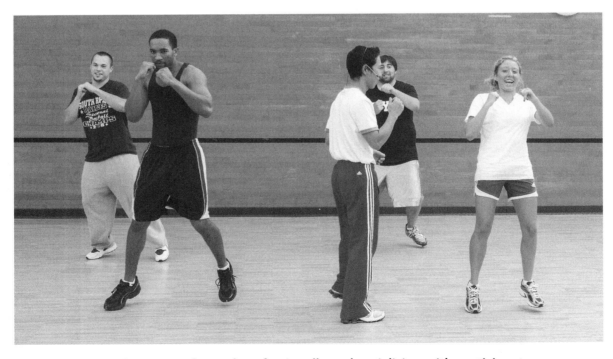

A group exercise instructor dressed professionally and socializing with participants.

Thus, instructors can help participants become more comfortable with their own bodies and help keep participants exercising by wearing modest exercise clothing. We live in a culture in which a thin and toned body is seen as the ideal. According to Ibbetson (1996), the idea that thinness is beauty is so well accepted that body-image dissatisfaction is remarkably high. Some researchers indicate that body-image disturbance is so prevalent that it can be considered a normal part of the female experience (Silberstein, Striegel-Moore, and Rodin 1987). Evans (1993) makes the following recommendations for enhancing participant and instructor body-image perceptions:

- Wear professional attire that is not too revealing and will make all participants feel comfortable.

- Display educational materials on body-image acceptance at strategic locations.

- Use positive motivational strategies. For example, encourage activity outside of class.

- Choose music that sends a positive message.

Student-Centered Versus Teacher-Centered Instruction

The motivational and inspirational aspect of instructing group exercise includes having new moves, catchy music, and state-of-the-art equipment as well as communicating and cueing movements effectively. The educational part of instructing group exercise involves knowing why certain moves are selected, incorporating current research and knowledge within a session, and making educated decisions about the information given to participants. It is important to be a teacher-centered and a student-centered instructor at the same time. An effective class begins with the attitude and atmosphere established by the instructor. A range of factors can influence a class environment. In the following discussion we focus on the professionalism of the group exercise instructor, who needs to be both a motivator and an educator (Claxton and Lacy 1991; Francis 1991; Kennedy and Legel 1992).

Let's compare a teacher-centered instructor with a student-centered instructor. The teacher-centered instructor focuses on developing relationships with students that are anchored in intellectual explorations of material; in group exercise, this means learning the movements and following along. The instructor focuses more on content than on student processing, and the approach is associated with the transmission of knowledge. Your focus while wearing the teacher-centered hat is to help students imitate your movements. The student-centered instructor, on the other hand, strives to establish an atmosphere of independence, encouragement, attainable goals, and reality. A student-centered instructor places the learning characteristics of all learners under the microscope and pays special attention to low-performing learners. Your goal when acting as a student-centered instructor is to clarify and individualize what is needed to create positive learning experiences to help your students enjoy success and the overall experience.

Learning to take responsibility for the health and well-being of participants starts with establishing a positive, professional attitude and atmosphere. Kandarian (2006) believes a group exercise instructor needs to be an instructor and not a performer. He advocates that instructors "leave their post up" positions at the front of the class and move around the room so they can get to know their participants (2006, p. 87). A purely student-centered instructor is often perceived as being there to make a difference in people's lives. A purely teacher-centered instructor can be mistaken as being there for his or her personal workout. Following are examples of how a teacher-centered instructor and a student-centered instructor perceive the learning experience. Having attributes from both of these styles will enhance the learning experience of students in a group exercise class. Recent observations of online learning experiences are beginning to demonstrate the importance of having both teacher-centered and student-centered learning experiences (Edmundson 2007).

Teacher-Centered Instruction

- Instructor's role is to give information.
- Emphasis is on getting the movement right and performing the correct patterns.

- Students are the only learners.
- Instructor teaches from a stage and does not leave the front of the room.
- Students passively reflect on the information and movements that are given to them.
- The overall class atmosphere is competitive and individualistic.

Student-Centered Instruction

- Instructor's role is to coach and facilitate the experience.
- The instructor and the students learn together.
- The instructor moves around the room and makes contact with all participants during the class.
- Emphasis is on moving and learning from errors rather than performing perfectly.
- Students are actively involved in the learning process, and the instructor carefully observes the students' progress before moving on to more difficult movements.
- The culture is cooperative, relaxed, and supportive.
- Partner exercises or countdowns of exercises bring the group together and make it less competitive.

When balancing your approach to teaching by focusing on students, another issue to consider is the way that a group exercise class fits into students' lives and overall health. Offering a variety of class times and activities is important for successful group exercise programs. At the beginning of the current century, public health experts (Hooker 2003) predicted that fitness professionals would begin collaborating to expand movement experiences, especially at the community level. This has come to fruition; one example is the way the group exercise experience is being moved outdoors in the form of boot camps, neighborhood walking groups, and stroller baby classes. Pate and colleagues (1995) endorsed the *Surgeon General's Report on Physical Activity and Health* and focused on the importance of increasing activity within daily living, such as walking the dog or taking the stairs more frequently. The

initial *Surgeon General's Report* stated that every U.S. adult should accumulate 30 minutes or more of moderate-intensity physical activity on most, preferably all, days of the week. Recently, the U.S. Health and Human Services Department (HHS) and the Centers for Disease Control (CDC) expanded this report into the *Guidelines for Physical Activity* (2008), advocating for 150 minutes of physical activity per week with less emphasis on frequency of exercise. Group exercise instructors cannot assume that people are getting 150 weekly minutes of physical activity due to the conveniences of daily living. In the 1970s and 1980s we could assume most Americans participated in 30 minutes of daily physical activity. Now, we can no longer assume this is the case. The research on sitting time reported in chapter 1 reminds us that we need to adapt differently to participants who come to classes for the first time.

Clapp and Little (1994) studied the physiological effects of participants and instructors who were performing three types of group exercise routines (low impact, high impact, and step). These researchers concluded that the participants consistently underestimated their level of performance. In other words, exercisers may often think they're doing more than they actually are. As instructors, we need to incorporate the evidence-based guidelines for exercise as well as focus on activities of daily living. For instance, a Zumba class may involve only moderate cardiorespiratory intensity movement and may not contain the other class elements such as muscular strength and flexibility. If you're teaching a Zumba class then, you'll want to encourage participants to also take classes with more of a muscular conditioning and stretching focus. (Note: Some facilities also offer Zumba Toning classes). Knowing your participants' physical activity patterns, as well as their fitness levels, is important in helping them meet their healthy lifestyle goals.

The challenge for group exercise instructors is to apply current research and information from the American College of Sports Medicine (ACSM) Guidelines for Exercise Testing and Prescription (ACSM 2014; see table 1.2) and the CDC *Guidelines for Physical Activity* (2008) in order to develop safe, effective, and highly motivating workouts that make a difference in participants'

Selected Obesity and Inactivity Research Findings

According to Blair (2009), physical inactivity could be the biggest risk factor for early death for all cause disease. Health experts suggest that if today's youth keep supersizing their meals while downsizing their physical activity, they risk becoming the first generation of Americans to live shorter lives than their parents lived, owing to obesity-related heart disease and diabetes (Weir 2004). In addition, the many health risks associated with obesity are economically costly. According to Bortz (2003), U.S. citizens ultimately will save money if they are healthy. Muller-Riemenschneider, Reinhold, and Willich (2009) performed a systematic review of the cost-effectiveness of programs that promoted physical activity; they found that these programs saved money in the long run. In a meta-analysis of the literature on costs and savings associated with workplace disease prevention and wellness programs, Harvard researchers (Baicker, Cutler, and Song 2010) reported that for every dollar spent on wellness programs, medical costs are reduced by US$3.27, and absenteeism costs are reduced by US$2.73. Ostbye, Dement, and Krause (2007) documented that obese workers filed double the number of worker compensation claims and lost nearly 184 days due to illness or injury per 100 employees. These statistics are a 13-fold increase over those from nonobese workers.

Exercise is an important part of maintaining a healthy body weight. Jakicic and colleagues (2003) found that a 12-month program combining exercise and diet resulted in significant weight loss and improved cardiorespiratory fitness for various durations and intensities of exercise. The study showed a direct relationship between total weekly energy expenditure and weight loss. So how does group exercise help create a healthy lifestyle? Grant and colleagues (2004) studied a group of 26 women in their 60s who were participating in a 12-week group exercise program. The study found that both functional and psychological improvements occurred as a result of participating in a 40-minute group fitness session twice a week. We know that beginning exercisers are often more comfortable with becoming informed about exercise when they are in the group setting. They like being instructed because they can learn correct exercise techniques and gain motivation to continue working out. Any activity that keeps people moving will make a difference in their health. Howley, Bassett, and Thompson (2005) advocate getting people moving as the first way to control obesity. If group exercise increases energy expenditure, then it will affect the health-related components of fitness that will be reviewed in chapter 3.

health and wellness. Enhancing quality of life is a theme that we need to carry throughout our group exercise classes. Franco and colleagues (2005) found that 30 minutes of walking gave older adults aged 50 years or older 3.5 more years of disease-free life. In addition, researchers at the University of Illinois reported that participating in 12 weeks of aerobic exercise for 3 hours a week significantly increased brain volume in older adults (Begley 2006). These studies, as well as many others, help validate the many benefits of exercise and physical activity. If we can provide these benefits to our group exercise participants, as well as include and role model healthy social interactions, then we are giving participants a valuable gift. The gift of health, happiness, and improved quality of life is more precious than any other gift a person can receive.

Chapter Wrap-Up

Fitness professionals need to be leaders in moving the industry from the aesthetic era of exercise toward more purposeful reasons for improving health and well-being. We can choose to buy into the ideal body image presented to us by the media and society at large, or we can set a normal, healthy example for our participants. A healthy body image is not something that we can take for granted as exercise instructors, as many of us are affected by our own body-image perceptions. However, feeling good about ourselves and projecting this confidence to our participants could be the most important health message that we have to offer. Representing health and wellness for participants can be an essential component of enjoying who you are when instructing group exercise. Group exercise can be powerful if participants feel welcome, learn new things, get to know others, are taught safely, and believe that their time is being well spent. The experience can not only make a positive change in their emotional outlook but also can improve their health and quality of living. One of the biggest challenges for the group exercise instructor is to balance all the health and emotional elements of the group exercise experience—this is, perhaps, the most difficult skill a fitness professional can master. Once we move beyond emphasizing quantized fitness gains and aesthetics, we can understand that the real power of exercise lies in the experience itself. Group exercise is definitely an experience, and the instructor makes or breaks that experience.

ASSIGNMENTS

1. Attend a group exercise class and evaluate whether the instructor has a student-centered or teacher-centered style. Give a minimum of three specific examples that support your analysis. Then, interview the class participants about the level of group cohesiveness. Ask whether they have met people through the experience and if that has helped their adherence. Write a 1-page paper on your findings.

2. Write a 250-word paper that describes your physical activity patterns from the time you started exercising until now. Tell how your exercise experience has changed for you over the years.

Foundational Components

Chapter Objectives

By the end of this chapter, you will be able to

- understand the integration of health components into group exercise class design,
- demonstrate how to create a positive preclass environment,
- understand basic health screening for group exercise leaders,
- learn important principles of muscle balance and terminology for muscle action,
- identify range of motion for major joints,
- investigate a 6-step exercise progression model, and
- analyze a group exercise tool for instructors to use in designing classes.

This chapter will review common principles of class design, class environment, and exercise selection and progression that apply to all group exercise classes. For example, the principles of muscle balance apply to all types of fitness classes, and selecting proper exercise progressions is also important. Learning the range of motion of different muscles and understanding how to select exercises for a group exercise setting are critical in order to help promote healthy lifestyles for your participants. Additionally, having an evaluation form, such as the one in appendix A that lists and reviews key concepts, allows the group exercise program director and the instructor to be on the same page regarding how to implement these principles in a class. Chapters 6 through 9 review in detail how to incorporate each of the health-related fitness components into a group exercise class. These components are cardiorespiratory fitness, muscular fitness (strength and endurance), neuromotor fitness (balance, coordination, agility, speed, and power), and flexibility.

Integrating Components of Health Into Class Design

Let's take a closer look at the basic segments of a workout in group exercise:

1. Warm-up
2. Cardiorespiratory activity
3. Post-cardio cool-down
4. Muscular conditioning, balance, and neuromotor exercises
5. Flexibility

Most types of group exercise, including step, stationary indoor cycling, sport conditioning, water exercise, yoga, Pilates, and older-adult classes, incorporate one or more of these segments. Most group classes begin with a preclass preparation followed by a warm-up that includes specific rehearsal movements to prepare for the upcoming workout. These movements are performed at a low to moderate speed and range of motion; they are designed to warm up the body for activity and increase blood flow to the muscles. If included, the cardiorespiratory segment follows the warm-up and is aimed at improving cardiorespiratory endurance and body composition; this segment therefore keeps the heart rate elevated for 10 to 45 minutes. After the cardiorespiratory stimulus, a gradual cool-down returns the heart rate to resting levels and prevents excessive pooling of blood in the lower extremities. The muscular conditioning segment may focus on resistance training, core training, balance, or other neuromotor exercises depending on the activity. The class typically ends with a flexibility component that includes stretching and relaxation exercises designed to further lower the heart rate, increase body awareness, and enhance overall flexibility.

Integrating the components of health into the group exercise program requires a look at the overall class format. There is no single class format that fits every type of group exercise class. In a step class, it is appropriate to warm up using a step; however, in a sport conditioning class, practicing sport-specific rehearsal moves in the warm-up is more conducive to preparing the body properly for the upcoming workout. In a water exercise class thermoregulation is important, so performing static stretches to enhance flexibility at the end of the workout may not be recommended. Static stretching may be beneficial in the warm-up and stretching segment of a low-impact class for seniors, but a 15-minute abdominal class may forego stretching because the purpose of the class is abdominal strengthening. All are examples of why the same class format may not be suitable for all group exercise classes.

Notice that the segments of a group exercise class are aligned with the health-related fitness components listed in the 2014 American College of Sports Medicine (ACSM) guidelines (see chapter 1). As mentioned in Chapter 1, when the first ACSM position statement was published in 1978 (ACSM 1978), it contained only cardiorespiratory guidelines. At that time there was little research on strengthening the musculoskeletal system. As clinicians and researchers began to realize that many people were experiencing back pain, the research focus turned to the musculoskeletal system. In the 1990 ACSM position stand, muscular strength and endurance were included along with cardiorespiratory fitness, but there was still no mention of flexibility.

Clinicians and researchers then discovered the importance of having flexible as well as strong muscles, and the 2006 ACSM position stand included flexibility. Group exercise classes have long included all these fitness components even though older ACSM guidelines were limited. The newest guidelines also recommend exercises for neuromotor fitness, which includes balance, agility, and proprioceptive training. The current ACSM position stand and guidelines (ACSM 2014) focus on all the health-related fitness components; these components are usually included in a general group exercise class.

The degree to which each of the health-related fitness components is developed in any particular individual can vary widely. For example, a person may be strong but lack flexibility or may have great cardiorespiratory endurance but lack muscular strength. Each component of fitness should be included in a program. We should understand the definitions of muscular strength, endurance, and flexibility so that we know that they're being properly included. Additionally, we need an understanding of the roles muscles play in various movements (see "Muscular Conditioning Terminology").

The 2014 ACSM guidelines were reviewed briefly in chapter 1. The emphasis that a group exercise class gives to each fitness component will vary depending on the objective of the class as well as the fitness level, age, health, and physical skill of the participants. Our goal as fitness professionals is to include all the components of fitness in our program but not necessarily all in one class. For example, a stretching class will enhance mobility, whereas a sport conditioning or boot camp–style

Health-Related Fitness Components Defined

cardiorespiratory fitness —The ability to perform repetitive, moderate-to-high-intensity, large-muscle movement for a prolonged period

flexibility—The amount of movement that can be accomplished at a joint

muscle strength—The maximum amount of force a muscle or muscle group can develop during a single contraction

body composition—The percentages of fat, bone, and muscle in a human body

Muscular Conditioning Terminology

muscle strength—The maximum force a muscle or muscle group can produce at one time.

muscle endurance—The ability to perform repeated muscle actions, as in push-ups or sit-ups, or to maintain a static muscle action for a prolonged duration.

muscle power—The ability of a muscle or muscle group to move a force quickly: (power = (force $\times$ distance) $\div$ time.

muscle stability—The ability of a muscle or muscle group to stabilize a joint and maintain a desired position. This is particularly important for postural muscles that stabilize the spine, pelvis, and shoulder girdle.

overload—Giving the body a challenge greater than it has had in the past. Overload may be accomplished by increasing the exercise frequency (number of days per week), duration (number of sets or repetitions), intensity (amount of weight lifted), or mode (type of exercise). The exercise mode can be modified by switching to a new exercise for the same muscle group; adding an unstable surface such as a stability ball, BOSU balance trainer, or foam roller; or changing from dumbbell to elastic resistance.

Various Roles of Muscles

Muscles can play different roles depending on the action they are performing. For example, in a triceps kickback, the triceps extends the elbow and is therefore the prime mover (agonist). In a biceps curl, the triceps acts as the antagonist while the biceps flexes the elbow (the biceps muscle is now the agonist). And in a bent-over low row, the triceps is only an assistor, assisting the action of shoulder extension (the latissimus dorsi are the prime movers). The triceps can also act as a stabilizer. Consider its role in maintaining the plank position—the triceps stabilizes the elbow joint, maintaining elbow extension. So, one muscle—the triceps—can play several different roles, depending on the exercise.

agonist—The prime mover, which is the muscle that is responsible for the movement that you see.

antagonist—The muscle acting opposite the agonist; it elongates and allows the agonist to contract and move the joint.

assistor—A muscle that assists in performing a movement but is not the prime mover.

stabilizer—A muscle that stabilizes a joint and helps to keep it from moving. When muscles perform a stabilizing role, they contract isometrically.

Terminology for Muscle Action

isometric movement—A static muscle action in which there is no change in the muscle length or the affected joint angle. Breathing is important when performing an isometric action; breath holding and straining, known as the *Valsalva maneuver*, can increase blood pressure and overload on the heart.

isotonic (dynamic) movement—A muscle action that is not held but instead involves movement. This is the most common type of muscle action for nonpostural muscles. There are two types of isotonic actions:

concentric action—The shortening contraction of the muscle as it develops tension against a resistance (often called the *positive phase*).

eccentric action—The lengthening action of the muscle as it develops tension against a resistance (often called the *negative phase*).

isokinetic movement—A muscle action performed using special equipment not generally found in fitness facilities. In this type of action, the speed of the movement is controlled, and any action applied against the machine results in an equal reaction force.

class will provide cardiorespiratory and muscular conditioning. Because our participants have busy schedules, we need to make the most of their exercise time by emphasizing the health-related fitness components in our programming.

Creating a Positive Preclass Environment

An effective group exercise class starts with appropriate preclass preparation. Most group exercise instructors arrive at least 15 minutes before a class starts in order to prepare equipment, set up the sound system, greet participants as they begin to arrive, and have some mental preparation time. Preclass preparation also involves getting to know your participants so you can design the class to improve their health and well-being.

A few common points must be considered when preparing for any group exercise class. As the instructor, you should know your returning participants and orient new participants, create a positive atmosphere, and begin class on time with equipment ready for use.

Reach Out to a Range of Participants

Teaching a class with both beginning and advanced participants can be challenging. A mixed class is usually the norm rather than the exception because of participants' schedules. Describing classes by duration is one way to help participants find a class at the appropriate level. An example is offering a sport conditioning class that lasts 30 minutes, one that lasts 45 minutes, and another that lasts 60 minutes. The participants can then choose a class based on their fitness level, endurance, and time constraints. The name of a class can be a key factor in attracting types of participants. Kennedy (2004) reported that members of a focus group who attended group exercise classes stated they stayed away from classes that included the words "turbo," "ultimate," or "extreme" in their titles. These names do not always appeal to the beginner. More descriptive names such as Step 30, Boot Camp 45, or Cycle 60 may appeal to a broader range of participants and will allow participants to choose their preferred duration. Offering 20- to 30-minute classes focusing on stretching or muscular conditioning will also help prepare some of the more sedentary participants for the longer classes that contain all the fitness components. Some participants, such as those who walk to work every day, may need only a flexibility or a muscular strength and conditioning class. Offering a variety of class options and venturing beyond the typical hour-long format that encompasses all the fitness components will help you meet the health goals of a greater number of people.

Know Your Participants

How do we individualize programs and protect participants during a group exercise class? By knowing the participants! You must know where people have been and what they want and need in order to lead them successfully. Knowing a participant's health issues is an essential part of providing excellent customer service and safety;

in addition, it may help decrease professional liability.

Although there are many ways of obtaining health information, the ideal is to have the participants fill out a written medical history form that you can review before they arrive for class. Unfortunately, a completed medical history is often the exception rather than the rule. All of us have been in the situation where our class is just getting underway, and a new participant appears. Using a short medical history form can help solve this problem. You can have a new participant fill out the short form upon arrival. Then you can quickly review the contents, clarify any vague information, and make a mental note of areas needing emphasis during class.

An example of a completed short form is included for your reference (see figure 3.1). Short and long health history forms and an informed consent form are in appendices B through D. These forms have been adapted from many sources and can be changed to fit your specific needs. The British Columbia Ministry of Health designed the Physical Activity Readiness Questionnaire (PAR-Q) to help identify individuals for whom exercise may pose a hazard. The PAR-Q can be used as a short form or can be conducted verbally. The developers of the PAR-Q suggest that participants who answer *yes* to any of the questions may need to postpone vigorous exercise or exercise testing and seek medical clearance. The PAR-Q is found in appendix E.

Orient New Participants

Using a health information form is the beginning of building a shared responsibility between the instructor and the participant and is one way to integrate new members into your class. On this form you also can ask participants about their birthdates, favorite rewards, and any other pertinent information that might enhance their performance. To further assist participants, you can provide written information about exercise, the facility schedule, or the program in general.

As exercise instructors, we want our participants to feel that they are responsible for their workout and to inform us of their personal physical limitations so we can assist them as much as possible. We can accomplish this by having the

Short Health History and Consent Form

Name __John Smith__   Date __8-15-14__

The following information will be kept strictly confidential and will be used only to help make your workout safe. Please check any conditions that may apply to you.

Have you ever been told by a physician that you have or have had the following?

	YES	NO
Heart attack	☐	☑
High cholesterol (>200)	☑	☐
Cancer	☐	☑
Arthritis	☐	☑
Seizures	☐	☑
High blood pressure	☑	☐
Diabetes	☐	☑
Osteoporosis	☐	☑
Stroke	☐	☑
Abnormal EKG	☐	☑
Lung problems	☐	☑
Gout	☐	☑

If you are currently taking any prescription or over-the-counter medications, please list them here:

__Beta blockers__

	YES	NO
Do you smoke?	☐	☑
Can you swim?	☐	☑
Do you exercise aerobically at least 3 or 4 times a week?	☐	☑

FIGURE 3.1 As an instructor, what would you consider if you received this completed short history form from a new participant?

Do you have any past injuries to, or current problems with, any of the following areas?

	YES	NO
Irregular heartbeat	☐	☑
Dizziness	☐	☑
Neck	☐	☑
Low back	☐	☑
Feet	☐	☑
Chest pain	☐	☑
Fainting	☐	☑
Hands	☐	☑
Midback	☐	☑
Ankles	☐	☑
Loss of coordination	☐	☑
Cramping	☐	☑
Hips	☐	☑
Shoulders	☐	☑
Knees	☐	☑
Heat intolerance	☐	☑
Shin splints	☐	☑
Calves	☐	☑
Other	☐	☑

I realize that there are risks, including injury and possible death, in all exercise. While every effort will be made to decrease any risk of injury, I take full responsibility for my participation in this class. Knowing that I may participate at my own pace and that I am free to discontinue participation at any time, I will inform the instructor of any problems—immediately.

Signature __John Smith_____ Date __8-15-14_____

FIGURE 3.1 > continued

participants read and sign an informed consent form. A sample of an informed consent form is in appendix D. Obtaining informed consent ensures that we have met an individual's right to know that there are risks associated with exercise. Participants also have the right to know how potential injuries may manifest themselves, how the risk of injury will be minimized, and what responsibility they have in reducing their risk.

You must use some type of medical history form or informed consent sheet since they are part of the legal standard of care in our profession. Also, these forms help establish the foundations of safety, responsibility, and communication, which are necessary elements of the group exercise experience.

Create a Positive Atmosphere

In chapter 2 we discussed many aspects of being a model instructor, from wearing appropriate attire to creating a healthy emotional environment. These points are all part of being an effective instructor and therefore need to be included in any evaluation process.

The following are ways to create a positive class atmosphere:

- Introduce yourself to the participants and have them introduce themselves to others in the class.
- Wear attire and footwear that is appropriate for the class but nonintimidating to members.
- Let participants know what equipment they will need for the workout.
- Explain the class format and review what participants can expect.
- Smile, give positive motivational cues, and be energetic with body language cues.

Creating a positive atmosphere begins with introducing yourself and having students introduce themselves before class begins, especially when you are teaching in a facility where different people come to class every week. These introductions help to establish the attitude of, "We're in this together." Also, if participants know your name and the names of others in the class, they will be more likely to ask questions and talk to one another. New people coming into a group exercise class are often afraid to ask questions and often feel out of place. Understanding this and asking for class communication will create a more open and safe environment for all involved.

The instructor's attire must be appropriate for the specific group exercise class. For example, when you are teaching a class for seniors, wearing a midriff-baring spandex outfit is inappropriate because it might be intimidating and cause members to feel uncomfortable. Observe what participants wear to class and try to match their style of clothing; this will help them to feel more comfortable with you. Ask what attire they prefer. At the same time, balance the comfort level of the class with functionality. Your spinal alignment and form should be visible with each movement you demonstrate. Make sure to notice what participants are wearing and discuss appropriate footwear and attire for the various group exercise classes you teach. For example, some indoor cycles have special clipless pedals that require a specific type of cycling shoe. Likewise, water exercise requires a swimming suit that can give the support needed to exercise effectively.

Finally, give an overview of the class format after introducing yourself. Because so many classes are being offered and so many unique instructional techniques are being used, participants need to know your class expectations. Tell them about water breaks, heart rate checks, expected intensity levels, and any other pertinent information that can help make the class a student-centered experience. For example, you might begin your class by saying, "This is a 30-minute stretching class. There will not be an aerobic component. The only equipment you will need is a mat. Please take your shoes off for the class." In some fitness centers, participants enter the class and see a dry erase board with the instructor's name, a welcome note, and a list of equipment needed for the session. The board informs participants about class expectations if they miss the verbal announcements. After previewing the class format, explain participant responsibilities. One such responsibility is exercising at the desired intensity. There is nothing worse than having a participant come to you after class and say, "This class was too easy for me." Intensity is the responsibility of the participant, not the instructor. You must suggest modifications that allow participants to pick an appropriate intensity level, but you are not responsible for choosing that intensity level.

 See online video 3.1 for a demonstration of beginning a class in a way that creates a positive atmosphere.

Principles of Muscle Balance

Instructors usually include base moves (moves that appear many times during the routine) within the cardiorespiratory segment. These base moves tend to use the quadriceps and hip flexor muscles. Examples include a basic march in place in cardio high-low classes, the basic step in a step class, the cross-country skier move in water exercise, and the flat-road medium resistance interval in stationary indoor cycling. The problem with these base moves is that many participants use the quadriceps and hip flexors extensively in activ-

ities of daily living; therefore, exercise routines that continue to use these muscles repeatedly can create muscle imbalance. Balancing daily spinal flexion and hip flexion with other movements is important. Understanding how the body functions in everyday moves can help you determine which muscles are naturally stronger and which muscles need extra attention during the group exercise session. For example, walking forward works the hip flexors, and so focusing on movements that use the buttocks and the hamstrings (the muscle groups opposing the hip flexors) helps participants achieve muscle balance. As another example, the abductors are important stabilizer muscles for the hips but are often weak in sedentary individuals. Thus, incorporating abductor moves into the cardiorespiratory segment is recommended in order to help with muscle balance and proper movement (see figure 3.2).

Water exercise provides an exception to the need to focus on muscle balance. In water exercise, muscle balance is achieved automatically because there is no gravity. When the hips are

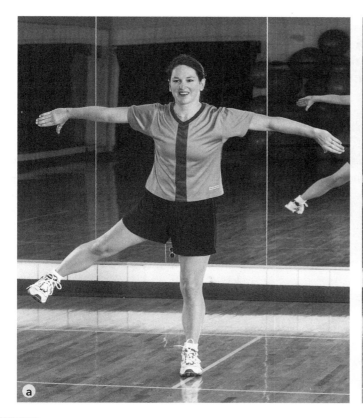 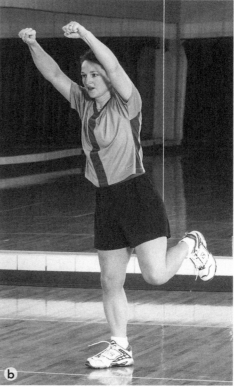

FIGURE 3.2 Working these muscle groups helps balance typical activities of daily living: (*a*) abductors and (*b*) hamstrings.

flexed in water, the iliopsoas and rectus femoris perform the work assisted by buoyancy. When the hip is extended, the hamstrings and buttocks perform the work. In the water, therefore, automatic muscular balance is more likely. With the exception of water exercise, it is important to analyze what movements work which muscles and vary the exercise selection to promote overall muscle balance as well as minimize repetitive movements.

Make the most of floor space to help minimize repetitive motions and be sure to select movements that work the muscle groups in opposing ways. Use different geometric configurations when using floor space (e.g., move in circles, diagonally, up and back) during the cardio segment to help increase safety and interest. Try performing figure eights, walking in circles, walking around a step or cone, or making letters such as an *A* or a *T* either on the floor or on a step to add variety and fun to the cardiorespiratory segment.

To ensure that your routines balance the muscles properly, let's take a moment to review where the major muscles are and what they actually do. Each joint has several muscles attached to it, and these muscles act in opposition to each other (see figure 3.3). Maintaining a balance of strength and flexibility in the muscles around the joints is an excellent way to prevent injuries and promote smooth functioning.

You will notice that many of your students have typical muscle imbalances attributable to activities of daily living, sedentary lifestyle, obesity, poor posture, or simply the natural tendency to perform activities in a forward direction. You need to know what these common muscle imbalances are and how you can help correct them by incorporating appropriate strengthening or stretching exercises into your class. Muscle imbalances left unchecked often lead to injury, especially when participants increase their frequency, intensity, or duration of exercise. Table 3.1 lists the most common muscle imbalances.

Because most muscle imbalances arise from a lack of muscular balance in activities of daily living, we need to keep in mind what participants do when they are not in an exercise class. Then we can analyze which muscle groups participants need to strengthen or stretch in order to counterbalance the muscle actions they use most often in daily activities. Think of the group exercise class

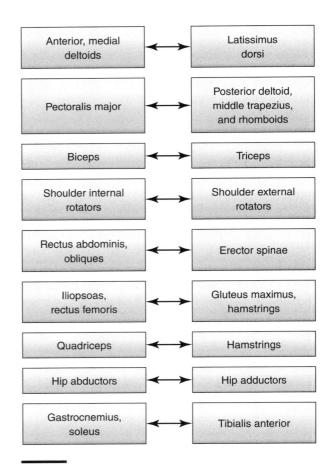

FIGURE 3.3   Opposing muscle groups.

as an opportunity to balance the work of daily living through functional training. Stretching and strengthening muscles that are not regularly used can help participants improve overall muscle balance. This approach brings the role of the group fitness instructor closer to that of an individualized trainer (Kennedy 1997). For a summary of which muscles generally need strengthening and stretching for improved health, see table 3.2.

Table 3.2 was created by conceptualizing muscle function during activities of routine living. For example, an object is normally picked up by performing elbow flexion, which works the biceps concentrically. The object is put down by working the biceps eccentrically against gravity. Because of the direction of gravity, the triceps are not often worked in daily living. The list in table 3.2 is designed to help enhance functional daily living skills for participants who are exercising for health and fitness. It is not meant to suggest that the stronger muscles should not be worked in a group exercise setting; however, we need to

TABLE 3.1 Common Muscle Imbalances

Muscle	Problem	Typical cause	Correction
Pectoralis major	Tight	Poor posture when sitting and standing	Stretch
Posterior deltoids, middle trapezius, rhomboids	Weak, overstretched	Poor posture when sitting and standing	Strengthen
Shoulder internal rotators	Tight	Poor posture, carrying and holding objects close to body	Stretch
Shoulder external rotators	Weak	Poor posture	Strengthen
Abdominals	Weak	Poor posture, obesity	Strengthen
Erector spinae	Tight (and often weak)	Poor posture, obesity	Stretch (and strengthen)
Hip flexors	Tight	Poor posture, sedentary lifestyle	Stretch
Hamstrings	Tight	Sedentary lifestyle	Stretch
Calves	Tight	Wearing high heels	Stretch
Shin	Weak	Not enough use in daily activities	Strengthen

TABLE 3.2 Muscle Balance for Functional Training

Body segment	Muscles that need strengthening	Stabilizers that need strengthening	Muscles that need stretching
Lower body	Anterior tibialis	Abductors	Gastrocnemius and soleus
	Quadriceps and hamstrings	Adductors	Quadriceps and iliopsoas
	Gluteals		Hamstrings
Upper body	Pectoralis minor and lower trapezius		Pectoralis major
	Triceps		Upper trapezius
	Shoulder external rotators (teres minor and infraspinatus)		Anterior and medial deltoids
	Rhomboids and middle trapezius		
	Posterior deltoids		
Core		Erector spinae	Erector spinae
		Abdominals	

focus on creating balance between the weaker muscle groups and the stronger muscle groups, especially if our goal is to create workouts that will benefit participants in their daily lives.

The strategy for correcting muscular imbalances is to strengthen the weak, loose, or small muscles and stretch the tight, short, or strong muscles. For example, since the abdominals typically are weak or loose, it makes sense to include strengthening and shortening exercises such as abdominal crunches in your class. Conversely, since the low-back muscles (the erector spinae) are commonly tight and tense, it makes sense to incorporate feel-good stretches such as the angry cat stretch on hands and knees to lengthen and relax the low back. If the muscle imbalance between the abdominals and erector spinae isn't addressed, the spine will gradually be pulled out of alignment, and this misalignment can lead to excessive lordosis, or swayback. Excessive lordosis is a contributing factor in low-back pain, a chronic disorder that 8 of 10 people in developed countries will experience at some point in their lives (Devereaux 2009; Frymoyer and Cats-Baril 1991).

The rectus abdominis can be trained dynamically through its full range of motion as a spinal flexor, while the oblique muscles can be similarly trained by performing spinal flexion with rotation. This type of training is especially important when the abdominals are weak and overstretched and are contributing to excessive lordosis. The abdominal muscles, including the transverse abdominis, also can be trained isometrically as stabilizers of the spine. In stabilization or core-strengthening exercises, a primary focus is contraction of the transverse abdominis to cause a hollowing or a sensation of navel to spine. In addition, some practitioners use the term *bracing* to help describe the action needed to keep the spine in a neutral position. In stabilization exercises, other joints and muscles may be moving, creating the challenge of maintaining a motionless spine throughout the duration of the exercise. A system of exercises designed to build a strong core is known as Pilates (developed in the 1920s by Joseph Pilates). This type of exercise has become very popular and promotes core strength, endurance, and flexibility. See chapter 16 for more information on Pilates.

Rounded shoulders and a hunched upper back (known as excessive kyphosis) can also become habitual over time, leading to neck, shoulder, and upper-back pain. Help your students prevent this problem by leading them in more posterior deltoid, middle trapezius, and rhomboid exercises than chest exercises and by emphasizing chest and anterior deltoid stretching.

 See online video 3.2 for a demonstration of training opposing muscle groups for balance.

Balancing Strength and Flexibility

Another aspect of balance is the relative balance that exists between the strength and the flexibility of a particular muscle group. If participants have a great deal of flexibility in a particular muscle group, you may need to emphasize strength exercises rather than stretching to avoid injury to joint structures and ligamentous tissues. If the participants have greater strength than flexibility in a particular muscle group, you may need to perform flexibility exercises to avoid strains to the muscles and tendons. Many people believe the misconception that more flexibility and more strength are always beneficial. In fact, it is the relative balance between flexibility and strength that creates a healthy system.

Both the athlete and the average adult with back problems require an appropriate emphasis on stretching or strengthening. Gymnasts, who are often the epitome of flexibility (especially of the spine), have high rates of back pain and injury. Their back pain can be associated with hyperflexible joint structures caused by overstretching the spinal ligaments as well as from the impact forces experienced in dismounting and hyperextending the spine. Strong muscles may be able to compensate for hyperflexibility, but without such strengthening exercises, pain and injury can continue to weaken the spinal structure. Thus, the extreme flexibility required in gymnastics makes lifelong back and abdominal strength exercises essential to any gymnast's program. After gymnasts leave the sport, they still must continue these strengthening exercises in order to maintain adequate function because the damage done while practicing the sport is likely irreversible.

People whose spinal ligaments might be overstretched due to a back injury from an accident or from repetitive motion of the spine have similar problems. As long as they perform their strengthening exercises, they may be able to control pain and maintain a reasonable level of function.

When they stop their strengthening exercises, the pain increases and reinjury may result. Much of low-back pain is caused by improper body mechanics often related to sedentary living. Fitness instructors can make a huge difference in back pain incidence by educating clients about proper posture in everyday tasks. A study (Kellett et al. 1991) on the effects of an exercise program on sick leave caused by back pain found that the number of sick leave days attributable to back pain decreased by 50% in the exercising group. Telling a person with back pain to rest may cause even more back problems because the muscle weakness and joint flexibility caused by inactivity are often the reasons for the onset of back pain. Literature on back pain (Cinque 1989) reminds us that a number of physicians recommend getting out of bed and into the gym. As the instructor, you need to recognize what muscle or muscle group is responsible for a specific action, and what muscle group works in opposition to that action. You need to consider what exercises you will choose to enable your participants to function optimally during exercise and daily life.

Range of Motion for Major Joints

Understanding joint range of motion (ROM) for each muscle group is another part of teaching safe and effective exercise technique. Why is understanding joint ROM important? Imagine you are teaching a standing hip abduction exercise. ROM for hip abduction is approximately 45°. If participants are abducting beyond 45°, they are probably using the hip flexor muscle group to perform the action since hip flexion has a ROM of 120° (the hip flexor group is a strong muscle group and has the largest ROM). If you do not know that ROM for the hip abductors is 45°, you will not be able to recognize when participants need to correct their technique so that they can get the most out of their workout. The following list gives the joint ROMs for the major muscle groups:

Hips and Knees

Knee extension: 5°-10°

Knee flexion: 130°-140°

Hip flexion: 90°-135°

Hip extension: 10°-30°

Hip abduction: 45°

Hip adduction: 10°-30°

Spine

Spinal lateral flexion: 30°

Spinal rotation: 40°

Spinal flexion: 30°-45°

Spinal extension: 20°-45°

Shoulders

Shoulder flexion: 135°

Shoulder adduction: 50°

Shoulder extension: 45°

Shoulder abduction: 80°-100°

Neck

Neck abduction and adduction: 40°

Neck hyperextension: 50°

Neck flexion: 40°

Neck rotation: 55°

Ankle

Plantar flexion: 45°

Dorsiflexion: 10°-15°

Note that range of motion (ROM) is a *range* and not an absolute number. Some participants will have greater ROM in a joint than others due to their overall flexibility and joint structure.

Progressive Functional Training Continuum

Used in the traditional sense, *progression* refers to progressively overloading the body's systems and increasing the training stimulus over time to gradually increase fitness adaptations. In resistance training, the muscles gradually become stronger or gain endurance as well as enhanced neuromuscular control, coordination, and balance. Gradual adaptation can be achieved by changing the variables of exercise frequency, intensity, duration, and mode. Our progressive functional training continuum specifically addresses mode, or type of exercise. Addressing this issue is important to group exercise because instructors have to decide what exercises they are going to teach in their classes. The progressive functional training continuum (Kennedy 2003; Yoke and Kennedy 2004) helps instructors make better decisions for their participants. Figure 3.4 outlines the continuum.

On the left end of the continuum are easy exercises that require less skill, balance, stability, proprioceptive activity, and motor control. Such exercises are safe for almost everyone and require the least amount of instructor cueing. Many of these exercises are performed in a supine or prone position, require isolated joint actions rather than total-body movements, and strengthen individual muscle groups. A few examples are the supine triceps extension, prone scapular retraction for the middle trapezius and rhomboids, and prone hip extension for the hamstrings and gluteus maximus. These exercises are low risk, easy to cue, and relatively safe for almost all populations.

At the right end of the continuum are exercises that need a great deal of skill and require an ability to maintain joint integrity, including integrity of the spinal joints and the joints involved in core stability (which is the ability to maintain ideal alignment in the neck, spine, scapulae, and pelvis no matter how difficult the exercise). These challenging exercises also place a high demand on proprioceptors and on the neuromuscular system for smooth coordination. As a result, the ability to perform these exercises safely depends on the exerciser's specific experience and overall fitness level. Many sport-specific exercises are categorized at this end of the continuum. A few examples of difficult and controversial exercises include deadlifts, plyometric lunges, handstand shoulder presses, and V-sits. Although these exercises are considered difficult and higher risk, a fit person with excel-

lent core stability might be able to perform them safely and appropriately. As a group exercise leader, you have to choose which exercises will be safe for your whole class. We also recommend selecting exercises that allow all participants to be successful. Exercises ranging from 1 to 4 on the continuum are most appropriate for group classes. Exercises in the 5 and 6 portion of the continuum ought to be reserved for advanced classes or personal training. A skilled instructor is adept at sliding back and forth along the continuum, always selecting exercises that best meet the needs of the class and the individual participants being taught. Always know how to progress an exercise (make it harder), as well as how to modify or regress (make it easier) the exercise. Let's look at the six levels of the progressive functional training continuum in more detail.

Level 1

Isolate and educate. This level focuses on muscular isolation and trains participants to contract individual muscle groups. Working at this level helps build confidence and body awareness and improves basic muscle functioning. Exercises are often performed in the supine or prone position, with as much of the body in contact with the floor or bench as possible, lessening the need for stabilizer muscle involvement. As a result, these exercises are generally quite safe; just about everyone can learn to do them effectively with minimal risk of injury. Also, many level-1 exercises are single joint and uniplanar, so they are usually easy to understand and perform correctly. Gravity is usually the main form of resistance applied at this level. Level 1 is perfect for almost all group exercise classes because all participants would be successful with these choices.

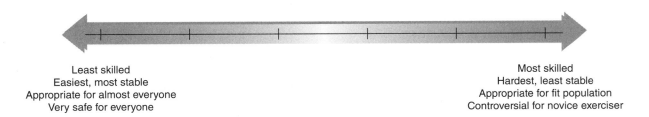

Least skilled
Easiest, most stable
Appropriate for almost everyone
Very safe for everyone

Most skilled
Hardest, least stable
Appropriate for fit population
Controversial for novice exerciser

FIGURE 3.4 Progressive functional training continuum.

Level 2

Add external resistance by adding weights, increasing lever length, or using elastic bands or tubes. In many cases, the actual exercise performed at this level is the same exercise performed at level 1—the difference is the added resistance. Notice that in both levels 1 and 2, the instructor typically needs to give minimal safety and alignment cueing; it's relatively easy for exercisers to perform these types of exercises safely and effectively while maintaining proper form because of the decreased stabilizer involvement and the isolated muscle and joint actions.

Level 3

Add functional training positions. Level 3 progresses the body position to sitting or standing, both of which are more functional positions for most people. Sitting or standing reduces the base of support and increases the stabilizer challenge. In most progressions, the targeted muscle group is still isolated as a primary mover, and the stabilizers are merely assisting. This is often the stage in which standing dumbbell exercises or standing exercises using tubing are introduced.

Level 4

Combine increased function with resistance. At this level, resistance from gravity, external weights, or bands and tubes is maximized, and overload on the core stabilizer muscles is increased. The exercises at this level are performed in functional positions; most are performed in a standing position to use the core stabilizer muscles. These exercises begin the process of overloading the muscles for the stresses of daily living.

Level 5

Work multiple muscle groups with increased resistance and core challenge. At level 5, the exercises use multiple muscle groups and joint actions simultaneously or in combination. Resistance, balance, coordination, torso stability, or multiplanar training are progressed to an even higher level. The primary emphasis at this level is on challenging the core stabilizers even more. For example, completing an overhead press with dumbbells while simultaneously squatting challenges the core more than simply performing a squat or an overhead press.

Level 6

Add balance, speed, and rotational movements. Exercises at this level may require balancing on one leg, balancing on a stability ball, plyometric movements, spinal rotation while lifting, or some other life skill or sport-specific maneuver. For example, training to clean your house requires power and rotation—not movements that work just a single muscle group. The risk of injury is increased at this level, so instructors must be cautious when introducing these exercises to a group. Although including speed and rotation is not as safe as performing simpler movements, it is how we live. Sensible progression to this level will transition into enhanced life skills. A sample progression is outlined in figure 3.5.

 See online video 3.3 for an application of the progressive functional training continuum. In this clip, the instructor demonstrates a range of exercise options to a class.

The Group Exercise Class Evaluation Form

The Group Exercise Class Evaluation Form can be found in appendix A. This form covers the principles that apply to most group exercise classes and is designed around the previously mentioned health-related components of fitness. We will review these principles here and in the Group Exercise Modalities section of the book (part III). You can use this form as an evaluation tool when you are observing classes and as a checklist to enhance your teaching and evaluating skills. Although it is difficult to generalize all group exercise classes onto one evaluation tool, we feel the principles included on this evaluation form apply to most group exercise classes. However, if you are teaching a 30-minute muscular conditioning and flexibility class, the warm-up segment and the muscular conditioning and flexibility segment may be the

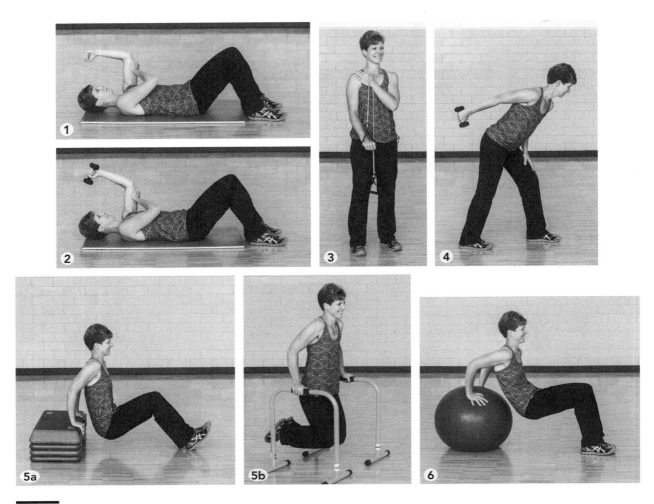

FIGURE 3.5 A sample progression for the triceps: (*1*) supine unilateral triceps extension, (*2*) supine extension with weights, (*3*) standing press-down with tube, (*4*) bent-over triceps kickback with weights, (*5a, b*) dips off a bench or using total body weight, and (*6*) dips using a stability ball. As you can see, level 6 is significantly more complicated and more challenging than level 1!

only ones you will use on the form. On the other hand, if you are teaching a 60-minute kickboxing class, then you can use all the components of the evaluation form. This form reflects the health-related fitness components, the ACSM evidence-based guidelines for exercise, and the basic research-based concepts of exercise physiology. As instructors, we need to keep these in mind when we are teaching group exercise classes so that we can make a difference in the health and wellness of our participants.

Safe, effective, and purposeful class design requires specific knowledge of fitness in order to provide the appropriate overload needed to achieve the desired gains. Therefore, one of the purposes of the Group Exercise Class Evalua-

tion Form is to provide a common language and an organizational system for discussing class format. We recommend that you use this form to evaluate a class before you attempt to teach. After you have completed this chapter and the Group Modalities segment of this book (part III), you will have a general understanding of what is needed to create a safe, effective group exercise experience. In an academic setting, the Group Exercise Class Evaluation Form in appendix A can be used to grade how well a student applies theory to application. In other settings, this form can be used to set expectations regarding what should be implemented in the formats of all group exercise classes, (e.g., step, kickboxing, or boot camp). Our hope is that program managers will require instructors to think about how they can best deliver the principles of exercise science in the group exercise setting. The Group Exercise Class Evaluation Form summarizes these principles and helps instructors put them into practical action. Following are sample evaluation forms completed by a group exercise leader in preparation for an evaluation and audition; the right-hand column includes what the instructor plans to do (figure 3.6). It is our hope that by sharing this form with you now, before we discuss all the concepts it covers, it will help you understand the big picture of where we are going as we put theory into practice.

Chapter Wrap-Up

The general concepts outlined in this chapter apply to all group exercise classes. As instructors, we need to integrate health-related fitness components into our classes, include preclass introductions and screenings, observe the principles of muscle balance, and learn proper progressions of exercises and appropriate ROMs for movements. This chapter also provided a general overview of the Group Exercise Class Evaluation Form (found in appendix A), which is an outline of the general principles applying to group exercise classes. You will be referring to this form throughout this book, and will also use it if you choose to complete the end-chapter assignments.

ASSIGNMENT

Attend a group exercise class of your choice. What type of class is it and which version of the Group Exercise Class Evaluation Form (appendix A) is most applicable? Write a 1- to 2-page paper addressing the following points:

- Were any health-screening procedures required by the front desk or by the instructor?
- Which health-related fitness components were addressed? How?
- Did the instructor address muscular balance issues? How?
- Did the instructor show or teach any type of exercise progression/regression? Describe.
- Did the instructor create a positive class atmosphere? How?

Group Exercise Class Evaluation Form

EXAMPLE 1

Instructor _____   Evaluator _____

Date: _____   Class: _Cyclefit 45_ _____

Time: _45-minute stationary indoor cycling class_ _____

Preclass Organization

Objective	For example
Knows participants and orients new participants	Notice new participants as they enter; show them the class whiteboard that outlines the workout for the day.
Has equipment and music (if using) ready for use	Play upbeat music in the background as participants arrive.
Introduces self and states class format	Begin class by stating the class format and your name.
Acknowledges class	"Welcome! Remember this is YOUR class. I will lead movement options. Feel free to take the movement option that works best for your fitness level."
Creates positive atmosphere	"I'm happy to be here and focused on helping you improve your fitness."
Wears appropriate attire and footwear	Bring cycling shoes and wear cycling shorts to Cyclefit class.

Comments

_____

_____

_____

Warm-Up

Objective	For example
Includes appropriate amount of dynamic movement	Have participants cycle slowly while waiting for class to begin.
Provides rehearsal moves	Review rebounding techniques and out-of-the saddle movements during the warm up. Count cadence by tapping knee for 15 seconds and multiplying by 4 to help participants understand the importance of cadence in stationary indoor cycling.

FIGURE 3.6 Two examples of the Group Exercise Class Evaluation Form, noting items an instructor could do to be successful for each of the form objectives.

Objective	For example
Stretches major muscle groups in a biomechanically sound manner (dynamic or static) with appropriate instructions	Have participants perform upper-body stretches while legs continue cycling; stretch triceps, deltoid, upper back (rhomboids).
Provides intensity guidelines for warm-up	Discuss with participants how cycling cadence and resistance interrelate to create workout intensity. Review procedures for increasing and decreasing intensity using the cadence and resistance knob on the bike.
Includes clear cues and verbal directions	Ask participants if they can hear cues and directions over the music volume and microphone.
Uses movements at an appropriate tempo and intensity	Include movement selections (out of the saddle, rebounding) that are 1 or 2 minutes in length with a low resistance; remind participants this is the warm-up and they are to progress into the workout.

Comments

_____

_____

_____

Conditioning

Objective	For example
Gradually increases intensity	State that the first two songs of the workout will focus on cadence training; low and medium cadences will be used.
Uses a variety of muscle groups	Have participants sit up tall on their bikes 2 times during the workout and focus on posture and core stabilization.
Provides muscular balance	Integrate single-leg (i.e., right-leg only and left-leg only) training to focus on core stabilization and emphasize proper posture while cycling.
Minimizes repetitive movements	Incorporate the following movement options: rebounds, out-of-the-saddle hill work, seated sprints, walking or jogging movements, and seated hill work.
Promotes participant interaction and encourages fun	During the seated sprints have half the room sprinting for 30 seconds while the other half is resting. Encourage resting participants to cheer on those that are sprinting.
Provides regular demonstrations and participation using good body mechanics	Before introducing the walking or jogging movement option, have participants practice proper technique. Model proper technique on the bike first, then dismount and walk around the room to check on participants.

> continued

FIGURE 3.6 > continued

> continued

Conditioning

Objective	For example
Continually offers modifications, regressions, progressions, or alternatives	Remind participants that this is their workout and to change the resistance on the bike for their personal fitness level.
Observes participants' form and provides constructive, nonintimidating feedback	Get off the bike during the group seated sprint and encourage individuals by moving around the room and acknowledging their effort.
Acknowledges and adapts class to participant preference for exercise selection or drills	For the last song of the workout portion, allow participants to pick a 3-minute segment of their choice. Have participants close their eyes and perform visualization of going up a hill they have driven on or biked outside on while performing hill work.
Gives motivational cues	Liberally uses upbeat, positive, and exciting cues such as, "Let's go team!," "We're all in this together," "Give it your best effort," and so on.
Educates participants about intensity; provides HR and/or RPE check 1 or 2 times during workout stimulus	In the middle of the cardio segment, allow for an HR (heart rate) and/or RPE (rating of perceived exertion) check; remind participants to monitor their intensity during the workout.
Uses appropriate movement or music tempo	During the seated flat-road segment, encourage participants to pedal at a cadence slightly faster than the music for 1 minute and then at the music cadence for another minute.
Gradually decreases impact and intensity at end of workout stimulus	Use a song that is less intense and more relaxing at the end of the cycling workout; encourage a complete cardiovascular cool down by reducing cadence and/or resistance.

Comments

_____

_____

_____

Cool-Down, Stretch, and Relaxation

Objective	For example
Includes static stretching for major muscles worked and for commonly tight muscles (e.g., hip flexors, hamstrings, calves, erector spinae, pectorals, anterior deltoids, upper trapezius)	Have participants stretch the upper body while cooling down the legs and cycling slowly; stretch triceps, deltoids, and upper back (rhomboids). Have participants get off their bikes and stretch quads, hamstrings, calves, glutes, and low back. Work on balance by having participants stand on one leg while stretching the quads.
Demonstrates using proper alignment and technique	Maintain excellent form during all demonstrations.

FIGURE 3.6 > continued

Objective	For example
Observes participants' form and offers modifications, regressions, progressions, and/or alternatives	Provide modification for participants unable to do a hamstring stretch with the leg up on the bike. Demonstrate modification or regression: Keep stretching leg and foot on floor with opposite support knee bent and hip hinge, hands on support leg. Give alignment cues: Stress proper posture and balance for standing quadriceps stretch by emphasizing shoulders back and down while engaging the core muscles.
Appropriately emphasizes relaxation or visualization	End with breathing exercises; use an instrumental song that is relaxing and a lower voice tone during cool down.
Ends class on a positive note and thanks class	End class with "Make it a good day!" and "Thank you."

Comments

_____

_____

_____

EXAMPLE 2

Instructor _____   Evaluator _____

Date:_____   Class: __**Step and Strength**_____

Time: __**60-minute step and strength interval class**_____

Preclass Organization

Objective	For example
Knows participants and orients new participants	Greet participants and notice new participants as they enter; show them class whiteboard that outlines the workout for the day.
Has equipment and music (if using) ready for use	Play upbeat music in the background as participants arrive.
Introduces self and states class format	Begin class by stating the class format and name.
Acknowledges class	"Welcome! Remember this is YOUR class. I will lead movement options for intensity and impact; feel free to take the movement option that works best for your fitness level."
Creates positive atmosphere	"I'm happy to be here and am focused on helping you improve your fitness!"
Wears appropriate attire and footwear	Wear professional-looking exercise attire, appropriate athletic shoes.

> continued

FIGURE 3.6 > continued

> continued

Comments

_____

_____

_____

Warm-Up

Objective	For example
Includes appropriate amount of dynamic movement	Use low-impact full-body movements.
Provides rehearsal moves	Use a floor-mix pattern that incorporates the step.
Stretches major muscle groups in a biomechanically sound manner (dynamic or static) with appropriate instructions	Provide dynamic stretches for calves, hamstrings, hip flexors, and erector spinae; provide static stretches for pectorals and upper trapezius.
Provides intensity guidelines for warm-up	Remind participants to begin by keeping intensity low and then gradually increase.
Includes clear cues and verbal directions	Ask participants if they can hear cues and directions over the music volume and microphone.
Uses movements at an appropriate tempo and intensity	Use music at a speed of 124 beats per minute.

Comments

_____

_____

_____

Conditioning

Objective	For example
Gradually increases intensity	Start with an easy, lower-intensity combo.
Uses a variety of muscle groups	During step work, use hip flexion, extension, abductor, and adductor moves. During strength intervals, provide exercises for legs, lats, deltoids, pectorals, middle trapezius and rhomboids, biceps, and triceps.
Provides muscle balance	Use supersets with opposing muscles for strength intervals. For step routines, evenly use both right and left lead legs.

FIGURE 3.6 > continued

Objective	For example
Minimizes repetitive movements	Limit repetitions of any one movement on the step.
Promotes participant interaction and encourages fun	Use call-and-response technique; ask participants to respond in rhythm.
Provides regular demonstrations and participation using good body mechanics	Participate during step portions; demonstrate several repetitions during strength portions.

Objective	For example
Continually offers modifications, regressions, progressions, or alternatives	Frequently give intensity and impact options on the step; during strength intervals present a more basic level, then say, "If you want a bigger challenge, do this . . ." If you notice a participant struggling with bilateral bent-over low row, provide a regression.
Observes participants' form and provides constructive, nonintimidating feedback	Balance general feedback to entire group with individual feedback to several participants during the strength intervals.
Acknowledges and adapts class to participant preference for exercise selection or drills	Ask class members for their favorite step move and incorporate it into a final drill.
Gives motivational cues	Liberally use upbeat, positive, and exciting cues such as, "Way to go!," "Give it to me NOW," etc.
Educates participants about intensity; provides HR and/or RPE check 1 or 2 times during workout stimulus	In the middle of a cardio interval provide an HR and/or RPE check; remind participants to monitor their intensity during the workout.
Uses appropriate movement or music tempo	Maintain an appropriate step tempo by using music at 128 beats per minute.
Gradually decreases impact and intensity at end of workout stimulus	For last segment before the stretch, include a strength segment (e.g., biceps, then supine abdominals) to allow HR to decrease.

Comments

_____

_____

_____

> continued

FIGURE 3.6 > continued

> continued

Cool-Down, Stretch, and Relaxation

Objective	For example
Includes static stretching for major muscles worked and for commonly tight muscles (e.g., hip flexors, hamstrings, calves, erector spinae, pectorals, anterior deltoids, upper trapezius)	On the floor, stretch all major muscles in supine, prone, side-lying, and seated positions.
Demonstrates using proper alignment and technique	Maintain excellent form during all demonstrations
Observes participants' form and offers modifications, regressions, progressions, or alternatives	Face class and offer modification during seated adductor (straddle) stretch with hands on floor behind body.
Provides alignment cues	Provide many cues for all stretches.
Appropriately emphasizes relaxation or visualization	End with soft, relaxing music and a brief visualization; have participants use seated cross-legged position, eyes closed.
Ends class on a positive note and thanks class	End class with "May you all have a fabulous, fantastic day!" and "Thank you."

Comments

_____

_____

_____

FIGURE 3.6   > continued

Traditional Concepts

Chapter Objectives

By the end of this chapter, you will be able to
- apply music skills in a group exercise class,
- build basic cardio combinations,
- apply the elements of variation,
- create smooth transitions,
- demonstrate additional choreographic techniques,
- apply cueing methods in a cardio class,
- demonstrate the ability to use visual cues and mirroring teaching techniques, and
- create and teach a 4-minute cardio routine with at least two 64-count blocks and proper cueing.

This chapter covers the elements you need to know in order to lead a great music- and choreography-driven class. We also discuss legal issues regarding music use as well as information about sound systems. Then we cover basic choreography issues, including performing the common moves, building combinations, teaching freestyle, and transitioning smoothly from one move to another. After that, we discuss cueing to music as well as various other types of cues. Finally, we describe how to give participants feedback in a nonthreatening way. Most of this information is important for leading any choreography-based class taught to music (on the beat), including cardio workouts, step, kickboxing, Zumba, and more. If you practice the drills we suggest and follow along with the online video resource accompanying this text, you'll be leading a class like a pro in no time!

Applying Music Skills in Group Exercise

Music is a vital part of almost all group exercise classes. Participants regularly report that they believe their exercise performance is better with music accompaniment. According to a 2007 literature review, music may facilitate exercise performance by (1) reducing feelings of fatigue, (2) increasing levels of psychological arousal, (3) improving motor coordination, and (4) promoting a physiological relaxation response (Harmon and Kravitz 2007). Music also appears to provide a motivational construct for exercise, buoying participants' mental state. In one study, students who listened to their favorite music while exercising reported feeling more comfortable and experiencing less fatigue (Yamashita et al. 2006). Numerous studies have revealed music's effects on mood, activity level, heart rate, blood pressure, and more; there is increasing evidence to suggest that the right music (however this might be defined) can lead to greater frequency, intensity, and duration of exercise behavior (Atkinson, Wilson, and Eubank 2004). An assessment tool has even been developed to help fitness professionals match music to participants' interests and level of motivation (Karageorghis et al. 2006). In cardio programs, step classes, and several other modalities, participants time their moves to coincide with the beat of the music. In Pilates, yoga, water exercise, sport conditioning, indoor cycling, and some equipment-based classes, participants can also use music to motivate themselves and make the movement experience enjoyable even if they don't necessarily move on the beat. Therefore, you have the option to use music to provide structure to your class or simply to set the mood.

You need to understand and work with the music you use in your group exercise classes. During the cardio segment, it feels especially good to move on the beat, and your students will feel more successful, positive, and energized when you lead them to move with the music. Additionally, because many people hear or feel the beat of the music, they unconsciously feel clumsy or uncoordinated when taking a class with an instructor who is off the beat. Participants in cardio and step classes expect their movements to flow with the music. Also, by using the music structure appropriately, you can reduce the need for constant cueing.

The next sections outline the basic elements of teaching to popular music. Practice the suggested drills until you can automatically hear the

Recommended Beats per Minute

Warm-up: 120 to 136 beats per minute

High-low impact cardio segment: 134 to 158 beats per minute

Step: 118 to 128 beats per minute

Muscle conditioning: Under 132 beats per minute

Flexibility work, yoga, and Pilates: Under 100 beats per minute or music without a strong beat

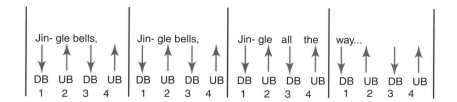

FIGURE 4.1 In simple songs such as "Jingle Bells," the upbeats (UB) and downbeats (DB) are easily identified.

musical components. Most skilled instructors have the beat, the downbeat, the 4-count measure, and the 8- and 32-count phrases in their heads at all times when leading class; hearing the music simply becomes second nature with practice. Note that there are certain tempos that fit well with the various segments and types of group exercise (see "Recommended Beats per Minute").

Beat

The beat is the smallest musical division of a phrase. Each regular rhythmic pulse is a beat, also known as a *count*. Beats are further organized into downbeats and upbeats. The downbeat is the stronger, more important or emphatic beat. The upbeat is the weaker, less important beat that immediately follows each downbeat. For example, figure 4.1 illustrates the downbeats and the upbeats in the song "Jingle Bells."

The downbeat falls on the most accented part of a word and usually on the most important words in a phrase, whereas the upbeat falls on the unaccented part of a word or the less important words. Also, when counting the beats forward in a measure, the downbeats are on the odd numbers (1 and 3) and the upbeats are on the even numbers (2 and 4).

Even though commercially mixed music for group exercise lists the beats per minute for each song, it's important to be able to identify the speed yourself, particularly if you're going to legally incorporate a favorite song or two into your playlist. Figuring the beats per minute is simple; while listening to a track, just count each beat forward while looking at a watch or clock. You can count for 15 seconds and multiply by 4 or, for greater accuracy, count for 30 seconds and multiply by 2. Alternatively, another method (Tendy 2010) has been identified: Count only

the first 16 beats, multiply by 60, and divide by the amount of time elapsed during the 16 beats (you'll need a stopwatch).

Measure

The measure is the basic organizational unit in music; it contains a series of downbeats and upbeats. In almost all popular music used in step and cardio classes, each measure holds 4 beats: downbeat, upbeat, downbeat, upbeat. Such music is said to be in *4/4 metered time,* which technically means that there are four quarter notes in each measure. In the example given in figure 4.1, the words *jingle bells* take up one measure.

Phrase

A phrase consists of at least two measures of music. Hence, it is common to speak of an 8-count phrase (two measures), a 16-count phrase (four measures), and a 32-count phrase (eight measures) in step or cardio music. A 32-count phrase contains four 8-count phrases grouped together and is ideal for building routines and choreographic combinations. Participants usually feel more successful and energized when new movement patterns are initiated at the beginning of each 32-count phrase; the first downbeat of the 32-count phrase is sometimes called the *top of the phrase.* Listen for the drumroll or other increase in musical momentum that comes at the end of each 32-count phrase (technically the seventh and eighth counts of the last, or fourth, 8-count phrase) and signifies the new 32-count phrase to follow.

Typically, the 8-count phrases within each 32-count phrase are divided into dominant and less dominant phrases, such as the following:

- First 8-count phrase: dominant
- Second 8-count phrase: less dominant

- Third 8-count phrase: dominant
- Fourth 8-count phrase: less dominant but with drum roll or other musical momentum during counts 7 and 8

 See online video 4.1 for the practice drill on counting out the beat (4 counts and 8 counts at 120 beats per minute and 132 beats per minute).

Make this learning process easier by selecting music that has a strong, easy-to-hear beat. You can also use commercial music that has been professionally premixed for step, kickboxing, and cardio classes. This music is blended (metered) into continuous 32-count phrases and is preferable to music found in music stores, which is not metered for group exercise and contains extra beats and bridges, making counting, choreography, and cueing much more difficult. See the "Music Resource List" for contact information.

Half Time and Double Time

When a movement is performed in half time, it is performed twice as slowly as normal. In other words, a box step (making a square pattern with your feet) usually takes 4 counts, but when performed in half time, it takes 8 counts. Performing in double time, then, means to perform a move twice as fast as usual.

Practice Drill

Using popular music with a strong beat, listen for the 8-count division within the music. Find the 8-count grouping with the strongest initial downbeat; this is the beginning of the 32-count phrase. To help integrate this information into movement, try this simple drill: (1) Leading with your right foot, walk eight steps to the right on the first 8-count phrase. (2) Make a sharp 90° turn to your right and walk eight more steps on the second 8-count phrase (always leading right). (3) Make another sharp 90° turn to your right and walk eight more steps on the third 8-count phrase. (4) Make another sharp 90° turn to your right and walk eight more steps on the fourth 8-count phrase, returning to your starting point. You should have made a large square pattern with your feet. Repeat to the right or try the same drill to your left, always leading with the left foot. Keep practicing this drill with different speeds and styles of music.

Musical Styles

One of the most enjoyable aspects of teaching to music is the availability of so many styles of music. Adapting the music to your participants' interests and ages will enhance their enjoyment and willingness to keep exercising. Dwyer (1995) found that when participants had a choice of music, they reported higher intrinsic

Music Resource List

Aerobeat Music and Video	www.aerobeat.com	800-536-6060
Burntrax Fitness Music	www.burntrax.com	800-672-8729
CardioMixes	www.cardiomixes.com	866-322-6868
Click Mix (custom mixes)	www.clickmix.com	800-777-2328
Dynamix	www.dynamixmusic.com	800-843-6499
GF Mix	www.gfmix.com	702-938-1700
Kimbo Educational	www.kimboed.com	800-631-2187
MusicFlex	www.musicflex.com	800-430-3539
Muscle Mixes Music	www.musclemixesmusic.com	800-833-1224
Power Music	www.powermusic.com	800-777-2328
Yes! Fitness Music	www.yesfitnessmusic.com	800-321-9379

motivation than did the participants who were not asked for input. Ask your participants what they like to listen to. Try new musical styles to stimulate creative energy and open up new opportunities for choreography. Keep an open mind and have a sense of play as you experiment with different music styles:

- Rock, Pop, Top 40
- House, techno, club, disco, electronica, Eurodance, Hi-NRG, trance
- Oldies, Motown
- Blues, jazz
- Classical
- Funk, rap, hip-hop, R&B
- Latin, salsa
- Reggae, ska
- Big band, swing
- Country
- Mind–body, new age
- Bollywood
- World beat (e.g., Irish, Peruvian, African, Asian, Middle Eastern)
- Holiday (e.g., Halloween, Valentine's Day, Fourth of July)
- Theme (e.g., beach, girl power, rainy day music)

Practice Drill

Listening to any piece of popular music; close your eyes and tap your feet, pat your knees, or clap your hands to the regular continuous beat. Write a list of 20 songs and their beats per minute and describe which portion of a workout each song would fit best.

Responsibilities for Using Exercise Music

The 1976 revision of the Copyright Law of the United States, which went into effect in 1978, made clear statements about the responsibilities of fitness instructors, studios, and centers regarding the music they use. Tested throughout the judicial system and upheld by the U.S. Supreme Court, the law states that copyright owners have the right to charge a fee for the use of their music in a public performance. A public performance is defined as a performance made in a place open to the public or any place where a substantial number of persons outside a normal circle of family and friends are gathered.

All exercise classes—whether they take place in a private club, public hall, exercise gym, or corporate fitness center—fall into the category of public performance. Because music is a copyrighted entity, corporations, studios, fitness centers, and instructors who use music during their exercise classes place themselves in jeopardy of violating U.S. or their local copyright law if they do not pay royalties to the people who write, publish, and distribute the music.

The American Society of Composers, Authors and Publishers (ASCAP); Broadcast Music, Inc. (BMI); and the Society of European Stage Authors and Composers (SESAC) are the main organizations that represent the artists who record the music used in group exercise classes. Together, these organizations represent more than 100,000 composers, lyricists, and publishers worldwide, with offices in places such as London, San Juan, and Puerto Rico, and partnerships with many national recording artists' organizations. They ensure that their members receive royalties and that the relevant copyright law is enforced. A few organizations offer music licenses to particular countries. For example, in the United Kingdom, MPCS-PRS for Music is an association that protects the rights of composers and musicians, and thus collects fees from businesses for the rightful playing of music at work.

Both ASCAP and BMI vigorously pursue violators and potential violators of the law. American Council on Exercise (2000) recommends that clubs and studios obtain a blanket license for their instructors. The license fees for clubs are determined by the number of students who attend classes each week, the number of speakers used in the club, and whether the club uses single or multiple floors. Independent instructors who teach in several locations may need to obtain a personal music performance license. Be sure to check with each club where you teach regarding music licensure. Also, know that you are much more likely to be protected from copyright infringement if you buy CDs or download songs that were specifically created and prelicensed for group exercise classes (see "Music Resource List"). According to industry experts, fitness music companies play by the rules and pay the licensing fees for you (Biscontini 2010); therefore, we strongly recommend that you use fitness music companies to help make your music selection process easy, fun, and legal. For more information on the costs of licensing and for further clarification of the U.S. Copyright Law, check out www.bmi.com, www.ascap.com, and www.copyright.gov. It is an instructor's responsibility to stay up to date on issues surrounding copyright law as opportunities for playing music increase with technological advances.

Greater numbers of fitness music companies are making it possible for customers to download prelicensed music directly onto an iPod or MP3 player. Doing so allows you to create your own playlist. Other new avenues for playing music include the music-editing software programs that let instructors mix songs, tracks, sounds, and music speeds. All these technological advances mean that an instructor's individual musical style and selections may become increasingly important in class popularity and exercise adherence. Be aware, however, that downloading material from popular online music sites for use in your class may put you in legal jeopardy. The terms of service for iTunes, for example, states that the purchaser is "authorized to use the products only for personal, noncommercial use." Strictly speaking, that means that downloaded music is covered under the same private-use restrictions as other forms of media, such as DVDs, and is not to be played in a commercial setting (i.e., group fitness class).

Sound System Fundamentals

A good sound system is essential for most group exercise classes. A basic sound system consists of one or more sound sources (wireless microphone headset, CD player with pitch control, iPod docking station, or digital music controller) connected to an amplifier and speakers. All systems, whether portable or fixed, contain these basic elements.

Products change so quickly that making specific recommendations for a sound system is unfeasible. It is worth your time to do some research to find a product that will sound good and also be easy to maintain. Try calling other fitness professionals and facilities to see what they have found to be successful in today's market.

Voice Care

Long and colleagues (1998) conducted a study on voice problems experienced by fitness instructors. Of the instructors who were surveyed, 44% experienced partial or complete voice loss during and after instructing. They also experienced more episodes of voice loss, hoarseness, and sore throat unrelated to illness after they became instructors. Heidel and Torgerson (1993) found that instructors experience a higher prevalence of vocal problems compared with individuals participating in group exercise. According to the National Institutes of Health (NIH), long-term vocal overuse, particularly when a microphone is not used, can cause nodules (small growths) to develop on the vocal cords and can decrease overall vocal quality with age (National Institutes of Health 2012). If you are instructing on a regular basis, using a microphone is essential for your long-term vocal health. You may feel that you don't need a microphone now because your voice projects well and is easily heard. However, if you instruct group exercise frequently, cumulative overuse will cause your voice to become hoarse in the future; so, preventive care is a must. Other recommendations for voice care include the following:

- Keep your head, jaw, neck, and shoulders relaxed when teaching.
- Face your class whenever possible; project your voice out rather than down or up.
- Use visual cueing as much as you can.
- Develop good breathing habits; learn to perform abdominal breathing.
- Try humming or yawning to relax the muscles of your face, neck, and throat.
- Keep your throat hydrated.
- Avoid irritants such as smoke, smog, or certain foods.
- Limit talking in noisy places.
- Keep your music at a reasonable volume level (see "Music Volume in Fitness Classes").

- Avoid clearing your throat frequently because doing so creates even more phlegm.
- Avoid screaming, yelling, or shouting when teaching—use that microphone.

To protect your voice you need a good sound system, a microphone with a headset and receiver, and high-quality speakers. These products will create a big difference in the quality of your group exercise instruction. After all, music is one of the main reasons why participants venture into the group exercise setting instead of exercising alone on a stair stepper or an elliptical machine. Monroe (1999) stated that music (along with the creative use of silence) is the heart of movement. She said, "If you love your music and have a passion for it, it will move you—and it will move the people you teach" (1999, p. 37).

Traditional Choreography

In a traditional cardio class, participants perform movements that work the large muscle groups to promote cardiorespiratory fitness and its benefits. These movements are generally dance-like and can be executed while jumping (high impact) or while keeping one foot on the floor at all times (low impact). Classes mixing high- and low-impact movements may be labeled as *cardio conditioning, aerobic dance,* or simply *high-low.* This type of class is versatile and requires no equipment. Learning the skills necessary for teaching a basic high-low cardio class is the foundation of group exercise instruction for many group leaders. The basic skills described in this chapter, such as anticipatory cueing, smooth transitioning, and choreography building, also apply to other forms of group exercise, including step, kickboxing, some forms of muscular conditioning and water exercise, slide, Zumba, and NIA. The elements of the Group Exercise Class Evaluation Form (appendix A) that pertain to cardiorespiratory classes are discussed in the following paragraphs.

To minimize repetitive stress on the joints and to prevent boredom (for both the leader and the participants), the best group instructors constantly vary their moves and movement

Music Volume in Fitness Classes

The IDEA Health and Fitness Association has published the following recommendations regarding safe volume levels for music played during group exercise classes in an "Opinion Statement" (2002). These recommendations are based on the standards established by the U.S. Occupational Safety and Health Administration (OSHA). Fitness professionals who work outside of the United States are urged to refer to the official volume guidelines established for their particular countries.

1. Because hearing loss is slow, cumulative, and often painless (though loud music does sometimes hurt!), group exercise instructors need to be aware that the intensity of their music and accompanying voice can put them and their students at risk without causing any apparent symptoms.
2. Health facilities and instructors have an obligation to their members and students to ensure safe music intensities during group exercise classes.
3. Music intensity during group exercise classes should measure no more than 90 decibels (dB).
4. Because the instructor's voice needs to be about 10 decibels louder than the music in order to be heard, the instructor's voice should measure no more than 100 decibels.
5. Fitness facilities are urged to place a Class 1 or 2 sound level meter (available from many electronics stores for less than US$100) on a stand near the center of the front of the room in order to measure sound levels during classes. Instructors or other staff members should check the meter regularly to make sure volume levels are safe. The volume control on the music amplifier is not an accurate means of measuring sound intensity.

patterns. Too much of any one move can create excessive wear on the joints. Movements must be balanced: forward and backward moves, right and left sides, and right and left leads. To protect the joints, avoid using too many high-impact movements, too many repetitive jumps on one leg (no more than 8 in a row), and too many repetitive moves that stress the musculoskeletal system. Moves such as jumping jacks, ski jumps, and scissors deliver large impact forces to the joints. To create the safest class, combine these types of moves with a totally different move, such as a march.

Demonstrate proper technique at all times to help prevent injuries. When performing high-impact moves, roll through the entire foot with each jump, bringing first the toes and then the heels to the floor. This toe-ball-heel landing pattern distributes the impact forces over the whole foot. Be careful with lateral foot movements such as grapevines and shuffles, especially on a carpeted surface. They increase the risk of a lateral ankle sprain, especially if participants perform them when fatigued. When performing lunges, keep the heel of the back foot up to prevent excessive eccentric loading of the calf muscles (potentially leading to Achilles tendinitis). It is also wise to avoid wearing ankle weights during cardio classes since doing so increases the risk of injury. If light hand weights are used, a slower music speed (such as 138 beats per minute) should be chosen to minimize the risk of upper-body injuries. Hand weights under 3 pounds (1.36 kilograms) have not been shown to significantly affect caloric expenditure in cardio activities (Yoke et al. 1988; Yoke et al. 1989). Hand weights over 3 pounds (1.36 kilograms) are not recommended during cardio activities because of the increased potential for upper-body injury. Given these findings, we generally do not recommend the use of hand weights during cardio activities. Avoid keeping the arms overhead for prolonged durations; in addition to increasing the risk of injuring the shoulder joint, keeping the arms up can elicit the pressor response by elevating the heart rate without creating a corresponding increase in oxygen consumption. Avoid knee and elbow hyperextension, both of which can result from excessive momentum during kicks or rapid press-outs.

In addition to considering joint health and injury prevention, good instructors are aware of potential safety issues caused by the difficulty of a movement or the participant's ability. Keep all movements fluid and under control. Be careful with sudden changes in direction; always provide clear, advance cueing to prevent falls and collisions. Finally, always provide an alternative to turning steps, such as pivot turns. Some participants become dizzy and disoriented with this type of move.

Technique and Safety Check

To keep your classes safe, observe the following:

Remember to
- provide a variety of moves (front to back, side to side, and right to left),
- roll through the entire foot with each jump,
- keep the back heel up when performing lunges,
- be careful with sudden changes in direction, and
- provide an alternative to turning steps.

Avoid
- too much high impact,
- too many repetitive jumps on one leg (no more than eight in a row),
- too many repetitive moves that stress the musculoskeletal system,
- excessive momentum,
- knee and elbow hyperextension,
- keeping the arms overhead for prolonged durations, and
- using ankle weights.

Basic Moves

A skilled cardio instructor has a large repertoire of moves that allows for endless variety and creativity. Most of these moves can be performed with low to moderate impact (one foot stays on the floor during the move) or high impact (both feet leave the floor during the move). For example, a grapevine can be performed by always having one foot on the ground (low impact) or by jumping from foot to foot (high impact). Research has shown that low- to moderate-impact cardio routines, when performed with full range of motion (ROM) and appropriate choreography, can provide a cardiorespiratory stimulus similar to that of high-impact routines (Clapp and Little 1994; Otto et al. 1986, 1988; Parker et al. 1989; Williford, Blessing et al. 1989; Williford, Scharff-Olson, and Blessing 1989; Yoke et al. 1988, 1989). Instructors may choose to lead routines or classes that are entirely high impact, entirely low impact, or a combination of both. Following is an introduction to basic lower-body and upper-body moves for cardio classes.

Lower-Body Moves

Lower-body moves and patterns can be divided into 2-count and 4-count moves, which are demonstrated on the accompanying online video. These moves have many variations as described in the next section.

 See online video 4.2 for a demonstration of basic 2-count and 4-count moves for the lower body.

An aerobic or cardiorespiratory exercise is one in which major muscle groups move repetitively through full ROM for a prolonged duration. Therefore, it is important to keep the lower body moving at all times during a cardio class. Lower-body muscles contain more muscle mass than upper-body muscles and will consume more oxygen, thus providing a stronger cardiorespiratory stimulus. Studies have shown that simply staying in one place with minimal lower-body involvement while vigorously pumping the arms brings up the heart rate but does not significantly increase oxygen consumption or caloric expenditure (Parker et al. 1989).

The following are basic 2-count and 4-count moves for the lower body:

2-Count Moves

- Walk, march, jog
- Step touch
- Hamstring curl
- Knee lift (front or side)
- Kick (front, side, or back)
- Heel dig (front or side)
- Toe tap (front or side)
- Jumping jack
- Heel jack
- Twist
- Pony
- Kick, ball change
- Lunge
- Pendulum (ticktock)
- Scissors
- Ski jump
- Plié

4-Count Moves

- Grapevine
- Walk front for 3, tap on 4 (also known as a hustle)
- V-step (also known as out, out, in, in)
- Mambo
- Box step (also known as a jazz square)
- Charleston
- Shuffle
- Power squat
- Cha-cha
- Rocking horse
- Jig

Upper-Body Moves

In many group exercise activities, the arms can move bilaterally (right and left sides perform the same movement simultaneously, as when performing biceps curls with both arms) or unilaterally (right and left sides move individually or perform different movements simultaneously, as when performing alternating biceps curls). In addition to being bilateral or unilateral, upper-body moves can complement or oppose the lower-body moves. For example, when performing knee lifts, the right arm can reach up when the right knee lifts (complementary arms), or it can reach up when the left knee lifts (opposition arms). Upper-body moves also can be categorized as low-, mid-, and high-range movements. Examples are biceps curls (arms at sides), front raises to shoulder height, and overhead presses, respectively.

See online video 4.3 for a demonstration of high-low arm patterns. These patterns can be used in other group exercise modalities as well.

Practice Drill

Practice both the low- and high-impact variations of the lower-body moves listed in this chapter. Then try adding different arm movements: low-, mid-, and high-range movements; unilateral and bilateral movements; and opposition and complementary movements. See the arm patterns clip in the accompanying online video for a demonstration of this drill.

Elements of Variation

Variation can help you get more out of your basic moves. Almost every basic move can be altered in numerous ways to create interest, additional challenge, and fun! Variations give the illusion of new moves and choreography, when in fact you are only tweaking moves that are already familiar to class participants. The primary elements of variation are the lever, plane, directional, rhythm, intensity, and style variations.

Performing a lever variation simply means changing from a move with a short lever to a move with a long lever, or vice versa. For example, progressing from a knee lift to a kick is a lower-body lever change; similarly, moving from a bilateral front raise to a bilateral biceps curl is an upper-body lever change. This element of variation does not work for all moves.

A plane variation means changing the plane of movement while performing essentially the same action. When you change a front kick to a side kick or a front raise to a lateral raise, you are introducing a plane variation. The basic planes are the frontal (abduction and adduction movements), sagittal (flexion and extension movements), horizontal (horizontal shoulder adduction and abduction or twisting movements), and diagonal planes. This variation does not work for all moves (see figure 4.2).

A directional variation can mean changing the direction of the movement. From facing front, the same move can be performed while facing the side or back; from traveling forward (e.g., as in a hustle), the direction can be

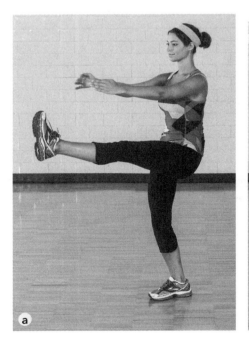 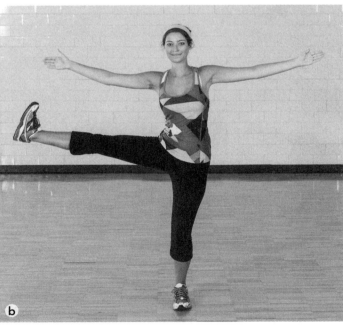

FIGURE 4.2 Moving from the (a) sagittal to the (b) frontal plane.

changed to travel diagonally instead. A directional variation can also mean traveling with the move instead of performing it in place. For example, alternating knee lifts can be performed while moving instead of remaining in one place. Varying the direction is an excellent strategy for increasing intensity and energy expenditure. It's amazing how familiar moves such as knee lifts can feel completely different when the direction changes! Some moves will naturally feel better when moving in a certain direction; jumping jacks, for instance, feel much more comfortable when moving backward rather than forward. A simple traveling combination might be four jumping jacks backward (8 counts) followed by a march or jog forward (8 counts); the move can be repeated for a complete 32-count phrase.

Rhythm variations involve changing the rhythm of the move or adding sound to the move. An example of a rhythmic change is switching from alternating single-knee lifts (a 2-count move) to alternating double-knee lifts (a 4-count move). Other moves that go easily from single to double and back again are hamstring curls, step touches, and lunges. Experiment with rhythmic sound variations: Try adding single and then double or triple claps to some moves. Snaps and stomps are also fun. Or ask participants to yell, whoop, or grunt at various points in the song; this technique has the potential to totally energize your class! Just keep your group's demographics and individual characteristics in mind; some people may be uncomfortable with making sounds, whereas others will enjoy it.

Variation in physiological intensity can be created in a number of ways, including

- increasing the lever length of the move,
- increasing the ROM of the move,
- increasing the speed of the move (or of the music itself),
- taking bigger steps when traveling as well as taking wider steps in stationary moves such as step touches, or
- changing the literal level of the move, which is also known as *vertical displacement.*

An example of vertical displacement occurs when a low-impact move is changed into a high-impact move. During a low-impact move such as a step touch, the center of gravity remains on the same level when the person steps side to side. However, in a high-impact move such as a side-to-side pony or triple step, the center of gravity moves up and down, and the movement involves more muscles , thus increasing the intensity. Vertical displacement can also occur in a downward direction, such as when bending the knees deeper during a low-impact step touch so that the emphasis is *down,* up (instead of *up,* down). A deeper bend shifts the center of gravity downward and requires more muscle-mass activation without jumping. Many low-impact moves lend themselves to this type of intensity variation, including hamstring curls, knee lifts, kicks, and lunges. Conversely, the intensity of these moves can be lessened by decreasing any of these variables (see figure 4.3).

Physiological intensity is not necessarily the same as complexity or psychological intensity. A combination built with simple choreography can be quite intense in terms of heart rate, oxygen consumption, and caloric expenditure. Ironically, performing a technical or complex combination involving many intricate foot and arm patterns can actually lower the exercise intensity because participants must focus on remembering what comes next and on not appearing clumsy. Sequencing and choreographic issues are discussed in greater depth later in this chapter.

 See online video 4.4 for a practice drill demonstrating the elements of variation (lever, plane, directional, rhythmic, intensity, and style variations).

One of the most enjoyable ways to alter moves is by playing with the style variation. A grapevine, for instance, can look and feel completely different when performed with a funky style versus a sporty style, even though it's essentially the same move! Other styles include Latin (salsa), hip-hop, dance, martial arts, country, jazz, Irish, or African. Expand your repertoire of styles and increase your fun potential!

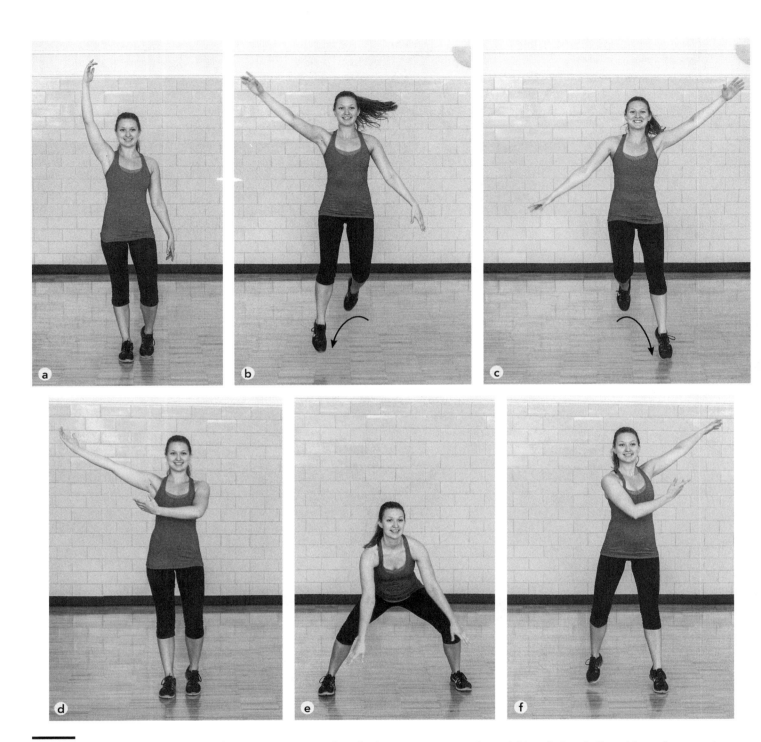

FIGURE 4.3 Intensity variations of the same move: (*a, b, c*) high-impact step touch, and (*d, e, f*) deeply flexed knee for more intense low-impact variation.

Practice Drill

Play your favorite music (pick a song with a strong beat) and perform a basic move, for example, a step touch. Add upper-body movements. On every 8th or 16th beat, change your move slightly by varying the lever, plane, direction, rhythm, intensity, or style. For example, go from a basic step touch with lateral arm raise to a front raise. Then try a direction change: Move the step touch (with front raises) diagonally to the front of the room and back again. Hold the basic move and then try changing the rhythm: Take 2 step touches to the right and then 2 to the left. Add an additional rhythm change by clapping on the 4th count each time. Return to the basic move. Have fun with a style change: Emphasize the upbeat by stomping the inside foot on the step touch while loosening the arms (allowing the elbows to flex slightly on the upbeat) and popping the torso slightly with an upbeat hip-hop style. When you feel you've exhausted the possibilities, go to another move, such as a march or grapevine, and try more elements of variation.

Creating Smooth Transitions

When skilled instructors teach, their moves flow seamlessly from one to the other, making the choreography easier to cue and easier for participants to follow, thus enhancing participant success. Spend some time on the drills in this section to build your skill at connecting moves. For the smoothest transitions, keep it simple. It's best if you change only one thing at a time—change only the arms or only the legs or only the lead foot.

Connecting End Points

Some moves just naturally transition into other moves. Most of the elements of variation provide for smooth transitions: Executing a plane change from a front kick to a side kick is an example of a smooth lower-body transition. The subtle change from a front kick with a front raise to a side kick with a lateral raise is easy for almost every participant to grasp and requires a minimum of cueing. Notice that each move has a starting point and an ending point. The smoothest transitions connect moves that have one of these points in common. For example, a bilateral front raise (a 2-count move) starts with the arms down and ends with the arms up at shoulder height in the sagittal plane. A lateral raise (another 2-count move) also starts with the arms down but ends with the arms up at shoulder height in the frontal plane. These two moves flow together well because they share a common starting point: arms down. It's easy and natural to go back and forth between these two moves; in fact, you could even create a combination 4-count upper-body move by putting these two moves together. You could then repeat the 4 counts over and over.

 See online video 4.5 for a drill demonstrating smooth transitions.

Practice Drill

Keeping your feet stationary, practice transitioning from one upper-body 2-count move to another, making sure that the two moves have a common denominator (starting point or ending point). Perform each 2-count move at least 4 to 8 times (for a total of 8-16 counts) and challenge yourself by connecting at least eight different upper-body moves sequentially. If necessary, pause briefly between moves to find a move with a common end point, but keep practicing until you eventually eliminate the pause. See the accompanying online video for an example of this drill.

Leading Foot

Another factor in creating smooth transitions and easy-to-follow choreography is to maintain an awareness of which foot is leading at all times (this is important!). In other words, you'll enhance your participants' success if you always lead with the same foot in each move throughout a combination. So, if you start with a step touch to the right (right foot leads off on count 1, or the downbeat), then you should also start your grapevine to the right if that's your next move. Starting a grapevine to the left after leading right in a step touch will confuse your participants

Practice Drill

Start with a simple lower-body move (e.g., a march) and add a simple upper-body move such as bilateral biceps curls. After 8 or 16 counts, change the upper-body move but maintain the lower-body move, experimenting until you find upper-body movements that share a common connecting point and flow smoothly and naturally (as in the previous drill). Notice if the transition feels right to your body. Continue for 8 or 16 more counts and then, maintaining your new upper-body move, smoothly transition to a new lower-body move. In this drill, only half the body changes at a time. Remember, you are working for smoothness; think of it as finding moves that flow so naturally that cueing is completely unnecessary. As you improve your skill, increase the speed of your transitions and switch to a new upper-body move or a new lower-body move every 4 counts.

---

and make the combination harder to follow. In addition to constantly hearing the downbeat in the back of your mind, stay aware of your lead foot and make sure it contacts the floor on the downbeats of the music. After performing a combination all the way through with the right foot leading, balance the body's neuromuscular and biomechanical systems by performing the entire combo with the left foot leading. (Note: In order to smoothly switch the lead foot, or leg, build a transition move or a connector move into the last 8 counts of the combination).

Connector Moves

You may have noticed that in some lower-body moves, both feet do the same thing at the same time; examples include pliés, jumping jacks, and double-time bouncy heel lifts (see figure 4.4). These symmetrical moves are valuable as filler moves and can help you switch your leading foot if you haven't built a lead change into your combination. Because both feet are doing the same thing at the same time, it's easy to start the next move on either the right foot or the left foot.

Another technique for changing lead legs (feet) is to use the single, single, double rhythm one time for the last 8 counts of your 32-count combination. If you've been leading right, you'll find that performing this rhythmic pattern (which takes 8 beats) will cause you to lead left. The single, single, double move works well with hamstring curls, knee lifts, and step touches.

 See online video 4.6 for a demonstration of how to use a single, single, double pattern to change the lead foot.

Other types of moves are so basic that they can be used over and over as fillers to ease transitions between other moves and to create participant security. A walk, march, or jog is a good filler. A good beginner combo might be walk 8 counts, perform 4 knee lifts (8 counts), walk 8 counts, step touch 4 times (8 counts), walk 8 counts, perform 4 hamstring curls (8 counts), walk 8 counts, perform 4 kicks (8 counts). This adds up to two 32-count phrases, or 64 counts. The 8-count walk inserted between all the other moves can enhance participant confidence and provide a psychological break from complex choreography. (Incidentally, these 8-count walks could be made more interesting by traveling, adding impact, changing the style, or adding arm variations.) Once participants become comfortable with the combination, try removing all the filler moves (the walks). What you'll have left is a 32-count combination that is more complex: 4 knee lifts, 4 step touches, 4 hamstring curls, and 4 kicks.

Every instructor needs filler moves as reliable standbys for those times when the brain seems to stop working and you simply can't remember what's supposed to come next! If this happens, you can always return to the safety of a walk, march, or jog.

Moves That Don't Fit Together Well

Some moves simply don't fit together well. When designing a combination, you may have to incorporate one or two transition moves to make the choreography smoother and easier to follow. For example, moving from a plié to a front kick is awkward; transition moves are needed for a more natural flow. A possible solution could be plié (8 counts), step toe touch side (8 counts), step toe touch front (8 counts), and then step kick front (8 counts).

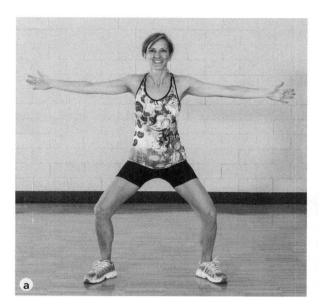
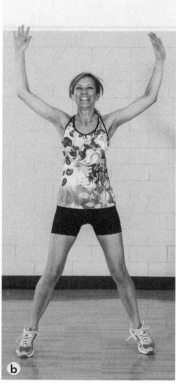
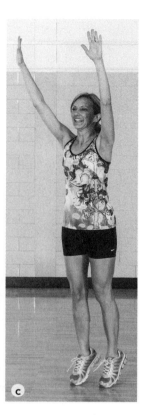

FIGURE 4.4 Connector moves: (*a*) plié (flex knees down, up, down, up), (*b*) jumping jack, and (*c*) bouncy heel lifts (flex knees down, up, down, up—may add a jump-shot action with the upper body).

Building Basic Combinations

Many instructors prefer to teach cardio classes with 32-count combinations of moves, sometimes referred to as *blocks*. Usually these combinations have been designed and practiced before class. Here are the typical steps used in designing a cardio combination:

1. Start with four lower-body moves that flow together. Make sure each move fills 8 counts for a total of 32 counts. Practice to find the smoothest arrangement of the four moves. Add transitional moves when necessary and eliminate moves that don't fit well but stay within the 32-count framework.

2. Find upper-body movements that go with the lower-body combination.

3. Check to see that your combination provides a balance of complex and simple moves, can be modified with appropriate intensity and complexity variations, flows smoothly, is easy to cue (see "Cueing Methods in Group Exercise" later in this chapter), and can be broken down easily (more about this later).

4. Repeat this process with another 32-count combination (sometimes referred to as a block). If you plan to link several blocks of 32-count combos together, you will need to see that they have common ending points and starting points for smooth transitions between blocks.

▶ See online video 4.7 for a demonstration of building a basic combination and introducing variation.

Showing Modifications, Regressions, and Progressions

Skilled instructors are adept at providing intensity and complexity modifications, thus making the routine easier or more suitable for a specific need, in order to accommodate skill and fitness levels among participants. If the class has fit participants, instructors need to offer intensity and complexity progressions, making the routine more difficult. Generally, instructors should teach at an intermediate level and demonstrate intensity variations for exercisers who are above or below that level. A group instructor should also occasionally incorporate an intensity drill into the class routine; with an intensity drill, participants will be more likely to take responsibility for themselves and modify or progress moves to fit their own needs. For an example of an intensity drill, see the practice drill that follows.

Practice Drill

To begin an intensity drill, show a basic move such as a hamstring curl and cue "Show me this move at low intensity." Watch the participants do the move for a moment and then say, "Now show me the same move at medium intensity." Finally, ask the participants, "Can you show me this move at high intensity?" It helps build participant confidence if you call out suggestions for increasing and decreasing intensity during the drill. Suggestions include taking wider steps; adding vertical displacement ("*Down*, up" or adding hops); increasing the range of motion of the arms; and traveling the whole move forward, backward, or in a turn. Once the participants have demonstrated high intensity, have them show both medium intensity and low intensity again so that they know how to increase and decrease the intensity of the hamstring curl. Repeat with other simple moves such as knee lifts, grapevines, or even a basic march.

The more complex your choreography is, the more important your ability to show modifications and break down your routines. This is particularly true with choreography that includes pivots or turns, as some participants tend to get dizzy or disoriented when turning. Always provide alternatives for pivots and turns. For example, a 4-count pivot turn can always be modified to a 4-count mambo or even a march.

Breaking Down and Building Combinations

A combination is broken down when an instructor takes the finished choreography and essentially works backward. In other words, many participants won't be able to grasp the final, most complex, most intense version of your routine the first time you show it. So instead of beginning with the final combination, start with the most basic, simplest moves of the combination and gradually build in intensity and complexity until participants are performing the final product. Breaking down a combination may take quite a while, depending on your choreography and your participants' skill levels. Design all your routines so that you can easily break them down into their basic components. Some practitioners call this the *part-to-whole method*. Practice teaching your routines as if you were leading novice participants through your combinations for the first time. Let's look at an example of how to break down a 32-count combination that contains a rather complex move. The final version of this combination is as follows:

1. Facing the left corner, perform 2 kick-ball-changes (right leg performs full ROM kick while right foot is leading) followed by 1 box step (jazz square). This is the complex move. The upper body performs alternating punches on the kick-ball-change, and the arms sweep backward on the box step—8 counts altogether. See the accompanying online video for a demonstration.

2. Repeat for another 8 counts.

3. Facing front, step touch right and left, and then repeat. The upper body performs a lateral raise through its full ROM—this move takes 8 counts.

4. Perform 4 jumping jacks, turning so that the last jack faces the right corner. The upper body performs overhead presses—this move requires 8 counts. You have now completed 32 counts altogether.

5. Repeat the entire combination on the other side, leading with the left foot.

Here's how to break down this combination:

1. Start by repeating the kick-ball-change over and over again, , right foot leading. Drill this move without arms until the majority of your class can perform it correctly. You could even break this move down further by teaching it in half time.

2. Now drill the box step, continuing to repeat the move until it appears that most of your participants are comfortable with it.

3. Next, combine the two moves: 2 kick-ball-changes with 1 box step. Again, repeat this two-move pattern over and over until participants have it.

4. Add on 4 sets of right and left step touches for a count of 16.

5. Perform 8 jumping jacks for a count of 16.

6. Now that your participants know the four movement patterns you'll be using, return to the beginning of the combo. At the top of the next 32-count phrase, lead your group in an expanded version of the final combination (still leading right): 4 sets of the 2 kick-ball-changes followed by 1 box step (32 counts), 4 sets of right and left step touches (16 counts), and 8 jumping jacks (16 counts).

7. Repeat this expanded version; this time, add the upper-body movements.

8. Repeat the combination again, asking for more energy and greater ROM during the kick part of the kick-ball-change.

9. Finally, reduce the combination to its intended version: 2 sets of the 2 kick-ball-changes followed by 1 box step (16 counts), 2 sets of right and left step touches (8 counts), and 4 jumping jacks (8 counts).

By this time, the participants should be familiar enough with the routine that they are ready to try it with the left foot leading. Because this routine is complex and it's best to balance left with right, it's probably wise to go through all 9 steps of the breakdown on the left side.

The combination we've just broken down illustrates the concept of balancing complex with simple moves. Because the kick-ball-change requires agility and feels complex to most participants, the simple step touches and jumping jacks provide a nice physiological and psychological balance. In addition, any decrease in intensity required by the complex footwork in the first moves can be balanced with the jacks at the end of the combination.

The teaching techniques used in this example include adding on and repetition reduction. Adding on is just as it sounds: After the class has learned a move, pattern, or short sequence, the instructor adds a new move or pattern to the existing sequence, gradually putting together the final product. Repetition reduction is useful because most participants need to repeat a move in order to learn it (particularly if it is complex). Thus, skilled instructors teach combinations in expanded versions that include many repetitions of each move. In other words, a combo that is intended to be 32 counts is drilled in a 64-count or 128-count version. In classes for beginners, the combo might remain expanded; it is not always necessary to reduce a combination to its most complex form. Repetition reduction, the process of reducing the number of repetitions to the most complex, 32-count version of a combination, is also called *pyramid building*: Start the sequence with large numbers of repetitions and gradually eliminate repetitions until the desired combination is achieved.

 See online video 4.8 for a sample choreography combination incorporating high-and low-impact moves.

 See online video 4.9 for a demonstration of the same combination at three different levels of intensity.

Writing Out a Combination

Knowing how to put your ideas down on paper is useful. Many instructors keep a file of moves, successful combinations, and routines. Note the following example:

	Lead leg	Movement	Counts
A	Lead R	4 marches in place	1-8
B	Lead R	4 alternating knee lifts, stepping w/R lead	9-16
C	Lead R	4 step touches	17-24
D	Lead R	4 alternating hamstring curls with "single, single, double" rhythm	25-32

Reprinted, with permission, from Lawrence Biscontini, 2010, *ACE Certified News.*

Note that A, B, C, and D signify different moves: The lead leg is designated, the numbers of each move and the moves themselves are described, and the numbers of counts are given. The chart helps make the combination clear and easy to understand. You can see that the final move, with the single, single, double rhythm, brings you to a left leg (foot) lead, so the entire combination can be repeated leading left, making a total of 64 counts. This combination could be one block of choreography, which can then be linked to other blocks, as you will see.

Additional Choreography Techniques

Although combination building is the most common way to teach cardio classes, it is not the only way. Other choreographic teaching techniques (in addition to breaking down a combination, adding on, and repetition reduction) include layering, using building blocks, and playing flip-flop. All of these techniques are usually planned and practiced in advance of the actual class. Another choreographic technique, called *freestyle* or *linear choreography,* is extemporaneous.

Freestyle Choreography

The freestyle method, also known as using *linear progressions,* is a valid and effective technique. Whereas combination-style choreography is usually planned and organized into patterns, freestyle choreography is spontaneous and delivered on the spot, without an emphasis on pattern development. In freestyle, one move flows smoothly into the next move, which flows into the next move, and so on. There is little repetition.

 See online video 4.10 for a practice drill on freestyle choreography.

Although freestyle demands skill on the part of the instructor, it is psychologically easier for participants, who don't have to remember complex moves and patterns. In well-led freestyle, exercisers don't have to worry as much about appearing clumsy or inept because they are always at least half right! This is because, ideally, the instructor changes only one thing at a time, either changing the upper-body movement while keeping the lower-body movement the same or changing the lower-body movement while maintaining the upper-body movement. This kind of linear progression allows participants to commit more fully to the moves and perform with greater intensity, which can result in a better training effect and higher caloric expenditure than might be achieved with combination choreography.

The best way to improve your skill at freestyle is, of course, to practice it. The drills described previously in the sections "Elements of Variation" and "Creating Smooth Transitions" are particularly useful for freestyle. Here's an example of freestyle choreography:

1. Start with a basic march.
2. Add arms pressing front.
3. Keeping the arm movement, change the march to a heel dig front.
4. Keeping the lower-body movement, change the arms to an overhead press.
5. Maintaining the upper-body movement, change the legs to a toe touch side.
6. Staying with the leg movement, change the arms to side press-outs.
7. Keeping the arm movements, change the lower body to heel digs to the side.
8. Keeping the heel digs, change the arms to long-lever lateral raises.
9. Maintaining the lateral raises, change the legs to a high-impact heel jack.

10. Maintaining the upper-body raises, change to a jumping jack.

11. Change the legs once more to a step touch (with same upper-body lateral raises).

12. Keeping the step touch, change the arms to unilateral overhead presses.

This example generally alternates upper-body changes with lower-body changes, but you may sequence your changes however you like as long as you provide variety and muscle balance and avoid excessive repetitions of moves that stress the musculoskeletal system. Each move can be performed for 4, 8, 16, or even 32 counts depending on your class (be sure to begin the cardio session on the first count of an 8-count phrase). As always, maintain an appropriate intensity level: Performing too many low-intensity moves in a row results in a low-intensity progression.

Notice that each move in the freestyle example transitions smoothly into the next. Not only is this easier for participants to follow—it's also much easier for you to cue! In fact, good freestyle requires a minimum of cueing; participants simply have to keep watching as they move, and they will naturally move with you. Freestyle choreography provides an ideal format for those times when you want to promote group interaction and sociability while working out or when you want to make class announcements or educational points. Because it's not as necessary to give anticipatory cues (cues that let exercisers know what move is coming next), you can talk about other subjects. Freestyle is especially useful during the warm-up and at any point in the routine when you sense that participants are experiencing brain strain from too much concentration on or memorization of complex choreography. Many instructors intentionally intersperse freestyle between choreographed routines to give their classes psychological breaks and to help boost intensity levels. The freestyle technique is also great for participants with less experience or coordination, because they don't have to remember specific sequences.

Layering

The layering technique is used to add more complexity to a move or combination. Each layer is repeated until participants appear confident, and then another layer of complexity is added. See the following example of layering:

1. Perform 3 counts of walking in place with a knee lift on count 4. Repeat, noting that the knee lift naturally falls on the other side on the second four counts.

2. Layer with a directional variation: Travel forward, repeating the move 2 times for a total of 8 counts, and then travel backward, repeating the move 2 times for 8 counts.

3. Increase the complexity by keeping only the pattern while performing the 8 counts forward; walk for 8 counts backward without any knee lifts.

4. Layer by adding a hop on counts 4 and 8 forward (on the knee lifts) while abducting the arms to shoulder height.

5. Layer by adding jazz style to the forward movements. While hopping and lifting the left knee, twist the spine and adduct the knee across the body, showing the left hip; while hopping and lifting the right knee, twist the spine and adduct the knee across the body, showing the right hip.

6. Layer the backward walk by performing a pivot turn on counts 5, 6, 7, and 8 (finish facing forward).

This example repeated the same 16 counts several times, but the patterns gradually became more interesting, stylistic, and complex.

Building Blocks and Linking

A *block* is a 32- or 64-count combination of moves. Instructors can create several blocks and then link them together for one long combination (e.g., block 1 + block 2 + block 3 + block 4). When linking several blocks together, try naming them or associating them with key words or numbers to help your students recall the different blocks. For example, you could cue your class with "Now let's do Carol's combo" (named after Carol) followed by "Next, the shuffle routine" (this routine has a shuffle in it) followed by "It's time for the traveler" (a combo with large traveling moves).

Flip-Flop

The flip-flop works well for combinations that have clearly defined elements such as high-impact and low-impact or stationary and traveling moves. After participants have become familiar with the initial combination, flip-flop the key elements; for example, change all the low-impact moves to high impact and all the high-impact moves to low impact. By using the flip-flop, you gain more variety from existing combos. You can also invert or change the order of the blocks. For example, if you've been combining your blocks as 1 + 2 + 3 + 4, try switching them and teaching the blocks in a different order, such as 2 + 4 + 3 + 1. This will add tremendous diversity to your choreography and make it feel fresh and new to your participants.

Cueing Methods in Group Exercise

Proper cueing is essential for a successful high-low cardio class. Class members will have different learning styles: Most will learn best by watching you, others will learn by hearing your verbal instruction, and still others will learn by doing the moves (visual, auditory, and kinesthetic styles, respectively). While most people combine the three types in order to learn, many people subconsciously have a preferred learning method (Faulkner and Faulkner 1996). Therefore, you'll want to use as many styles as possible and expand your teaching vocabulary so that you can say the same thing in multiple ways. Several types of cues are necessary, including anticipatory, movement, motivational, educational, alignment, and safety verbal cues, plus visual cues. In this section we describe these types of cues as well as discuss the advantages and disadvantages of mirroring your class.

Anticipatory Cueing

An anticipatory cue tells your participants when to do the next movement and what that next movement will be. Learning to deliver timely and appropriate anticipatory cues often takes considerable practice, so be patient and practice the drills given in this book, and eventually you will become an instructor who is easy to follow.

To give good anticipatory cues, you must understand music structure and be able to hear the beat, the downbeat, and the 4-, 8-, and 32-count phrases as discussed earlier in this chapter.

It's easiest for your class if you count backward when cueing an upcoming new move or transition. If you count, "4, 3, 2, and _____," your participants know that after "_____" (where the 1 would be) there will be a new move. This helps them pay attention and be ready to change and move with the rest of the class. If your anticipatory cue is short (e.g., "step touch"), only one beat might be needed, as in, "4, 3, 2, step touch." Longer cues (e.g., "grapevine right, arms up") take more time to say and therefore will need more beats: "4, 3, grapevine right, arms up."

Instructors don't usually speak on every single beat for anticipatory cueing; doing so is too wordy and confusing—and it's also hard on your voice! Instead, count backward on every other beat of your 8-count phrase as shown in figure 4.5. Practice this example by clapping your hands on every beat while speaking in rhythm at the suggested times. This method of counting on every other beat works well when you are performing 2-count moves.

Cueing 2-Count Moves

Starting without music, march, feeling your lead foot (e.g., right foot) coming down on every other beat (a march is a 2-count move). Begin to practice the cue given in figure 4.5 ("4, 3, 2, step touch"), saying "4" when your lead foot strikes the floor (this is a downbeat and the first beat of an 8-count phrase). If all goes well, you will be ready to step touch to the right at the end of the 8 counts, beginning the new move (step touch) with your right foot (lead foot) on the downbeat. Notice the paradox: You are saying one thing while your body is doing something else. This probably won't feel natural at first, but keep practicing—it's a skill worth acquiring if you want your participants to all do the same thing at the same time and feel satisfied with your class!

After mastering the transition from march to step touch while cueing, see if you can continue the step touch and, when ready, cue back to a march. Note that you may continue step touching for as many counts as you like, starting the anticipatory cue "4, 3, 2, _____" when you are ready to change (see figure 4.5). Be sure to

Counts	8		7	6	5	4	3	2	1	8
Footstrike	(March) R		L	R	L	R	L		R	L	(Step-touch) R
Cue	"4,			3,		2,	step	touch"		

FIGURE 4.5 Cueing 2-count moves. Practice transitioning from the march to the step touch while cueing.

say "4" when your lead foot (e.g., right foot) is striking the floor and stepping right. Always be mindful of your lead foot.

When you return to the march, your right foot is still leading, and the foot strike occurs on the downbeat or the actual first count of the 8-count phrase (which, as explained, is counted backward in 4s to make it easier for your participants). Be aware that to finish the 8 counts of the step touch, your right foot performs a tap or touch (the last movement of the 8-count step touch) immediately before leading right in the march. This is called *finishing the movement phrase* and is a key component in staying on the downbeat. If you forget to perform this tap or last touch, you will no longer be moving with the music, and your participants will eventually become confused. Finishing the phrase is much simpler than it sounds; performing these moves to music will feel quite natural. You don't even need to mention this final tap or touch to your students; they'll do it unconsciously as long as you're moving with the downbeats.

Before trying this drill with music, go back and forth between marching and step touching, continuing each move as long as necessary for you to collect your thoughts and cue properly. Practice leading with your left foot as well. Another basic pattern to practice is to go from a march to a wide march and then back again to the march, cueing "4, 3, march it wide" and "4, 3, march it back in." Experiment with speaking in rhythm. You want to hear the ticktock of the constant rhythmic beat at all times in your head while teaching. Eventually, you can expand this drill to include a wide variety of 2-count moves (see the "2-Count Moves" list earlier in this chapter).

Practice these drills with a friend who will pretend to be your student. Your friend's responses can give you instant feedback about the timeliness and effectiveness of your cues.

Then, repeat the entire drill with music. Pick popular music (preferably commercially mixed group exercise music) with a strong, easy-to-hear beat. At first, these drills and speaking in rhythm may have a slightly robotic feel. This is appropriate in the early stages of learning to cue, when hearing and moving on the downbeat may not yet be habitual and spontaneous for you.

Cueing 4-Count Moves

Learning to cue 4-count moves is similar to learning to cue 2-count moves; however, instead of counting on every other beat, you count on every fourth beat. For example, perform grapevines, first to the right and then to the left continuously, leading with the right foot. When you are ready to change to the next move, such as a march, begin counting backward, starting with 4 when the right (lead) foot initiates a grapevine to the right. This time, however, count each individual grapevine, or every fourth count, as shown in figure 4.6.

Finish by marching right, which should be your lead foot. Notice again the final tap of the right foot just before the march; this tap finishes the last grapevine and is essential for staying on beat with the music. While marching, return to the 2-count cueing you have already learned, saying, "4, 3, 2, grapevine" to cue the grapevine, at which point you'll again switch to the 4-count cueing (see figure 4.6). Practice moving back and forth between 2- and 4-count moves until the anticipatory cueing feels comfortable. A grapevine is a perfect move to practice visual cueing simultaneously, which we'll discuss shortly. Participants will be grateful if you point in the direction of the initial grapevine (to help them get started) and if you hold up fingers (4, 3, 2, 1) to let them know when the next change will occur.

 See online video 4.11 for a practice drill on anticipatory cueing for 2-count and 4-count moves.

Another drill that entails switching from 2-count to 4-count anticipatory cueing involves moving from singles to doubles and back to singles again. Several moves work well for this drill, including knee lifts, hamstring curls, lunges, and step touches. Start with single hamstring curls, for instance, and cue on every 2 counts: "4, 3,

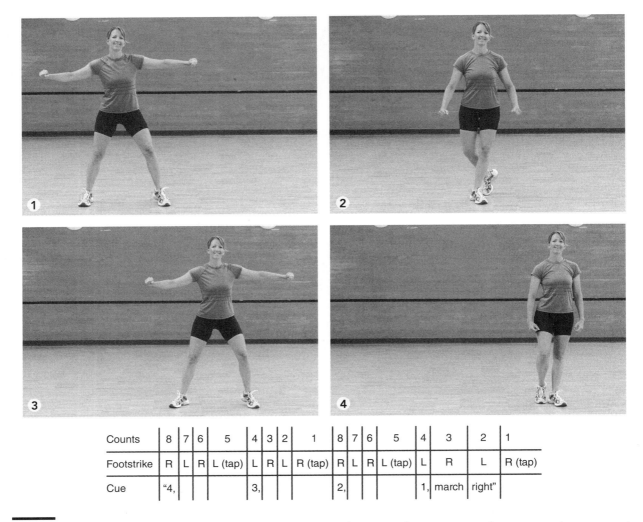

Counts	8	7	6	5	4	3	2	1	8	7	6	5	4	3	2	1
Footstrike	R	L	R	L (tap)	L	R	L	R (tap)	R	L	R	L (tap)	L	R	L	R (tap)
Cue	"4,				3,				2,				1,	march	right"	

FIGURE 4.6 A basic grapevine is a four-count move. The chart shows cues for transitioning from a grapevine to a march.

2, now doubles." Once you are doing doubles, each hamstring curl requires 4 counts. When you are ready to return to singles, cue on every 4 counts: "4, 3, 2, 1, now single."

Writing Out a Combination With Anticipatory Cues

When you're first learning, it's good practice not only to put your combo on paper, but also to write out the anticipatory cues. Using the combination presented earlier, your written anticipatory cues might be as follows:

	Lead leg	Movement	Counts	Anticipatory cues
A	Lead R	4 marches in place	1-8	"4, 3, 2, knee lifts"
B	Lead R	4 alternating knee lifts	9-16	"4, 3, 2, step touch"
C	Lead R	Stepping with R lead 4 step touches	17-24	"4, 3, hamstring curl pattern"
D	Lead R	4 alternating hamstring curls with "single, single, double" rhythm	25-32	"single, single, double—march left!"

Let's review the cueing for this pattern. As the chart illustrates, the cue for the next move happens while you're actually doing the current move. For move A, marching, you cue backward from 4, and say, "Knee lifts" where the word "one" would be—while you're still marching. For move B, knee lifts, use the same technique, cueing the next move, "Step touch" where the word "one" would be. During move C, however, the next anticipatory cue is longer and more complicated, so it must take place where the words "two and one" would be. You could say, "4, 3, hamstring curl *pat*tern," with the accent on "pat" (where the "one" would be). In other words, you'd speak in rhythm, which helps participants to hear the beat better. Move D then, is even more complex, so you'll probably need to give a movement cue in rhythm *plus* an anticipatory cue; this means there's no time to count. The cue would then sound, "*Single, single, double*—march *left*." This may sound complicated, but with a bit of practice you can master anticipatory cueing. The result is worth it: Your class will eventually label you as a "good cue-er and easy to follow." This skill alone can make you an in-demand teacher because everyone will feel more confident and have more fun.

Technique and Safety Check

When cueing, be sure to

- hear the downbeat and the 8-count phrase,
- initiate new moves at the top of the 8-count phrase on the downbeat,
- initiate new moves with your lead foot,
- finish all moves (e.g., the last tap or touch),
- cue backward starting with "4,"
- speak in rhythm (at least initially), and
- cue the next move while you're still performing the current move.

Movement Cues

A movement cue verbalizes what is seemingly obvious. Many participants need this verbal reinforcement to enhance their confidence and success. A movement cue can point out footwork, either with rhythmic counts, as in a cha-cha ("the feet go 1, 2, 1, 2, 3—1, 2, 1, 2, 3"), or with rights and lefts, as when lunging ("right foot back, left foot back, right foot back, left foot back"). It can also provide basic directions, as in a double lunge ("feet go down, up, down, switch—down, up, down, switch"). Such cues may be repeated over and over with appropriate rhythmic emphasis until participants perform the pattern correctly. Movement cues also include naming the move (e.g., "pivot turn" or "twist") and stating an actual direction, as in "grapevine right." We recommend always accompanying the words *right* and *left* with the visual cue of pointing. Some participants experience confusion and anxiety when suddenly asked to move right or left, but these feelings can be eased or eliminated with pointing, which is a visual cue.

Motivational Cues

Motivational cues increase your participants' self-confidence and enjoyment and encourage a sense of play! Your speech should be liberally sprinkled with encouraging words and phrases: "Great," "Super," "Well done," "Fantastic job," "You people look terrific," "Outstanding." Some instructors give motivational cues every 8 to 16 counts—no wonder their classes are so popular! Additionally, many instructors cut loose with whoops, trills, yahoos, hup hup, and other noises just for fun. If you have a good time in class, the chances are good that your students will too!

Educational Cues

An educational cue delivers relevant information about the workout or about other topics related to fitness and wellness. Reviewing the benefits of aerobic training while leading simple freestyle moves is an excellent way to incorporate education into your teaching. And, of course, it's essential to give intensity recommendations throughout your class. Identifying muscle groups ("These are your hamstrings") and providing hydration information are other examples of educational cueing.

Alignment and Safety Cues

Skilled instructors constantly deliver pointers on alignment and safety. Common misalignments observed during cardiorespiratory training include a forward head (chin jut), rounded and hunched shoulders, shoulders that elevate when reaching overhead, hyperextended elbows and knees, and a lack of spinal and pelvic stability (particularly during knee lifts and kicks). When participants perform lunges or repeaters, the hips, knees, and toes all need to point in the same direction. Safety cues include reminding participants to bring the heels down when jumping, avoid excessive momentum, stay in control, keep the fists relaxed, listen to their bodies, work at their own pace, and stay hydrated. It's nearly impossible to give too many of these types of cues! Remember to word your cues positively by avoiding the use of the word "don't" whenever possible. For example, it's much better to say, "When reaching overhead, keep those shoulder blades down," rather than "Don't hunch your shoulders." The first cue specifically tells participants what to do, whereas the second, negative, cue tells them what not to do but can leave some members at a loss as to what you're asking them to perform. In addition, using lots of negative "don't" cues can make you sound threatening, bossy, and unpleasant.

Visual Cues and Mirroring Techniques

Do everything possible to ensure your participants' success. If the majority of the class members consistently have trouble following or grasping new moves, their difficultly probably has more to do with the instructor than with them. Such problems can be traced to the instructor's moves, transitions, sequencing, ability to work with music, and ability to cue correctly. Thus, you will want to work hard to make your cueing crystal clear. One major way to help participants move with you at all times is to use visual cueing in conjunction with verbal cueing. Adding visual cues is essential when you work with large groups or without a microphone, and in addition it can save your voice. A number of visual cues have been developed and are used commonly by cardio instructors (Webb 1989). These include hand signals for counting, showing direction, turning, holding a move, indicating the lead leg, calling for everyone's attention ("Watch me!"), and pointing

to various parts of your own body to indicate proper alignment (see figure 4.7).

Most people are visual learners. Without really thinking about it, they tend to copy the instructor's body language, including alignment, physical energy, and movement style. This is good if you have excellent alignment and physical energy; however, it can be problematic if you use incorrect alignment or technique.

When you face your class while moving, you are using the technique of mirror imaging. Mirror imaging is another valuable group leadership skill that takes practice. The advantages of mirror imaging include more personal and direct eye contact with your students, better vocal projection, and less temptation to become mesmerized by your own image in the mirror. Facing your class shows that you are a student-centered instructor and makes your job seem less like a performance. We recommend facing your class as much as possible, especially during the warm-up, during times you are leading freestyle choreography, and during the muscle conditioning and flexibility portions of your class. The major disadvantage of facing your class is that if your combinations are relatively complex, they'll be more difficult for your class to follow. In other words, your participants are more likely to be successful if you face away from them during intricate choreography.

Mirroring takes practice. When you want your class to move right, you have to point left with your left hand, even as you are saying "right." If you want your participants to march forward, you'll need to move backward as you motion them to come toward you. Your directional cues will be reversed for you but not for your class. For practice, repeat all the drills described in this chapter while facing a partner.

Movement Previews

When you are teaching more complex choreography, sometimes a movement preview is useful. While having your participants continue with a familiar move, you can demonstrate (preview) the new move or the more complex variation for them so that they can see it before they do it. For example, while your participants perform grapevines, you can preview the next, more complex layer by demonstrating grapevines with a turn.

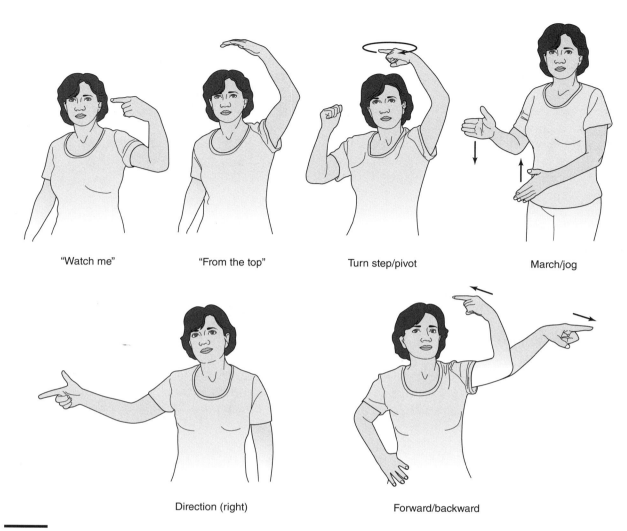

"Watch me"   "From the top"   Turn step/pivot   March/jog

Direction (right)   Forward/backward

FIGURE 4.7 Visual cues.

Practice Drill

Play your favorite music—pick something with a strong beat. Face a partner and begin a familiar move (such as a walk or step touch). Try not to speak at all; use only visual cueing to communicate with your partner. This includes having an animated face and conveying lots of enthusiasm! Your partner should follow along according to your visual cues. Continue the move for 4 to 16 counts and then transition through several moves (this works best if your transitions are smooth and natural, and you use the elements of variation). Note how well your partner follows your visual cues. Is there any way you could improve your visual cueing to enhance your partner's success?

Constructive Corrections

We must not underestimate the importance of the participant's overall experience in a group exercise class. How participants are treated and whether they are comfortable can make or break their attendance in your class. Bain and colleagues (1989) compared the dropout rate of group exercise participants who were overweight with the rate of those who were at their recommended weight and found that the dropout rate of the overweight participants was higher. They dropped out not because they did not like the music or the routines but because they were concerned about being embarrassed and judged by others. Wininger (2002) found that an instructor's ability to communicate is an important aspect of the participant's overall enjoyment. Therefore, how you give your participants feedback is important. If you have observed improper technique in your group exercise classes, take action but make sure you are kind. Some instructors find this the most challenging part of teaching because it's often hard to be a strong motivator yet also a soft encourager when a participant needs correction. Figure 4.8 provides a cueing example, but first, here are suggestions on how to cue the participant on correct position or technique without being threatening or critical.

- **Deliver general statements to the whole group.** "Stop for just a moment—look at your back foot to see if your toes are facing straight ahead. The toes must be straight ahead for the most effective calf stretch." Or, "I see people having difficulty—let me demonstrate what I want you to do."

- **Make corrections by moving the person into the proper position.** During a wall stretch for the calves, give the following instruction to people experiencing difficulty: "I would like to turn your foot so it is straight. Is that OK? Can you feel a difference in the stretch?" Always ask permission before touching a student.

- **Exercise next to the participant.** Stand beside the person having trouble and demonstrate what you want done. Perhaps he

or she cannot quite see or hear you well enough to comply. If the person you are correcting is down on the floor, get down next to that person to demonstrate. A person on the floor is more vulnerable than a person standing, so you must get down on the same level to instruct in a non-threatening way.

- **Move around the room.** If you stay at the front of the class, only the people in the front row will be able to observe your technique. If you are teaching step, put several benches around the room so you can move around during the cardio segment. Try teaching in the middle of the class instead of the front or regularly move from the front to the back, or to the side of the room.

- **Catch people doing it right.** Most people respond much better to positive rather than negative reinforcement. If a participant is having difficulty with a movement or series of movements, point out someone performing well in class for him or her to watch or pair them together. Always demonstrate and instruct good alignment to keep a focus on correct technique.

- **Always appeal to a person's need for safety and give your rationale.** Compare "You must have your foot in this position" with "Place your foot in this position because it will prevent you from falling forward and will make this exercise easier." Or, "Don't bounce while stretching; that's the wrong technique" versus

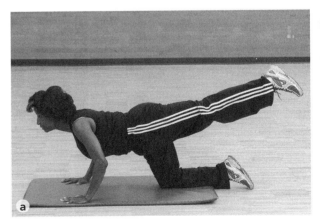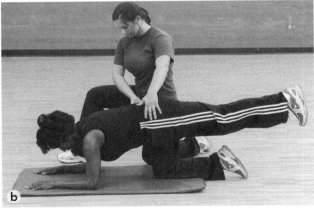

FIGURE 4.8 Cueing example: (a) poor technique and (b) instructor correction. You may imagine that the instructor is telling the participant, "Please bring your forearms down to the mat. Let's move those hips back so they are directly over your knees. Also, please keep your gaze down so that your head is in line with your spine."

"If you bounce while stretching, you might pull or tear a muscle—I don't want you to get hurt. Try holding the stretch instead." Which statement would you rather hear? All the statements tell the participant how to correct the actions; however, the second statements include a rationale and helpful alternatives.

- **Use positive descriptions rather than labels.** Words such as *good, bad, right,* and *wrong* are emotionally loaded and judgmental. Instead of saying, "Joe, you are doing this movement wrong," try, "Joe, you seem to be having trouble with this movement. Let's try this . . . I think it will help."

Find ways to make your class a positive experience for all. Correcting and recommending alignment changes in a polite and nonthreatening way makes the exercise experience more comfortable for participants. If they are comfortable, they will be more likely to come back. If students are ill at ease, they may miss some of the wonderful therapeutic benefits that come from group exercise (Choi et al. 1993; Estivill

1995), such as a positive mood and increased self-esteem. The mental and emotional benefits derived from group exercise can be just as beneficial as the physical gains.

 See online video 4.12 for a practice drill on correcting alignment for a stationary lunge.

Technique Check

Here are the key points for cueing:

- As much as possible, cue both verbally and visually.
- Use a microphone whenever possible.
- Avoid endless counting. Instead, use your time whenever possible to deliver other types of cues (e.g., alignment, motivational).
- Always count down instead of up.
- Keep cues relatively short and to the point.
- Initiate cues on the downbeat and time them so that new moves are also on the downbeat.

Chapter Wrap-Up

Our goal as group exercise instructors is to make classes fun in order to enhance the health and well-being of our participants. One way to do this is by using quality music played on a good sound system. This chapter covered music fundamentals as well as practical techniques for leading a traditional high-low cardio group exercise class. Most of the topics and techniques described in this chapter apply to several other types of group exercise, including step, slide, Zumba, NIA, and kickboxing.

When developing your cardiorespiratory segment, check yourself against the Group Exercise Class Evaluation Form (appendix A) to be sure you've met the basic criteria for leading cardio segments. To become proficient at leading group exercise, practice, experiment, and keep challenging yourself. The rewards are worth it: You will soon lead a class that your participants will want to take again and again!

ASSIGNMENTS

1. Attend a group exercise class and observe an instructor getting ready to teach a class. Write down all the steps she or he takes to set up the music and microphone and how equipment is set up. Research the Web or contact one vendor from the "Music Resource List" and create a price list of a complete sound system for use in a group exercise setting. Write a one-page summary of your findings.

2. Create a 4-minute high-low impact cardio routine with proper cueing. Practice the routine until you are ready to teach it. (Very few classes are entirely high impact or entirely low impact. Therefore, always provide BOTH options for all moves.) Use at

> continued

> continued

least two 64-count blocks of simple choreography (32 counts leading R; 32 counts leading L). Incorporate anticipatory cueing (on the downbeat), visual cueing, and at least one other cueing technique. Write out the routine according to the example in the "Writing Out a Combination" section of this chapter.

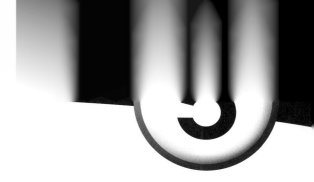

Coaching-Based Concepts

Chapter Objectives

By the end of this chapter, you will be able to

- understand coaching-based concepts as they apply to a group exercise class,
- generate and apply motivational strategies while working with class participants,
- create dynamic team environments in the group exercise setting,
- create rapport with participants to empower and connect them with individual and group preferences,
- apply exercise modification and progression skills for participant injury prevention,
- demonstrate proper alignment and give a variety of cues appropriate for classes that are not beat driven, and
- apply and program music for a class that is not beat driven.

This chapter addresses a major trend in group exercise—that is, classes that are non-beat, and sometimes non-music, driven. In this type of class, the instructor is no longer constrained by having to keep participants on the beat, or by having to ensure that everyone moves together while doing the same choreography at the same time. As such, the instructor does not necessarily have to physically perform all the moves, sets, or repetitions with the class. The instructor typically functions more as a coach, moving around the room, providing encouragement, motivation, and safety cues, and occasionally demonstrating or participating. In coaching-based group exercise, the focus is generally less on the instructor leading the movement experiences and much more on the participant. Evaluate your coaching competency level by using the self-evaluation tool (figure 5.1); this form can help you pinpoint areas where you need improvement.

The *2013 IDEA Fitness Programs and Equipment Trends Report* (2013) found that 89% of facilities offered group strength training, 80% offered core conditioning, 67% offered indoor boot camp classes, 58% offered sport-specific training, 76% offered circuit training, 63% offered body-weight leverage training, 32% offered outdoor boot camp classes, and 32% offered small-group classes on machines. Additionally, 55% offered indoor cycling-based classes, while 44% offered water-fitness classes. In all these modalities, the instructor is less likely to be continuously participating with the participants during the class. Class members are less likely to perform each move synchronized with each other; there is little to no choreography. Sometimes classes are even performed outdoors. In short, a coaching-based class is an altogether different model for group exercise than the traditional, choreography-driven model that requires, among other things, skillful anticipatory cueing on the part of the instructor.

However, a distinction needs to be made between coaching for a sport team and coaching in a group exercise class; when coaching a sport team, a primary focus is on competition, winning, and choosing the best athletes. In group exercise, though, we believe in participation by all, not just those with elite levels of fitness and skill. The primary goal of coaching-based classes is to improve the health-related aspects of fitness and lead purposeful exercise experiences in order to improve the quality of life for participants. It's important to remember that elite athletes and extremely fit individuals make up a very small percentage of the population, and obviously, they are motivated by outcomes such as running a faster race or starting in the next ball game. Athletes will exercise with or without a group exercise instructor. Although

Traditional Versus Coaching-Based Group Exercise

Traditional group exercise	Coaching-based group exercise
Staying on the beat is emphasized	Staying on the beat is not necessary
Music is key	Music may or may not be used
Typically highly choreographed	No choreography
Often dance oriented	No dance moves
Instructor performs all or most moves with class	Instructor demos only occasionally
Anticipatory cueing is essential	No anticipatory cueing is needed
Participants expected to move precisely together	Participants may move individually or together; precision not expected
Instructor unable to give much individual attention	Instructor able to work more one on one with participants
Modalities include step, high-low impact, kickboxing, Zumba, and hip-hop	Modalities include boot camp, water exercise, indoor cycling, trekking, body leverage classes, and sport conditioning

What Is Your Coaching Competency Level?

	Needs work	OK	Excellent
Physical skills			
Ability to provide an appropriate warm-up and cool-down			
Injury prevention and safety			
Risk management			
Ability to give modifications and progressions			
Time management and punctuality			
Ability to educate participants			
Interpersonal communication skills			
Leadership ability			
Team-building skills			
Self-control			
Sense of humor and fun factor			
Genuine interest in all participants			
Ability to learn everyone's name			

FIGURE 5.1 Self-evaluation tool for coaching-based instruction.

some extreme conditioning programs (ECPs) emphasize competition, believing this is the best way to motivate participants, research shows this may not be effective for everyone (Garcia and Avishalom 2009). Read more about ECPs in chapter 1. In fact, in a phenomenon known as the N-effect, more competitors (and competition) may be tied to a lessening of motivation for some participants. Competition apparently has the potential to both enhance and reduce interest (Epstein and Harackiewicz 1992). If winning is the primary focus, intrinsic motivation may be undermined. Competitive programming may discourage the people who need us the most—those who are unfit, sedentary, obese or overweight, and those who've had negative experiences with

exercise or competition in the past. We therefore encourage you to be an inclusive coach, not an exclusive coach, in group exercise leadership.

In a coaching-based class, participants may be performing all moves together (as in stationary indoor cycling), or they may be rotating through stations in small groups (typical of a sport conditioning class). These modalities, and many others, are discussed in later chapters. If you're leading a class with stations, we strongly recommend that you create professional-looking placards to clearly identify what participants will do at each one. Professional-looking, interesting placards help let participants know that you have a plan and a goal for the class. Read more about creating placards in chapter 13.

Motivational Strategies for Coaching-Based Group Exercise

What does a coach do? According to Martens (2012), a coach is in the "positive persuasion" business. A coach is a leader and motivator of others, someone who brings out the best in people. A coach has a vision of what can be and is able to communicate that vision to others. Specifically, a leader, or coach, helps participants develop an "I can" attitude. When you lead a group exercise class, you want to create enthusiasm for whatever goals are being set; you may need to articulate the goals many times (in varying ways) in order to sustain participant motivation. Most people are motivated when things are fun and exciting; they are also motivated when they feel successful. Positive experiences motivate future behavior. A good leader or coach is also a good salesperson who can sell a class on the benefits of fitness, wellness, and self-improvement. Helping participants buy into the benefits in order to work hard enough to get results is the key.

Here's a 5-step plan for leading people (DuBois and Hagen 2007) that may be helpful: (1) Tell participants what you want them to do, (2) show them what good performance looks like, (3) let them do it, (4) observe their performance, and (5) praise their progress or redirect (provide a modification they *can* do well). Remember that since you'll have a wide variety of participants, you'll need a variety of strategies. Different strategies are needed for different people. In general, beginners need much more support and encouragement, whereas those who are already dedicated to exercise may need more of a challenge. An example of the 5-step plan put in action during the warm up for an indoor cycling class is as follows:

1. Tell participants what to do: "Today we'll be performing 'jumps' during the cardio segment. Some of you who might be new to indoor cycling might not know how to perform these."

2. Show them a good jump movement: Demonstrate a jump movement, explaining how it's properly performed.

3. Let them do it: "Now let's all practice this movement together so we don't interrupt our cardio segment."

4. Observe their performance: Walk around the room during this practice session and give individual feedback.

5. Praise their progress or redirect: "Good job everyone; I see many of you performing this correctly. Make sure your buttocks brush your bike seat for good 'jumping' form." You might also point out a participant who has good form to the entire group.

It should be obvious that a primary motivational strategy is to liberally use genuine motivational cues. A motivational cue excites, stimulates, praises, inspires, and creates a sense of fun. An affirmational cue is similar to a motivational cue, except that an affirmational cue specifically mentions something a participant is doing well—in other words, catches the participant doing it right (see "Examples of Motivational or Affirmational Cues").

Creating Dynamic Team Environments

As the leader of a coaching-based class, it's important to build a psychological and social environment that will help all participants work together and feel successful. As a saying goes, "When you smile at life, half the smile is for your face, the other half for someone else's". Helping participants feel successful can be achieved partly by creating a group culture where all members feel accepted and able to contribute. Many people take group exercise classes because they're looking for a sense of belonging and connection with others. You can help foster connection by using participants' names and facilitating introductions. It's also important that you simply pay attention to all participants; studies have shown that respectful attention from a leader promotes group cohesion and motivation (Veach and May, 2005). One way to put this into practice is to notice when a participant is doing well and give a positive affirmation, such as, "Wow, Scott, you are having

Examples of Motivational or Affirmational Cues

- Pick it up, guys!
- You only have (amount of time, e.g., 1 minute) left!
- Finish strong!
- You're almost there!
- This is the hardest part!
- Dig in!
- Crank out this last portion!
- Let's stay in this together!
- We can do this!
- This is it!
- You've got this! I know you do!
- Push it!
- Come on!
- We are strong!
- How bad do you want this?
- It's just 3 minutes out of your day; you can do it!
- I believe in you!

- We are all in this together!
- Focus on the finish!
- Great form, Allison, way to keep your chin up and shoulders back!
- Move those legs quick!
- Make it happen!
- You keep this up, and you're on your way to being healthy and fit!
- Come on, team, stay with me
- Just a little more!
- Every second is a second closer to a better you!
- You're already here—Why not make the best of it?
- Look at the person next to you and give them some encouragement!
- We are unstoppable!
- Show me what you're made of!
- Stay positive!

a GOOD day today! Way to go!" You could even encourage the group to shout, "Way to go, Scott!" Group cohesiveness is enhanced when participants give each other positive feedback. Positivity is powerful; it draws members to your class and increases adherence. And a dynamic team environment is more likely when participants help each other grow and succeed.

Another important aspect of making participants feel like a team is to ask for their input. For example, you could ask for music suggestions or, in some classes (e.g., sport conditioning or boot camp) for their favorite moves, which you can then incorporate into stations or drills. Accepting feedback and incorporating participants' ideas promote the concept that everyone is in this together. In an extensive literature review conducted by Burke and colleagues (2006), multiple team-building strategies were found to increase participant adherence and participation. In addition to the suggestions discussed previously, developing collective group self-efficacy is key. This means promoting a "we can" attitude

in addition to an "I can" attitude in your class members. Gavin (2007) believes coaches need to be experts in communication and change. He suggests they use positive psychology and the power of commitment to challenge participants' self-limiting beliefs, which in turn enables participants to appreciate their strengths. By acquiring coaching skills and changing the nature of your dialogue during class, you can activate participants' capacities for sustainable change. A group exercise class, coached well, can lead to long-term life changes for participants if you take responsibility for the energy and education you give to your class.

Exercise Modification for Injury Prevention

One of the key concepts in a coaching-based class is the idea of individualization. Instead of being labeled as a beginner, intermediate, or advanced class, which may be necessary in a

Motivational Tips

- Greet people as they enter.
- Develop an "I can" attitude for yourself and in others.
- Create enthusiasm.
- Keep class fun and exciting.
- Help participants have positive experiences.
- Smile!
- Be empathetic.
- Mingle with your class.
- Reach out to everyone: Give high fives, fist bumps, handshakes, and so on.
- Use people's names; recognize them.

- Give each participant specific feedback.
- Challenge members to progress beyond their comfort zones (not too much for beginners, though); set challenging but realistic goals.
- Encourage effort, not results.
- Be genuinely interested in all your participants.
- Make each participant feel important; recognize those who seldom get attention.
- Avoid words, actions, or attitudes that could cause negative consequences.

choreography-driven class, a coaching-based class can more easily accommodate all levels. That is, *if* the instructor has the skill to individualize and provide appropriate modifications and progressions for each class participant. In this text we have chosen to use the word *modification*, which implies that an exercise is modified to fit a particular issue, such as back pain, knee pain, or shoulder pain, thus making the exercise safer. Generally, but not always, a modification makes the exercise easier, so the term is sometimes confused with regression. When an exercise is regressed, it becomes easier; when an exercise is progressed, it becomes harder. In 2004 we developed a progressive functional training continuum that visually illustrates the principles of regression and progression (see figure 5.2; Yoke and Kennedy, 2004). We originally assigned 6 levels to the continuum, but, in fact, if you know 70 ways to perform a push-up (or any other exercise), you could organize 70 levels along the con-

tinuum from easiest to hardest. Our continuum can be applied in two ways: (1) to organize all the possible variations of one exercise from easiest to hardest, or (2) to organize all the exercises for a particular muscle group or purpose from easiest to hardest. You can find more information on this exercise continuum in chapter 3.

Being able to move back and forth along the continuum is an essential skill for the coaching-based group exercise instructor. With this skill you can accommodate all participant levels in one class. Of course, doing so requires that you know a large number of exercises and modifications and have a thorough understanding of what makes an exercise easier or harder. Thus, if you see a participant is struggling (or, conversely, is not sufficiently challenged), you can quickly and easily provide a more appropriate variation or exercise. It's important to select exercises that you know you'll be able to readily modify or progress, if necessary.

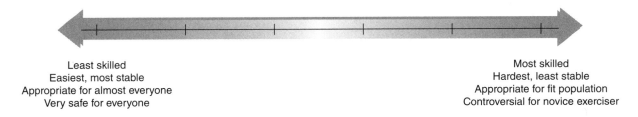

Least skilled
Easiest, most stable
Appropriate for almost everyone
Very safe for everyone

Most skilled
Hardest, least stable
Appropriate for fit population
Controversial for novice exerciser

FIGURE 5.2   The progressive functional training continuum.

As you can see, the exercise continuum helps organize exercises in terms of safety, from low risk to high risk. In order to practice injury prevention and risk management, you'll want to use lower-risk exercises the majority of the time. Look at joint stresses to determine whether an exercise is low risk, high risk, or somewhere in between. For example, a popular boot camp exercise is the burpee, which involves doing a toe touch while squatting, springing back into a plank, doing a push-up, springing forward into a squat, quickly standing up and performing a jumping jack, and rapidly repeating the whole movement from the beginning (see figure 5.3). Is the burpee an exercise that would be easy for all participants to perform? Or is it an exercise that would require a modification to be shown,

in case it's too difficult for some individuals in the class to perform? A burpee can put stress on the wrists, spine, shoulders, knees, and feet. Since the burpee is intended to be performed quickly, momentum and sudden impact forces can increase joint stresses. In addition, for some people, there may be cardiovascular stresses as the heart is suddenly dropped below the head and back up again; for some participants this may create a dangerous situation due to the sudden shifts in blood-flow patterns. The issue here is not whether the burpee exercise is good or bad—it's a question of appropriateness for a class full of participants with varying fitness levels. The burpee is probably appropriate for those participants who do not have any joint pain in their wrists, shoulders, spine, hips, or

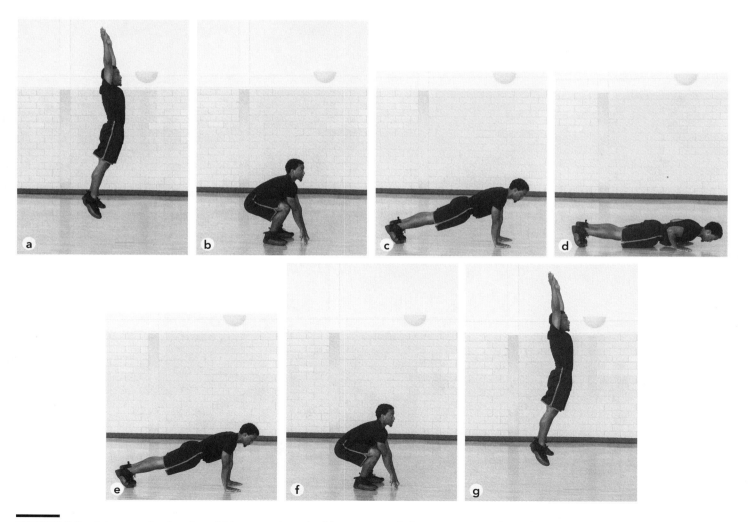

FIGURE 5.3 A burpee, broken into (a) jump and reach, (b) squat, touch floor (c) jump tuck to plank, (d) push-up, eccentric phase (e) push-up, concentric phase (f) jump to squat, (g) jump and reach.

knees and who are familiar with the exercise. If you lead a mixed-level class, it will be important to demonstrate a modification. Be ready to provide modifications and regressions for the burpee as shown in figure 5.4. Reassure less fit participants and those with joint or cardiovascular issues that it's fine for them to go at their own pace (more slowly) and modify as necessary.

Safety is your first priority from a legal and health perspective. Knowing how to modify an exercise for safety and injury prevention, and how to maximize your risk management, is important. Err on the side of caution when selecting exercises and know that violating the principle of progression by doing too much,

too soon, is a major overall cause of injury and dropout in group exercise classes. If the intensity of the exercise is high, the duration is long, or there is too much impact, injuries are more likely. For example, a class that contains several high-intensity moves in a row, such as jumping jacks, full squats, rope jumping, tire slams, and hops across the room on one leg, followed by multiple repeats of the entire sequence, may simply create too much overload for some participants. This type of sequence not only has a predominance of high-intensity moves; it also asks members to perform a high number of repetitions (long duration), and includes mostly high-impact moves. Proper progression means gradually increasing the workload (fre-

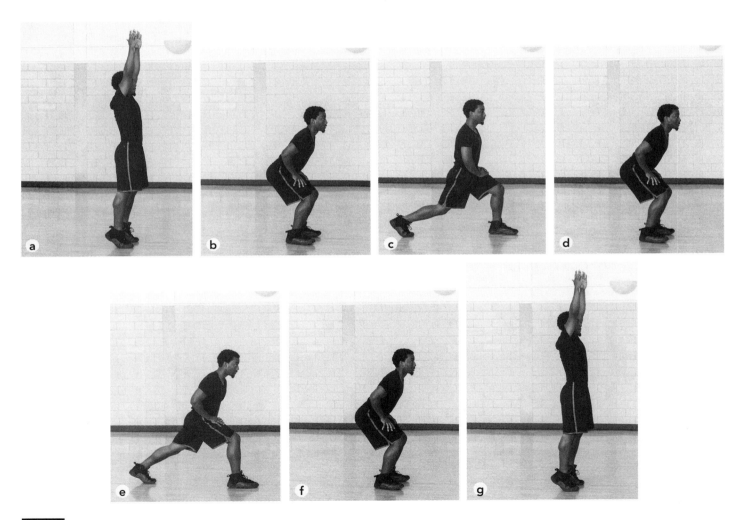

FIGURE 5.4 A modified burpee, (a) start position, reach and lift, (b) modified squat, (c) lunge back with right leg, (d) modified squat, (e) lunge back with left leg, (f) modified squat, and (g) reach and lift.

quency, intensity, duration, or modality), in small enough increments that the body is able to safely adapt and grow stronger, as shown in figure 5.5. Additionally, all instructors need to be familiar with the common mechanisms of injury for major joints; this knowledge allows you to analyze and avoid exercises that put the body in potentially unsafe positions. See "Major Mechanisms of Injury for the Shoulders, Back, and Knees" for a list of common mechanisms of injury.

Demonstrating Proper Alignment and Giving a Variety of Cues

In a coaching-based class, demonstrating the correct performance of the desired move or exercise to participants is key. Even though the instructor generally does not participate as the class continues on to perform all the repetitions, good form by the instructor is important.

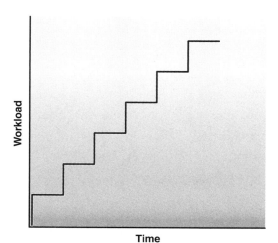

Time
Improper progression—too much, too soon. Injury and drop-out result.

Time
Proper progression—gradual increases in frequency, duration, intensity, or mode. Gradual adaptation occurs.

FIGURE 5.5 Increasing the workload through proper progression.

Major Mechanisms of Injury for the Shoulders, Back, and Knees

Shoulders

- Extreme horizontal shoulder abduction while in external rotation
- Internal rotation while abducting in the frontal plane
- Muscle imbalance between the powerful internal rotators and the weaker external rotators
- Muscle imbalance between the scapular elevators and the scapular depressors
- Uncontrolled eccentric phase in bench presses and flys

Back

- Unsupported spinal flexion
- Unsupported spinal flexion with rotation
- Extreme lumbar hyperextension
- Long-lever traction creating shearing forces (e.g., double straight leg lifts)

Knees

- Hyperflexion (> 90°) while weight bearing
- Torque (twisting)
- Hyperextension

Since a majority of people are primarily visual learners (Knowles, Holton, and Swanson 2011), they need to see a demonstration with optimal alignment and technique in order to perform the exercise well themselves. It is important that you walk the talk, embody excellent posture throughout your class, and use ideal form during all exercise demos. Make sure to demonstrate each exercise or move, including any modifications or variations, at least once for your participants.

What cues are important in a coaching-based class? Since no anticipatory cues are needed (these are discussed in chapter 4), the instructor has more time to deliver other types of cues, which include

- alignment cues,
- safety cues,
- educational and informational cues,
- breath cues,
- motivational and affirmational cues,
- imagery cues,
- visual cues, and
- tactile cues.

These cues are discussed in depth in chapter 8 under "Cueing Muscular Conditioning Exercises" and "Cueing Flexibility Exercises and Ending a Class Appropriately". Skilled instructors constantly challenge themselves to give better cues—cues that participants "get" and can use to make their workouts safer and more effective. You will find that you need a large vocabulary, and you'll need to be able to say the same thing in multiple ways, using different words. For example, imagine you see a participant with his or her shoulder blades elevated while reaching up (see figure 5.6). You might say, "Keep your shoulder blades down" (an alignment cue), but what if the participant doesn't make the correction? Repeat the same cue in a different way. Possible alternatives include these: "Press your shoulder blades down toward your back pockets," "Lower your shoulders away from your ears," "Shrug your shoulder blades down," "Pretend there's a large space between your ears and your shoulders," "Make sure you can see the sides of your neck in the mirror," or "Pretend you're wearing long, dangling earrings, and you don't want them to touch your shoulders" (an

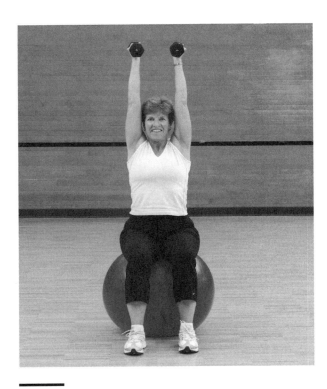

FIGURE 5.6 In order to correct the movement, how would you cue a participant whose shoulder girdle elevates whenever the arms are lifted?

image cue). Or you may want to perform an obvious visual cue, first hiking your own shoulders up and then pressing them all the way down in an exaggerated fashion. With permission from the participant, you may need to do a tactile, or touch, cue: Stand behind the person and gently hold the scapulae down while the participant raises the arms. Be creative! Different cues will work for different participants.

Programming Music in a Class That is Not Beat Driven

Traditional and dance-based group exercise classes such as Zumba require mixed music in which the music tempo is uninterrupted. Music for a coaching-based class, however, can be taken right off an iPod or MP3 player since there is no need to have a consistent, metered music tempo. (Be sure to consider copyright laws, however.) Music can be in the foreground (e.g., participants change from a squat segment to a burpee segment when the music changes) or in the background (music is not consciously acknowledged in any way) and is used to enhance the overall experience of the workout. For example, using the theme song from *Rocky* for cardio intervals can motivate participants to be strong like Sylvester Stallone when he portrayed Rocky. The music on the *Jock Jam* CDs used on ESPN or for introducing sport teams can take participants back to their glory years when they were introduced with their athletic teams.

Music helps you as the instructor by providing motivation beyond your encouragement and instruction. It also can help you time your workout session. For example, if you want to perform 3 minutes of cardio followed by 3 minutes of strength work, you can create a music play list that helps guide your overall plan. Some instructors also have music play lists that include beeps every 30 seconds for intense cardio segments and when a rotation of stations is needed. Using music to help structure the class gives you more time to assist participants with correct movement form. If music is in the foreground, it needs to fit the workout segment in order to help with motivation. For example, a song matched to a muscular conditioning and flexibility segment may be less intense with less bass so that participants are able to hear the specific instructions for the exercises. Some segments, such as a relay race or competition, may even be better without music so that participants can interact with one another. Matching music to workout segments can be a challenge for the instructor. Poll your participants and see what music they prefer, or even ask them to bring in motivating music they would like to hear while exercising. With a coaching-based class almost any music will work, so you have an ideal opportunity to ask for and use participant input and music suggestions.

Chapter Wrap-Up

A coaching-based class requires slightly different skills than a traditional group exercise class led to music. Instructors participate and exercise less themselves and instead put more focus on individualizing and personalizing participants' workouts; this is somewhat similar to a group personal training session. Mingling and interacting with as many class members as possible is emphasized. The coaching-based instructor has excellent motivational skills and creates a team-oriented environment where all participants feel acknowledged and able to contribute. Keeping participants safe is key, so giving appropriate modifications, regressions, and progressions, as well as a large variety of safety, alignment, educational, and motivational cues, is essential. In this group exercise paradigm, music is optional, but when skillfully used to motivate and enhance participant experience, it can help create positive change for participants. Learning to teach this type of class will broaden the impact you can have on the health and wellness of all participants.

ASSIGNMENTS

1. Describe how you would regress (make easier) each of the following:

   - Bear crawl
   - Bottom-out squat
   - Power clean
   - One-legged hop across the gym
   - Traveling (walking) front lunges
   - TRX push-ups
   - Tire throws

2. Look online for another example of a challenging or level-6 exercise from the progression model. Describe the exercise and write how you would regress the exercise for a novice, deconditioned participant.

Part II

Primary Components of Group Exercise

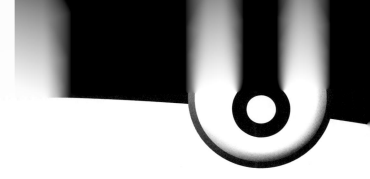

Warm-Up and Cool-Down

Chapter Objectives

By the end of this chapter, you will be able to

- formulate a preclass introduction,
- design a warm-up segment,
- create rehearsal moves for a warm-up,
- evaluate the timing of stretching in a group exercise class, and
- create and present a cool-down segment.

Group Exercise Class Evaluation Form Essentials

Key Points for Preclass Segment

- Knows participants and orients new participants
- Has equipment and music (if using) ready for use

- Introduces self and states class format
- Acknowledges class
- Creates positive atmosphere
- Wears appropriate attire and footwear

Key Points for Warm-Up

- Includes appropriate amount of dynamic movement
- Provides rehearsal moves
- Provides dynamic or static stretches for at least two major muscle groups

- Provides intensity guidelines for warm-up
- Includes clear cues and verbal directions
- Uses movements at an appropriate tempo and intensity

Key Points for Cool-down, Stretch, and Relaxation Segment

- Includes static stretching for major muscles worked and for commonly tight muscles (hip flexors, hamstrings, calves, erector spinae, pectorals, anterior deltoids, upper trapezius)
- Demonstrates using proper alignment and technique;
- Observes participants' form and offers

modifications, regressions, progressions, or alternatives
- Provides alignment cues: includes many cues for all stretches
- Appropriately emphasizes relaxation or visualization
- Ends class on a positive note and thanks class

An effective group exercise class starts with appropriate preclass preparation. In chapter 3 we discussed the importance of preclass preparation for setting the atmosphere of the overall class. We recommended that group exercise instructors arrive at least 15 minutes before a class starts in order to prepare equipment and set up the music system and microphone. After completing setup procedures, the next focus is on building class cohesion, which was discussed in Ch. 2. We recommend greeting participants as they arrive and letting them know what equipment they'll need. Some instructors use a white board where the class format and class equipment can be listed; if used, this board should be in a visible place for participants to see as they enter the class. Other instructors lay out their own equipment in a noticeable spot and ask participants to find the equipment they'll need based on what they see. In chapter 2 we also discussed the importance of getting to know your participants so you can design the class to improve their health and well-being. Knowing by name your returning participants and orienting new participants is

important for creating a positive atmosphere. Beginning class on time with equipment ready for use is also important. These two points in combination help establish a professional atmosphere. And, in chapters 2 and 3, we discussed many aspects of being a model instructor, from wearing appropriate attire to creating a healthy emotional environment.

An important part of the preclass preparation phase is to acknowledge your class by briefly describing the class format and reviewing what participants can expect during their workout. For example, you might say, "Hello, my name is Kayla, and I'm excited to be your instructor today in this 45 minute core–strength class. There will not be a cardio segment to this class; we will be focusing on strength and flexibility exercises. I hope you can also find the time to include some cardio exercises in your day so you get the benefits of all the health-related components of fitness." Every class needs an introduction by the instructor even if all participants are aware of the class format.

After the preclass period, the first concern for instructors is the warm-up. A warm-up has several important functions, including producing mental and physiological neuromotor changes to help get the body ready for a workout. In this chapter we will discuss how to design a warm-up that is evidence-based and gets your class off to a good start. We will also discuss when during a class to incorporate stretching and rehearsal moves and how to create a cool-down for the end of class. See the "Group Exercise Class Evaluation Form Essentials," which overviews the important points for the preclass, warm-up, and cool-down segments of a group exercise class. You will be using the Group Exercise Class Evaluation Form (see appendix A) to evaluate a class, as well as to make sure you're incorporating these important segments in your own class. Most group exercise formats involve some form of preclass period, a warm-up, and a cool-down segment.

Designing a Warm-Up

A warm-up typically begins by setting the atmosphere with engaging music and energy. If you are using music, the first song sets the tone for your class and gets people ready to begin moving. During the first portion of the warm-up, create movements that are dynamic and use large muscle groups. The second portion builds on the first and combines warming up and stretching if appropriate. A class tends to flow better if the second portion is upbeat and if stretching (when used) is performed in a standing position so that the class can move right into the cardiorespiratory segment.

Energetic music can be one of the keys to a successful and fun warm-up. Using music with a tempo of 120 to 136 beats per minute and positive lyrics is recommended for most group exercise classes and is essential in traditional modalities such as step, high-low, or dance-based classes. Songs that motivate and inspire, such as the theme to *Rocky* or fun instrumental music by Avicii that is used when introducing players at the start of a basketball game, bring energy to the room and create a dynamic, interactive aspect in a group exercise class. In essence, the music selection sets the stage as much as the movement selection does. For music resources, see chapter 4.

Goals of a Warm-Up

The warm-up prepares the body for the more rigorous demands of the cardiorespiratory and muscular strength and conditioning segments; one way it does so is by raising the body's internal temperature. For each degree of temperature elevation, the metabolic rate of cells increases about 13% (Astrand and Rodahl 1977). In addition, at higher body temperatures, blood flow to the working muscles increases, as does the release of oxygen to the muscles. Because these effects allow more efficient energy production to fuel muscle contraction, the goal of an effective warm-up is to elevate internal temperatures by 1 or 2 degrees Fahrenheit ($0.5°$-$1°C$). You may notice that sweating results. Increasing body temperature has other effects that are beneficial for exercisers; see the section, "Physiological Benefits of Warming Up." Many of these physiological effects may reduce the risk of injury because they have the potential to increase neuromuscular coordination, delay fatigue, and make the tissues less susceptible to damage (Alter 2004). According to Neiman (2010), a warm-up will enhance the activity of enzymes in the working muscle, reduce the viscosity of muscle, improve the mechanical efficiency and power of the moving muscles, facilitate the transmission speed of nervous impulses augmenting coordination, increase muscle blood flow and thus improve delivery of necessary fuel substrates, increase the level of free fatty acids in the blood, help prevent injuries to the muscles and various supporting connective tissues, and allow the heart muscle to adequately prepare itself for aerobic exercise.

There was much confusion in the stretching literature due to a misinterpretation of research on warming up. For years a group exercise session began with static stretching exercise followed by dynamic movements. We now know that dynamic movements are essential for the warm-up period before performing any stretching exercises. Herbert, deNoronha, and Kamper (2011) found that warming up by itself has no effect on range of motion (ROM), but that when warming up is followed by stretching, ROM increases. Many people interpreted this finding to mean that stretching before exercise prevents injuries, even though the clinical research is inconclusive on this issue. McHugh and Cosgrave (2010) state that stretching

Physiological Benefits of Warming Up

The physiological benefits of warming up are as follows:

- Increased metabolic rate
- Higher rate of oxygen exchange between blood and muscles
- More oxygen released within muscles
- Faster nerve impulse transmission
- Gradual redistribution of blood flow to working muscles
- Decreased muscle relaxation time after contraction
- Increased speed and force of muscle contraction
- Increased muscle elasticity
- Increased flexibility of tendons and ligaments
- Gradual increase in energy production, which limits lactic acid buildup
- Reduced risk of abnormal electrocardiogram
- Joint lubrication

does not reduce the risk of sustaining injuries, but it does reduce the risk of muscle strain. Much of the stretching research has been performed on athletes and is related to sport performance. However, the 2014 American Council on Sports Medicine (ACSM) guidelines for exercise prescription remind us that flexibility exercises are most effective when the muscles are warm, so it is safe to say that group exercise participants should warm up before stretching to gain the benefits of stretching. A thorough overview of stretching principles, guidelines, and exercises is provided in chapter 8; the section "Evaluating Stretching in the Warm-Up" later in this chapter discusses the factors involved in deciding when to include stretching in a group exercise class. What we do know is that warming up may prevent injury, whereas stretching apparently has little or no effect on injury prevention. Therefore, the focus during the warm-up needs to be on dynamic movements that increase core body temperature (see figure 6.1).

Focusing on Dynamic Movement

Most warm-up segments of group exercise classes last 5 to 10 minutes. The sport literature recommends that the majority of this time be spent on warming up rather than stretching. What would dynamic movements look like in a group exercise setting? Examples include walk-ing while performing arm circles to warm up the legs and shoulders and then walking on toes and heels to warm up the calves and shins. Another example might be shuffling sideways to warm up the abductor and adductor muscles or walking while circling the hip joints to loosen up the gluteal muscles. Dynamic movement performed at a lower intensity and impact is the preferred mechanism of getting the body ready for work. Dynamic movement is especially important if participants are coming from sedentary jobs or from sitting in their cars.

Remember that the diaphragm, the major muscle involved in breathing, is like any other muscle group and needs time to shift gears. A rapid increase in breathing that doesn't give the diaphragm enough time to warm up properly can result in side aches and hyperventilation (rapid, shallow breathing). Sudden increases in breathing mean that the transition into the cardiorespiratory segment was not gradual enough. Incorporating a few deep breaths into the dynamic warm-up will assist in warming up the diaphragm.

Incorporating Rehearsal Moves

Rehearsal moves make up the majority of the warm-up, preparing participants for the challenges of the workout to come (Anderson 2000). Blahnik and Anderson (1996) defined rehearsal

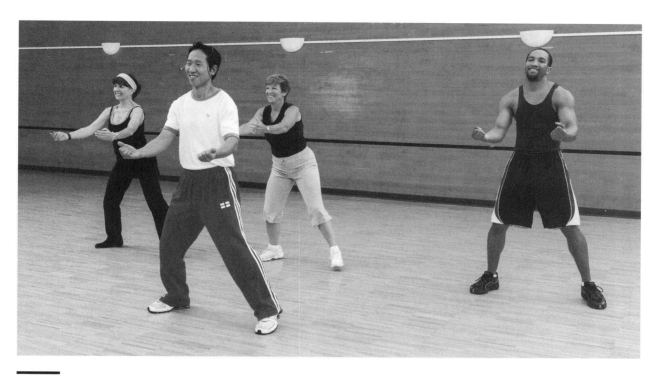

FIGURE 6.1 According to research, the warm-up segment focus is on dynamic movements that increase core body temperature.

moves as "movements that are identical to, but less intense than, the movements your students will execute during the workout phase" (1996, p. 50) For examples of rehearsal moves, see "Rehearsal Move Suggestions for Various Group Exercise Formats." Appel (2007) feels that the right rehearsal move warms up participants mentally as well as physically. She encourages instructors to focus on dynamic flexibility rather than static stretching and to emphasize exercises that improve balance, coordination, postural control, and joint stability. With the 2014 ACSM guidelines' inclusion of neuromotor movements as a component of fitness, balance and

Rehearsal Move Suggestions for Various Group Exercise Formats

These suggested movements preview actions that will be used in the cardio segment after the warm-up.

- Boot camp: Use slow side shuffles, partial squats.
- Sport conditioning: Use the ladders and walk through, walk around cones.
- Step: Use the bench during the warm-up.
- Stationary indoor cycling: Teach participants how to climb a hill properly.
- Water exercise: Practice an interval segment (30 seconds rest, 30 seconds work) using a cross-country skier movement.
- Muscle conditioning: Use muscle-specific movements, including biceps curls, triceps kick-backs, and squats.
- Kickboxing: Use shuffles, kicks, and punches.
- High-low impact class: Review a 32-count series.

proprioceptive moves, such as standing alternating hip abduction, also belong in the warm-up.

The concept of using rehearsal moves in the warm-up relates to the principle of specificity of training. This principle states that the body adapts specifically to whatever demands are placed on it. We know that specificity applies not only to energy systems and muscle groups but also to movement patterns. Because the motor units used during training demonstrate the majority of physiological alterations, movement patterns must be specifically trained. In a group exercise class, one of the main reasons participants become frustrated is that they are not able to perform the movements effectively. Introducing movement patterns in the warm-up helps wake up associated motor units and ensure that participants perform those patterns with success later on in the workout.

Using rehearsal moves in the warm-up not only specifically prepares the body for the movement ahead but also helps groove neuromuscular patterns by introducing new skills. For example, a carioca-type movement (referred to as a grapevine in a traditional high-low or step class) might be broken down into a walk, cueing "walk, step front, walk, step back" (while traveling to the side). This move could be introduced slowly in the warm-up, preparing the body to perform it quickly later on. If groundwork is laid during the warm-up, when a carioca (grapevine) is referred to in the cardiorespiratory segment, class participants will know what to do. The same idea applies to complex choreography movements in a Zumba or Jazzercise class. The movement combination can be practiced slowly in the warm-up, when maintaining a higher level of intensity is not the focus. When this movement comes up later in the cardio portion, it will have been rehearsed, and this will make it easier for participants to maintain their intensity level. Rehearsal moves, specific to the class format, are what make up a large part of the warm-up.

 See online video 6.1 for an example warm-up for a high-low impact group exercise class.

 See online video 6.2 for a sample step warm-up. Note that this warm-up is also outlined in appendix F.

The warm-up for a sport conditioning or a boot camp class, much like that of any other group exercise format, involves activities that will be used in the cardiorespiratory segments. A typical coaching-based class uses a different style warm-up than what you might see in a more dance-based class. Its warm-up is more like what you would do if you were warming up to play tennis, soccer, volleyball, or other sport activities. This type of warm-up typically includes general calisthenics performed at a lower intensity than in the workout stimulus. A coaching-based warm-up can be performed in an open or circle format, much like what you may have experienced in your physical education classes. A sport conditioning warm-up segment might involve the following movements:

- Walking in a circle on the toes to warm up the calves
- High-knee walks to warm up the quadriceps and hip flexors
- High-knee walks with hip rotation to warm up the abductor and adductor muscles
- Heel kicks to the seat to warm up the hamstrings while walking or jogging
- Large shoulder circles while walking to warm up the shoulder joint
- Lateral movements such as a grapevine (carioca) to enhance coordination
- Rehearsal moves such as a brief walk or jog around cones to increase lateral movement and balance, which will both be challenged at a higher intensity during the conditioning segment.

 See online video 6.3 for an example of a warm-up for a sport conditioning or boot camp class.

Evaluating Stretching in the Warm-Up

Whether to stretch during the warm-up is a debated issue, one on which the literature has not yet agreed. There are two exercise goals involved in this debate—that of creating a warm-up that reduces the risk of injury and that of improving flexibility, an important component of fitness.

Taylor and colleagues (1990) found that flexibility gains were most significant when a stretch was held for 12 to 18 seconds and repeated 4 times per muscle group. Another study (Walter, Figoni, and Andres 1995) found that stretching the hamstrings for 30 seconds produced significantly greater flexibility than stretching for 10 seconds. If these two studies were the complete story, we would probably recommend not stretching in a group exercise warm-up because it is impossible to stretch a muscle group 4 times and hold each stretch for 30 seconds and still accomplish the goals of increasing heart rate and core temperature. Another study (Girouard and Hurley 1995) on strength and flexibility training in older adults found that stretching before and after training did not increase flexibility. Convincing research on runners (Lally 1994; Shrier 1999; Van Mechelen et al. 1993) demonstrated that static stretches performed during the warm-up did not prevent injury. These studies encouraged injury prevention through dynamic warm-up rather than stretching.

The 2011 ACSM position stand (Garber et al. 2011) on exercise addresses flexibility, recommending that each major muscle group be stretched a total of 60 seconds per exercise on more than 2 days per week with 5 to 7 days being ideal. The ACSM position stand was based on a review of many research studies on stretching. It is generally agreed that flexibility exercises are beneficial, but questions remain about where to put them in the class format for group exercise. New research suggests that stretching doesn't prevent muscle soreness after exercise. In a systemic review and meta-analysis of 10 previously published studies on stretching, Herbert, deNoronha, and Kamper (2011) concluded that stretching before exercise doesn't prevent postexercise muscle soreness. They found little support for the theory that stretching immediately before exercise can prevent either overuse or acute injuries. Meroni and colleagues (2010) compared hamstring active stretching with static stretching and concluded that active stretching was more time efficient and needed a lower compliance to produce effects on flexibility.

Most prominent exercise physiology textbooks (McArdle, Katch, and Katch 2009; Howley and Thompson 2012; Kenney, Wilmore, and Costill 2011) and stretching books (Anderson and Anderson 2010) recommend an active warm-up that includes rehearsal moves followed by brief stretching; these books recommend that most flexibility work be done during the cool-down segment of the workout. However, these books are written with the individual, and often the athlete in mind, and they are not necessarily specific to working with a group. Generally, these sources also include some stretching within the warm-up, and they all advocate that a warm-up precede any stretching so that muscles experience the benefits of warm-up before they are stretched. Thacker and colleagues (2004) determined there is not sufficient evidence to endorse or discontinue routine stretching before or after exercise to prevent injury among competitive or recreational athletes.

Static stretching exercises have been a common part of the warm-up routine for athletes and group exercise instructors. However, static stretching appears to decrease muscle-force production capacity. For instance, static stretching before competition has been shown to decrease leg press 1 repetition maximal (1RM) tests (Bacurau et al. 2009), 20-meter sprint performance (Nelson et al. 2005), and knee-extensor concentric torque (Cramer et al. 2005). In addition, Fowles, Sale, and MacDougall (2000) reported a residual effect in which maximal plantar flexion torque remained depressed even 60 minutes after the stretching routine. Finally, McHugh and Cosgrave (2010) determined in a meta-analysis of stretching articles that an acute bout of stretching will decrease the ability to generate a maximal force in the muscle. In essence, these decrements in performance may be attributed to greater stress relaxation of the muscle tissue, which leads to lower muscle-tendon stiffness and strength (Kubo, Kanehisa, and Fukunaga 2001, 2002). These effects are extremely important to athletes, but for the average exerciser, it appears that an active warm up is the best way to begin a group exercise session with the focus on enhancing flexibility through stretching being performed at a time that meets the needs of the individual participant. Are you beginning to see that the issue to stretch or not stretch in the warm up segment of a group exercise class is not an easy question to answer?

Studies do support the finding that ROM can be increased by a single 15- to 30-second stretch for each muscle group per day. However, some people require a longer duration or more repetitions to increase their flexibility. Research also supports the idea that the optimal duration and frequency for stretching may vary by muscle group (Witvrouv et al. 2004). The long-term effects of stretching on ROM show that after 6 weeks, people who stretched for 30 seconds per muscle each day increased their ROM much more than those who stretched for 15 seconds per muscle each day. No additional increase was seen in the group that stretched for 60 seconds per muscle per day (Shrier and Gossal 2000). Overall, we support the ACSM guidelines for flexibility that recommend 60-second stretches at least 2 times per week (and ideally 5-7 times per week) as part of general conditioning to improve range of motion. See chapter 8 for specific stretching movements for all the major muscle groups.

Different forms of stretching, such as proprioceptive neuromuscular facilitation (PNF), have been touted as creating greater increases in ROM compared with static or active stretching. However, PNF stretching is usually not appropriate for a group exercise setting since it requires detailed explanation and lots of individual attention to participants. Static stretches are easier to perform than PNF stretches and appear to have good results. However, using seated static stretches, held for 30 seconds or more, in the warm-up is not recommended since doing so disrupts the flow of the group exercise class. We recommend brief lengthening of the muscles in the warm-up by holding stretches for 5 to 10 seconds in a standing position to increase ROM for the activity to come. Most experts believe that ballistic stretching, or bouncing while stretching, is dangerous because the muscle may reflexively contract, triggering the myotatic stretch reflex and potentially leading to injury.

In addition to improving ROM, static stretching can be extremely relaxing. One of the biggest benefits of stretching may be something that research just can't quantify: It feels good. Given that there is no conclusive evidence showing any inherent benefit to stretching during the warm-up and that there are a few studies suggesting that it might be dangerous, our overall recommendation is that the warm-up contain mostly dynamic movements with the possibility of some light preparatory static stretches held briefly (5-10 seconds), particularly if this is the only place flexibility is included in the format. Prolonged, deeper stretches that meet the ACSM guidelines of static stretching for 60 seconds or more would be performed at the end of the group exercise experience, where seated stretches fit better into the class format. It's important to include stretching somewhere in your class format, depending on the class structure.

When you are designing the warm-up segment for your group exercise class, it's best to focus on rehearsal movements. If you are including light preparatory stretches, such as the one shown in figure 6.2, try to focus on active movement as well as stretching. For example, while performing a standing calf or hamstring stretch, keep the arms moving up and down to stay warm (see figure 6.2). Likewise, when you are designing a warm-up for a stationary indoor cycling class, keep the legs pedaling while performing upper-body stretches.

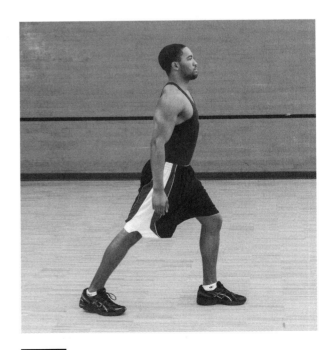

FIGURE 6.2 Standing calf stretch appropriate for warm-up and cool-down.

If you are teaching a 30-minute class, it may be better to save the stretching for the end, when it will be most beneficial for enhancing flexibility. In a short class, we recommend light preparatory stretching in the beginning. On the other hand, when you are teaching a group of seniors, you might find that they prefer performing several minutes of static stretching at the end of their warm-up and before the actual workout. After they have warmed up, they can hold a stretch for increased flexibility and balance. By the end of the class, fatigue may prevent them from performing static stretches appropriately.

Only instructors who know their participants well will know which warm-up format fits best. We know that flexibility is a health-related component of fitness and should be included in the overall workout; warming up and performing rehearsal moves before performing any static stretching are important no matter what group exercise format is being taught. We also know that flexibility is enhanced best at the end of class. Therefore, save the stretching for the end of the workout for optimum health benefits to your participants.

Designing a Cool-Down

The first 5 minutes and the last 5 minutes of class can make or break the experience for your participants. We review specific stretches appropriate for the final cool-down, as well as additional information on the end of the class, in chapter 8. During your class, participants have been working hard increasing the blood flow of nutrients and oxygen to their exercising muscles. Most likely, they feel less stiff and less tense than when they started class. As each minute of the class has progressed, you hope they've let go of anxieties, worries, and stressors of the day. While the music was playing, their brains probably switched from logical and calculating functions and began operating with spontaneity and fluid thought. The hardest part of coming to your class was getting there, and now they have come to the end of the workout. The mindset is typically quite different than it was at the beginning of class. They have taken the time to care for themselves. They have taken another step toward healthier living. Now is the time for you to help your participants complete their journey. Take the last 5 minutes of class to let participants experience a few moments of increased relaxation, or to reenergize before returning to their duties and commitments. These relaxation moments can be structured or free flowing, philosophical or quiet.

Silence or quiet, calming music (90 beats per minute or under) might be enough. Storytelling, guided imagery, or creative visualization might help deepen their relaxation as you describe quiet forests, gentle breezes, a warm fire, or a cozy room. Starbursts, bright, intense sunlight, the power of a wave or waterfall might suggest the energy necessary for continuing on with the day's activities. Partner massage or group stories, deep breathing, or progressively tightening and releasing muscle groups may help your participants find that any remaining tensions, areas of pain, or resistance to change melt away. While your audience is receptive, you might use the time to compliment them on their hard work and reinforce their positive lifestyles, or help them perform a mental exercise to increase their self-esteem and personal power. You might read inspirational quotations or poetry, or make announcements about upcoming events. Use the last few minutes to end the exercise experience on a positive note; allow participants to take their encounter and remember that the true power of the experience of exercise lies within.

Chapter Wrap-Up

This chapter outlined the variables that are common to the preclass, warm-up, and cool-down segments of group exercise classes; these variables are listed on the Group Exercise Class Evaluation Form in appendix A. Whether you are teaching a cycling, boot camp, step, or kickboxing class, including an appropriate amount of dynamic movement, providing rehearsal moves, stretching major muscle groups in a biomechanically sound manner, and ending with a relaxation and static stretching segment are important.

ASSIGNMENTS

1. Attend a group exercise class in a format of your choice. Using the Group Exercise Class Evaluation Form, evaluate the instructor's preclass, warm-up, and cool-down segments of the class. Record your observations on the form.

2. In outline form create a detailed warm-up segment for a class that has a cardio component (for 4 or 5 participants) that integrates the concepts discussed in this chapter. Prepare to present your warm-up segment to a group.

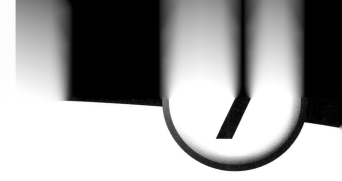

Cardiorespiratory Training

Chapter Objectives

By the end of this chapter, you will be able to

- understand cardiorespiratory training systems specific to group exercise,
- investigate appropriate intensity levels,
- formulate movement options and verbal cues for the cardiorespiratory segment,
- demonstrate methods of intensity monitoring,
- understand the principles of muscle balance in cardiorespiratory programming,
- address safety issues as well as proper alignment and technique for cardiorespiratory classes,
- understand the importance of participant interaction,
- demonstrate how to gradually reduce impact and intensity during the cardio cool-down segment, and
- understand the importance of having an automated external defibrillator (AED) on site.

Group Exercise Class Evaluation Form Essentials

Key Points for the Conditioning Segment

- Gradually increases intensity
- Uses a variety of muscle groups
- Minimizes repetitive movements
- Observes participants' form and provides constructive, nonintimidating feedback
- Continually offers modifications, regressions, progressions, or alternatives
- Provides alignment and technique cues
- Gives motivational cues

- Educates participants about intensity; provides HR (heart rate) or RPE (rating of perceived exertion) check 1 or 2 times during the workout stimulus
- Promotes participant interaction and encourages fun
- Provides regular demonstrations and participation with good body mechanics
- Uses appropriate movement or music tempo

A few common principles apply to the cardiorespiratory segment of group exercise classes. These principles are listed in the conditioning segment of the Group Exercise Class Evaluation Form (appendix A) and repeated in "Group Exercise Class Evaluation Form Essentials." Including regression and progression options, determining the format for the conditioning segment (i.e., interval or steady state), and having fun remain essential components of this segment of the workout. During the cardiorespiratory segment of a group exercise class, you will need to monitor exercise intensity, thus requiring participants to "check in" with how they are feeling so that they enjoy the exercise stimulus. Important details for learning and teaching these techniques are discussed in this chapter.

Cardiorespiratory Training Systems

The major training systems used in cardio classes are continuous training (also known as *steady-state training*); interval training, which may be timed or sporadic; interval training using different cardio modalities (usually timed); and interval cardiorespiratory and strength training (sometimes known as *supercircuit training*).

In continuous, or steady-state, training, movement techniques are used to produce one long, continuous endurance workout with few intensity variations. Generally, during steady-state cardiorespiratory exercise, the overall physiological effect is steady; participants are encouraged to monitor their exercise intensity without major fluctuations (see figure 7.1).

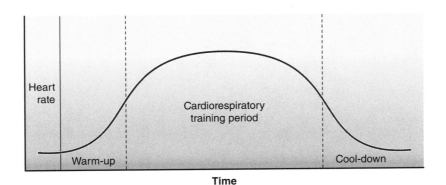

FIGURE 7.1   Steady-state training.

In interval training, intensity levels fluctuate between high, low, and moderate. The instructor provides high-intensity moves or short, intense drills for an anaerobic (power) interval. During this interval, which may last for 15, 20, 30, or 60 seconds, participants are encouraged to challenge themselves, perhaps pushing into the top range of their target heart rate zone (or even beyond, for advanced participants). Patterns used during the intervals may include plyometric, sprinting, or power moves. The cardiorespiratory conditioning segment can be organized into regular timed intervals (e.g., a 4-minute song with a moderate-intensity combination followed by a 1-minute power interval, with this sequence repeated 5 times), or the intervals can be interspersed randomly throughout the cardio portion of the class.

Interval training with varying cardiorespiratory modalities is a great way to incorporate cross-training and alleviate boredom. It is also more appropriate for beginners than HIIT (Tabata) workouts. A typical format might involve 4 minutes of general cardio movements, such as modified jumping jacks or knee lifts, followed by 4 minutes of hopping up on the step (alternating legs), and repeated with other combinations of cardio or power moves for 32 minutes. Modalities to consider for interval training include kickboxing, boot camp, sport conditioning, and jumping rope (see chapter 13).

Another popular system is to alternate timed intervals of cardiorespiratory training with strength training. For example, you might lead the class in 4 minutes of cardio, 4 minutes of squats and lunges, 4 minutes of cardio, and 4 minutes of triceps and deltoid exercises. Regardless of which type of cardiorespiratory training is selected, Foster and Porcari (2010) suggest that the higher-intensity elements take place fairly

High-Intensity Interval Training

High intensity interval training (HIIT) has become popular; another buzzword for this type of program is metabolic training. A well-known version of HIIT was developed in Japan by Izumi Tabata. He conducted tests on two groups of athletes, comparing training that was of moderate-to-high intensity with high-intensity interval training. Tabata found that the athletes who used high-intensity interval methods improved both their aerobic and anaerobic cardiorespiratory systems. However, the athletes who performed the training methods that were moderate-to-high intensity predominantly improved the aerobic cardiorespiratory system with little to no increase in the anaerobic system. Hence, Tabata designed a program that promoted changes in both aerobic and anaerobic cardiorespiratory pathways. A sample Tabata workout generally involves 20 seconds of all-out, near-maximal effort followed by 10 seconds of recovery. This pattern is typically repeated 8 times.

HIIT training, although time efficient (participants can get in a 30-minute workout with this type of training equivalent to a 60-minute steady-state workout), is not for the beginner. Tharrett and Peterson (2012) write in their fitness management textbook that in the past 10 to 15 years, the health club industry has served only 12% to 14% of the U.S. population. HIIT training is for participants who are already quite active (the 12%-14%), and who have progressed to a level of fitness where they can train at a high intensity without as much risk of injury or dropout. A beginner, on the other hand, needs to be cautious when working out in HIIT-type programs. Muscle fatigue and soreness are much more common with high-intensity training, particularly in the beginning. Interval-style training has been a training option since intentional exercise came on the scene in the 1970s. It has been proven in the literature to be an effective way to improve cardiorespiratory fitness. However, we often see fit instructors promoting HIIT programs to challenge participants who are not yet at an appropriate level of fitness. It's key to consider the principle of progression and gradually create overload for participants. Too much, too soon is the major cause of injury and dropout.

early in the conditioning phase, and that the conditioning phase conclude with more steady-state exercise, even if the intensity is still in the range likely to serve as a stimulus.

Beginning Intensity

Even though the human body adapts efficiently to exercise, gradually increasing intensity at the beginning of an exercise session is necessary for many reasons:

- Blood flow is redistributed from internal organs to the working muscles.
- The heart muscle gradually adapts to the change from a resting level to a working level.
- The respiratory rate gradually increases.

The most dangerous times for changes in the heart's rhythm are in the transitions from resting to high-intensity work and from high-intensity activity back to resting. At rest, the cardiorespiratory system circulates about 1.3 gallons (5 L) of blood per minute. Imagine the contents of 2 and a half 2-liter water bottles circulating through your body every minute. At maximal strenuous exercise, as much as 6.6 gallons (25 L) per minute must circulate to accommodate working muscles in a fit person—that's 12 and a half 2-liter water bottles per minute! Going from rest to strenuous exercise takes time and requires a gradual increase in intensity during the cardio segment. If your participants are out of breath in the first few minutes of the cardio session, you have not allowed enough time for the redistribution of blood flow to occur. Use verbal cues such as "Keep your arms low!" You can also begin with, "We are just starting out, so let's give our bodies time to adapt to this new level of intensity."

To gradually increase intensity within a group exercise setting, start with moves that use small ranges of motion (ROM), a short lever length, and limited traveling. Keep moves less intense by not using jumping or propulsion moves at the beginning of class. In a water exercise class, use moves that have a smaller ROM or shorter lever length as well. Finally, in a stationary indoor cycling class, make sure participants keep the flywheel tension set at a lower resistance for the first few minutes of cardio training.

Appropriate Intensity Levels

No matter what type of class you're leading, it is impossible to be everywhere at once or help everyone simultaneously. Each participant is working at a different intensity level and has different goals. Ideally, all classes would be organized according to a given intensity and duration. The reality is that many participants come to a class because the time is convenient and not necessarily because the class length or intensity level is suitable. If participants try to exercise at the instructor's level or at another participant's level, they may work too hard and sustain injuries, or they may work too little and not meet their goals. A few ways to promote self-responsibility are to encourage participants to work at their own pace, teach them how to make the moves harder or easier, demonstrate HR monitoring or RPE checks, and use common examples to inform participants how they should feel. For example, during the peak portion of the cardiorespiratory segment, ask participants if they feel out of breath but are still able to talk. During the cool-down after the cardio segment, ask them if they can feel their HR slowing down. Be as descriptive as possible concerning perceived exertion. Demonstrate high-, medium-, and low-intensity and impact options in order to reach participants at various levels. Pointing out participants who work at higher or lower levels while you yourself demonstrate several intensity levels can also help. The main ways to increase intensity are these:

- Increase the ROM.
- Increase the lever length.
- Use multiple muscles and joints.
- Increase traveling and locomotor movements.
- Increase vertical displacement, either by adding jumping and propulsion or by bending and straightening the knees and hips more (emphasis is on DOWN-up, rather than UP-down).
- Increase the speed of movement.

- Increase the weight that is being moved.

To decrease intensity, teach participants to simply do the opposite.

 See online video 7.1 for an example of appropriate conditioning intensity options and effective verbal cueing.

Help participants achieve the level of effort they need to reach and continually remind them that reaching this point is their responsibility. It is not your job to be responsible for participants' exercise intensity, but it is your job to present movement options of varying intensity so participants can understand the importance of making good intensity choices for themselves. Instructing a class at your own intensity level will not allow for examples of intensity options. We recommend you maintain a medium intensity most of the time and present other options and intensities as needed. A practical example of this is to demonstrate a modified jumping jack using a heel dig right and left, while encouraging those who want more intensity and impact to perform a regular jumping jack. For those who want even more impact or a higher intensity, you can suggest a power squat or even a fly jack.

(See figure 7.2.) Being able to teach several levels and abilities is the true art of group exercise instruction and the reason why group exercise can be more difficult to lead than one-on-one instruction.

It is also important to monitor intensity and present intensity options during interval training. This approach may be slightly different than for steady-state training. Interval training involves varying the exercise intensity at fixed intervals during a single exercise period. The duration and intensity of the intervals can be varied depending on the goals of the training session and physical fitness level of the client. For example you can work hard for 1 minute and rest for 1 minute or work hard for 30 seconds and rest for 30 seconds. Some instructors use a progressive model of interval training. This would involve engaging in 20 seconds of work followed by 20 seconds of rest, then progressing to 30 seconds of work and 20 seconds of rest followed by 45 seconds of work and 20 seconds of rest. Whatever timed series you decide on, it's important to let the participants know the options ahead of time so they can plan their own intensity output. There is no hard and fast way to perform interval training for a group. Interval

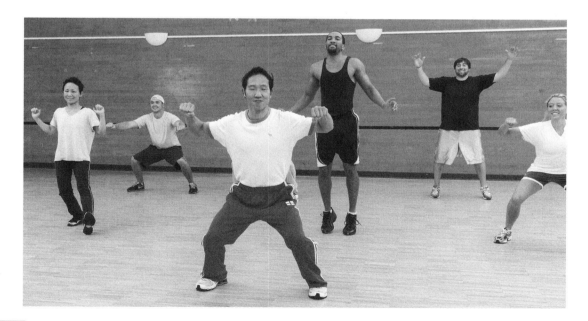

FIGURE 7.2 For cardiorespiratory training, demonstrate the low- and high-intensity options but continue moving at the middle option. In this example, the instructor performs a power squat while participants are demonstrating the step tap (lower intensity) or jumping jack (higher intensity).

training can increase the total volume and average exercise intensity performed during an exercise session. Improvements in cardiorespiratory fitness with short-term (i.e., 3 months) interval training are similar to or greater than those with single-intensity exercise (steady state) in healthy adults and individuals with metabolic, cardiovascular, or pulmonary issues. The use of interval training appears beneficial, but the long-term effects and the safety of interval training remain to be evaluated.

Intensity Monitoring

Monitoring exercise intensity during the cardiorespiratory segment is one of the most important duties of a group exercise leader. It is also one of the most difficult elements of leading a group exercise class. There are numerous methods by which a group exercise leader can progress and monitor exercise intensity. There is also no one measurement that works for all group exercise participants (see the section, "Applying Intensity Monitoring in the Group Exercise Setting"). Many group exercise instructors have stopped using manual HR monitoring because it disrupts the flow of the class, although using a HR monitor is always an option. There are no firm rules for monitoring intensity other than it is important that it be done. Using methods to check in and monitor intensity shows concern for the participants. A summary of how to use target HR, RPE, and the talk test follows.

Measuring Heart Rate

Proper instruction on how to measure HR is the first step in monitoring intensity effectively. There are many sites on the body to monitor heart rate. The potential sites that are the easiest for measuring heart rate are shown in figure 7.3.

- The carotid pulse site is on the carotid artery, just to the side of the larynx. Use light pressure from the fingertips of the

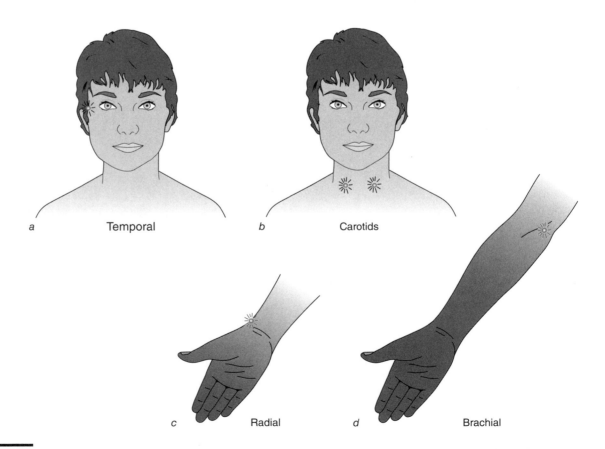

FIGURE 7.3 Anatomical locations for measuring HR: *(a)* temporal, *(b)* carotid, *(c)* radial, and *(d)* brachial.

first two fingers, not the thumb, to take your pulse. Never palpate both carotid arteries at the same time and always press lightly.

- The radial pulse site is on the radial artery at the wrist, in line with the thumb. Use the fingertips of your first two or three fingers to take your pulse. Keep your hand below your heart. Many people find a pulse in this location right where they wear their watchbands.

- The temporal site is just to the side of the eye right above the ear. This site can often be felt without palpating a pulse. Marching lightly and paying attention to this area can allow the pulse rate to be felt.

- The brachial site is on the inside of the arm where blood pressure would be measured. This is a difficult one to palpate and is the least used in a group exercise setting.

Be careful when using the carotid site for checking your pulse. Near the carotid site are baroreceptors that are sensitive to pressure. When the carotid artery is pressed, these baroreceptors send a message to the brain to decrease HR and increase blood pressure to allow the brain better access to oxygen. If you press too firmly and cut off the oxygen going to your brain, you will quickly find yourself horizontal on the ground. Instruct participants to press lightly whenever they use the carotid artery site. Also discourage the use of this site by older adults since they may have plaque buildup in these arteries. Additionally, older adults may obtain an incorrect reading and also can decrease blood flow to the brain.

Heart Rate Reserve and Target Heart Rate

A method for determining target HR is the HR reserve method, commonly known as the *Karvonen formula* (see "Using HR Reserve to Determine Target HR"). The recommended intensities when monitoring with the HR reserve method (40%-85%) correspond to similar recommended percentages of maximal oxygen uptake. The HR

reserve method takes into account resting HR when determining target HR. It is estimated that a participant's maximal heart rate (MHR) equals 220 beats per minute minus the participant's age. Currently, there are many equations for predicting MHR that take into account variables other than age, but these may contain large standard errors of estimate, which may result in inaccuracy when applied to general populations (Roberg and Landwehr 2002). Foster and Porcari (2010) recommend the MHR formula suggested by Gellish and colleagues (2007): 206.9 - (0.67 × age) = estimated MHR. Tanaka, Monahan, and Seals (2001) have also recommended a 208 - (0.7 × age) formula using a percentage of maximal heart rate. Both of these formulas are recommended by the American Council of Sports Medicine (ACSM) (2014), although the simple Karvonen formula may still be used for convenience.

The bottom line is that one specific formula for measuring intensity using heart rates is no longer acceptable nor recommended by the ACSM. There are also population-specific prediction equations (i.e., equations designed for people who smoke, who are obese, who are elderly, and so on) that may provide more accurate estimates of MHR (Miller, Wallace, and Eggert 1993; Whaley, Kaminsky, and Dwyer 1992; Grant et al. 2002).

Keep in mind that 220 minus age provides only an estimate of MHR. It is based on a regression equation, which means that 220 minus age will not be appropriate for everyone. Participants taking prescribed HR-altering medications who want to use the HR method should use a MHR measured during an actual stress test. The HR reserve method involves taking a percentage of the difference between MHR and resting HR and then adding that percentage to the resting HR in order to identify the target HR. See "Using HR Reserve to Determine Target HR" for a sample calculation of target HR using the HR reserve method. Keep in mind that using a variety of measurements to inform participants of exercise intensity levels is recommended. Later in this chapter we review alternate methods such as RPE and the talk test as two other options that can be effective for measuring exercise intensity in a group exercise setting.

Using HR Reserve to Determine Target HR

A 40-year-old participant with a resting HR of 60 beats per minute wants to exercise at 50% to 70% of her HR reserve. What is the range of her target HR?

Step 1: Estimate MHR.

- Estimated MHR = 220 - age
- Estimated MHR = 220 - 40
- Estimated MHR = 180 beats per minute

Step 2: Find HR reserve.

- HR reserve = estimated MHR - resting HR
- HR reserve = 180 - 60
- HR reserve = 120 beats per minute

Step 3: Find 50% to 70% of the HR reserve.

- 50% of HR reserve = HR reserve × 0.50
- 50% of HR reserve = 120 × 0.50

- 50% of HR reserve = 60 beats per minute
- 70% of HR reserve = 120 × 0.70
- 70% of HR reserve = 84 beats per minute

Step 4: Find target HR range (50%-70%).

- Target HR range = % of HR reserve + resting HR
- 50% target HR = 60 + 60 = 120 beats per minute
- 70% target HR = 84 + 60 = 144 beats per minute
- Target HR range = 120 to 144 beats per minute

Since many participants will palpate the pulse and may not have a heart rate monitor, it's helpful for them to divide the target HR by 6 in order to get a 10-second count.

Rating of Perceived Exertion

Rating of perceived exertion (RPE) is another common method of determining exercise intensity. Participants use their subjective perceptions of intensity to rate their level of steady-state work on the 6 to 20 RPE scale or the 0 to 10 RPE scale developed by Borg (1982). Many methods rating perceived exertion have been invented by instructors since the inception of the Borg RPE scale. Interestingly, RPE is both valid and reliable (Dunbar et al. 1992; Robertson et al. 1990) and is closely associated with increases in most cardiorespiratory parameters, including work, maximal oxygen uptake, and HR. In a group exercise setting, RPE can be used with or without HR to monitor the relative exercise intensity of most participants. Participants taking medication that alters HR can use RPE to monitor their relative exercise intensity. Foster and Porcari (2010) state that RPE works well for about 90% of the population; extremely sedentary individuals and individuals with significant muscular strength apparently have the most difficulty using this formula. The verbal description of each level of the RPE scale is important when using RPE. The descriptions must give participants a clear idea of the intensity that each level represents. For example, if using the 6 to 20 Borg scale, a rating of 6 or 7 could be described as the intensity of standing still, 11 could be walking to the store, 13 could be breathing hard during an interval conditioning activity, and 15 could be running after the dog down the street. Relating real-life tasks to RPE helps participants understand how they should feel at each rating.

Talk Test

The talk test is another subjective method of gauging exercise intensity and can be used as an adjunct to HR and RPE. When participants exercise, their breathing should be rhythmic and comfortable. Particularly for newer clients, talking while exercising can indicate whether they are achieving an appropriate intensity. As the intensity increases, breathing rate will become faster and shallower. If a participant needs to gasp for breath between words when conversing, then the exercise intensity is too high and should be reduced. The talk test may work well for those with higher fitness levels, but it can be confusing for beginners who do not know their bodies well enough to understand the talk test concept.

Applying Intensity Monitoring Research in the Group Exercise Setting

Research shows that the best method for monitoring exercise intensity varies depending on the mode of exercise. Parker and colleagues (1989) performed a research study on intensity monitoring in group exercise, in which they determined that HRs taken during high- and low-impact group exercise reflected a lower relative exercise intensity (% of $\dot{V}O_2$max) than HRs taken during running. This is apparently due to the pressor effect, in which vigorous upper-body moves can elevate the HR without a corresponding increase in $\dot{V}O_2$. Other research (Roach, Croisant, and Emmett 1994) on forms of group exercise (step, interval, high- and low-impact, and progressive treadmill training) concluded that HR may not be an appropriate predictor of exercise intensity, and that RPE is the preferred method of monitoring intensity. Grant and coworkers (2002) compared RPE and physiological responses for two modes of aerobic exercise (walking and aerobic dance) in men and women aged 50 years and older. They found that aerobic dance was a bit more intense than walking was for this age group. However, both modes of exercise met the ACSM requirements for exercise intensity. Finally, research by Frangolias and Rhodes (1995) suggests that using HRs when the chest is submerged in water during water exercise is not appropriate. Janot (2005) suggests that it is best to combine methods of intensity monitoring in order to maximize effectiveness in a group exercise setting. Many research studies on HR were performed on runners and cyclists, not on participants in group exercise. Therefore, in a treadmill class or a stationary indoor cycling class, HR monitors can be effective, while in a kickboxing class in which the arms are moving in many directions, RPE might be a better choice.

Galati (2010) and the American Council on Exercise created a model for cardiorespiratory training that has four phases and uses the talk test, which they have incorporated into their integrated fitness training (IFT) model. Each phase of the IFT model is designed to facilitate specific physiological adaptations to exercise. Not every client starts in phase 1; each client has a unique entry point into the cardiorespiratory training phases based upon his or her current health, fitness, and goals. Programming in each phase is based on a three-zone training model (see figure 7.4). The exercise intensities in each zone are based on client-specific intensity markers that include heart rate (HR) at the first and second ventilatory thresholds (VT1 and VT2), the talk test, and RPE. Traditional intensity markers such as percentages of maximal HR (% MHR), HR reserve (% HRR), or $\dot{V}O_2$ reserve (% $\dot{V}O_2$R) are not the recommended methods for monitoring cardiorespiratory exercise intensity in the ACE IFT model because they require actual measurement of MHR or $\dot{V}O_2$max to provide accurate individualized data for programming. Most group exercise instructors do not have the equipment to assess $\dot{V}O_2$max, and there is little or no reason to find a client's actual MHR unless $\dot{V}O_2$max is also being assessed. Group exercise instructors using these traditional intensity markers must estimate MHR and $\dot{V}O_2$max using equations with large standard deviations. Exercise guidelines based upon predicted MHR or $\dot{V}O_2$max can help clients reach their goals, but such guidelines have a lot of room for error and do not account for each client's unique metabolic response to exercise. Therefore, using the talk test or the ACE IFT four phases is a practical option for monitoring intensity in a group exercise setting.

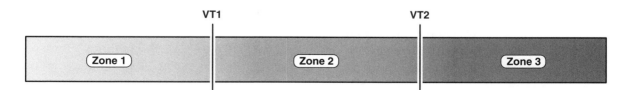

FIGURE 7.4 ACE three-zone model for cardiorespiratory training monitoring.

Reprinted, by permission, from T. Galati, 2010, "ACE IFT model for cardiorespiratory training," part 4, *ACE Certified News*. Available: www.acefitness.org/certifiednewsarticle/709/ace-ift-model-for-cardiorespiratory-training

Whether you are using target HR, RPE, or the talk test to monitor exercise intensity, there are a few points of practical application to remember and share with the group:

- When measuring HR, turn off the music so the beats do not influence the counting of the pulse rate.

- Encourage use of the radial pulse rather than the carotid pulse; if you are using the carotid pulse, remind participants to press lightly to avoid reducing blood flow to the brain.

- Check intensity toward the beginning, middle, and end of the workout so it can be modified if necessary.

- Keep participants moving while checking intensity to prevent blood from pooling in the lower extremities.

- Use a 10-second pulse count if using target HRs and start counting with 1. Count each beat and multiply this number by 6 to get beats per minute. Many group exercise facilities have charts in the group exercise area that do the multiplication for you.

- When measuring RPE, ask participants to rate how they're feeling. If an RPE chart is in the room, direct participants to the numbers on the chart. If there is no chart visible, simply ask them how hard they think they're working on a scale of 1 to 10, explaining that 1 is like standing still, and 10 is equivalent to maximum. Encourage your participants to work at a 5 (moderate or medium level)—or at a 6 or a 7 (hard level) if they're having a good day.

- Give modifications based on HR or RPE results and encourage participants to work at their own levels.

 See online video clip 7.2 to observe how an instructor puts the concepts of monitoring exercise intensity into practice. Notice how the participants are kept moving, the instructor suggests modifications, and HR and RPE are used to help the participants check their exercise intensity in two ways.

Principles of Muscle Balance in Cardiorespiratory Training

In leading any cardiorespiratory segment, remember to balance the stresses applied to the muscles and joints. For example, if the class consists entirely of front martial arts–style kicks, muscle balance is not promoted. Many martial arts moves and sport conditioning classes involve a large amount of forward movement; hips, spine, cervical spine, and shoulders are repetitively flexed for long durations throughout a class. To counterbalance the bias toward flexed movements, incorporate a sufficient amount of hip, spine, and shoulder extension moves as well as scapular retraction exercises. In a stationary indoor cycling class where hip and low-back flexion is the standard position, have participants sit up several times during the class and extend the spine, depress the shoulders, and retract the scapulae. Correct and give cues on posture during the cardiorespiratory segment of a workout anytime you can; these help remind participants of the importance of posture in their lives. As group exercise instructors, we want to positively affect and educate participants whenever possible. Regarding muscular balance, consider how participants move each day, and how we can help them move better. Generally speaking, we walk forward and move predominantly in the sagittal plane with most of our daily movements. Incorporating standing hip abduction and hip extension movements into workout sessions helps participants balance the movements they perform on a daily basis with life tasks. Walking or running forward in a sport conditioning class and then following that with a backward walk or run helps promote muscle balance. Discussing muscle balance during the cardiorespiratory session helps participants find a sense of purpose in the workout that is greater than the movements themselves. Taking time to point out muscle imbalances and how you are working to correct them adds an educational component to the class that is essential for a positive group exercise experience.

Safety Issues, Good Alignment, and Technique

As always, safety is the number one priority in cardiorespiratory training. In order to minimize repetitive stress, avoid large numbers of high-stress moves in a row. For example, a jumping jack is considered a high-stress move. How many jumping jacks are too many? There is no definitive answer—it depends on your class and your participants. It's always wise to intersperse high-stress moves (e.g., jumping jacks) with moves that provide a lower or different kind of stress to the muscles and joints, such as marches, kicks, or agility drills. In general, avoid too much repetition of any move, particularly high-intensity or high-impact moves. Other high-stress moves include rope jumping, skier hops, high kicks, deep squats, burpees, lunges, and continuous hops on one leg. Another safety and technique recommendation is to bring the heels all the way down when performing high-impact and jumping moves; avoid jumping on the balls of the feet—roll through the entire foot. Also, encourage participants to move through full ROM without hyperextending the elbows or knees; always keep a slight bend in the knees and elbows in order to protect the joints.

What are the signs of serious medical problems during exercise? According to the ACSM (2014), symptoms that warrant stopping exercise or consulting with a physician include chest pain, unreasonable breathlessness, dizziness, fainting or blackouts, sudden ankle swelling, and heart palpitations. In order to obtain a national fitness certification, group exercise leaders need to be CPR and AED certified and aware of the facility's emergency procedures. According to Riley (2005) and Bates (2008), many states require the use of AEDs in fitness facilities. States also recommend that fitness facilities coordinate their AED program with the local emergency management system (EMS). The reason for this requirement is to ensure smooth communication and an integrated response with EMS providers. A survival rate as high as 90 % has been reported when defibrillation is achieved within the first minute of collapse (Balady et al. 2002). Survival rates decline 7 % to 10 % with every minute that defibrillation is delayed; a cardiac arrest victim without defibrillation beyond 12 minutes has only a 2 % to 5 % chance of survival. The American Heart Association (AHA) and ACSM's joint position statement on AEDs (2002) in health and fitness facilities makes recommendations for the use and purchase of AEDs in both clinical and fitness settings. Once a facility is equipped with an AED, it becomes part of a more comprehensive "chain of survival" that can improve the recovery odds for a victim in need of cardiac resuscitation.

Automated External Defibrillators (AEDs)

An AED is a computerized medical device that can check a person's heart rhythm, recognize a rhythm that requires a shock, and advise the rescuer to deliver that shock. Fitness facilities in several U.S. states are required by law to provide AEDs, and most CPR classes now include AED training. It is important to determine if your facility is in a state that requires an AED to be present for the safety of the participant. According to Wolohan (2008), a fitness facility may be considered negligent if it does not have an AED on site. The International Health, Racquet & Sportsclub Association (IHRSA) encourages health club operators to consider the advantages of installing AEDs in their facilities. According to Schroeder and Donlin (2013) the number of health club members aged 35 years and older is steadily increasing. In fact, this population currently accounts for more than 55 % of facility memberships. The number of members with some form of cardiorespiratory disease is also on the rise (AHA & ACSM, 2002). Having an AED on site shows that your primary concern is the safety of your participants. We suggest all facilities have an AED on-site and believe that eventually the AED will be required in all states and in all workout areas.

Importance of Participant Interaction and Enjoyment

As we discussed in Chapter 2, involving your participants in interpersonal interaction lets them feel good about exercise and your class in general. This camaraderie makes up for the hard work of exercise. Although social connection techniques require motivation on your part, they can make you an extraordinary instructor and can keep your students coming back. If you believe in yourself and the power of exercise and wellness, it will be easy for you to project fun and enthusiasm to all who attend your class.

Goleman (2006), in his book on social intelligence, discusses what he has called "mirror neurons" and the importance they play in human interaction. "Mirror neurons make emotions contagious, letting the feelings we witness flow through us. We 'feel' the other in the broadest sense of the word: sensing their sentiments, their movements, their sensations, and their emotions as they act inside us" (2006, p. 40). Such interaction may be extremely important to the whole exercise experience in terms of making a difference in participants' health. Group cohesiveness does not just happen, however—it needs to be fostered through your leadership skills. Here are some suggestions for promoting participant interaction in a cardiorespiratory training class:

- Talk to people and call them by name.
- Have people choose partners and perform hand-slap activities while moving, or have people introduce themselves to one another.
- Play musical themes and schedule special activities on holidays.
- Use partner exercises in muscular conditioning.
- Devise circuit classes where participants work together in small groups.
- Form circles and have participants demonstrate or lead their favorite moves.

Cool-Down After the Cardio Segment

It is suggested that the last few minutes of any group cardio session be less intense to allow the cardiorespiratory system to recover. Lack of a cool-down after the cardio segment is correlated with an increased risk of heart arrhythmias (American Council on Exercise 2011). Because metabolic waste products can get trapped inside the muscle cells if the intensity is not decreased gradually, many people experience increased cramping and stiffness if they do not cool down. A proper cool-down enables waste products to disperse and the body to return to resting levels without injury. The cool-down also prevents blood from pooling in the lower extremities and allows the cardiovascular system to make the transition to more gradual workloads. This is especially important if muscle work will follow the cardiorespiratory segment. During the cool-down, encourage participants to relax, slow down, keep their arms below the level of the heart, and put less effort into their movements. Klika (2012) uses partner stretches at the end of boot camp classes in order to help participants cool down and also feel welcome and accountable to the group. She feels that this accountability also helps them show up for class again. Shechtman (2008) has participants use noodles in her water exercise class to stretch and cool down at the end of a cardio water workout. For example, while standing in shallow water, she puts a water noodle under one leg, balances on the other, and allows the supported leg to rise to the surface with the noodle for an effective hamstring stretch while working on balance at the same time. During the cool-down, use calmer music, change your tone of voice, and verbalize the transition to the participants to help create this atmosphere of cooling down and allowing blood flow to readjust after a cardio segment. For more information, see chapter 6, "Designing a Cool-Down" and chapter 8, "Recommendations and Guidelines for Flexibility Training."

 See online video 7.3 for a demonstration of a cool-down after a cardio segment.

Chapter Wrap-Up

This chapter outlined the variables that are common to the cardiorespiratory segments of most group exercise classes. Whether you are teaching a cycling, water, step, or boot camp class, we recommend you increase intensity gradually, vary the muscle groups used, provide movement options, interact with participants, monitor intensity, and lead a cool-down after the cardio segment. Later chapters on various group exercise classes (in Part III) will refer you back to these principles.

ASSIGNMENT

Attend (and participate in) a group exercise class that contains a cardiorespiratory segment. Observe how the instructor monitors intensity. Monitor your own intensity every 5 minutes, switching between HR and RPE. Record your values. Describe in a one-page paper which method worked better for you and why. Also, reflect on your observations regarding the instructor's ability to monitor exercise intensity during the cardio segment.

Muscular Conditioning and Flexibility Training

Chapter Objectives

After reading and practicing the information in this chapter, you will be able to

- explain recommendations and guidelines for muscular conditioning;
- cue muscular conditioning exercises with skill;
- demonstrate exercises with proper form and alignment;
- demonstrate exercise progressions, regressions, modifications, and alternatives;
- understand safety issues in muscular conditioning;
- use equipment in group muscle conditioning;
- explain recommendations and guidelines for flexibility training;
- cue flexibility exercises and end a class appropriately;
- understand safety issues in flexibility training; and
- identify and demonstrate muscular conditioning and flexibility exercises.

Group Exercise Class Evaluation Form Essentials

Key Points for Conditioning Segment: Muscular Conditioning

- Provides alignment and technique cues
- Gives motivational cues
- Uses a variety of muscle groups
- Minimizes repetitive movements
- Observes participants' form and provides constructive, nonintimidating feedback
- Continually offers modifications, regressions, progressions, or alternatives
- Gives clear verbal directions and uses appropriate music volume
- Provides regular demonstrations and participation with good body mechanics
- Uses appropriate movement or music tempo

Key Points for Conditioning Segment: Flexibility Training

- Includes static stretching for major muscles worked and for commonly tight muscles (hip flexors, hamstrings, calves, erector spinae, pectorals, anterior deltoids, upper trapezius)
- Demonstrates using proper alignment and technique
- Observes participants' form and offers modifications, regressions, progressions, and/or alternatives
- Provides alignment cues
- Appropriately emphasizes relaxation and/or visualization
- Uses appropriate movement and/or music tempo
- Ends class on a positive note and/or thanks class

The development of muscle strength, endurance, and flexibility is essential for overall fitness and is an integral part of any group fitness program. To be a competent group instructor in muscular conditioning and flexibility, it's important to understand basic anatomy, kinesiology (joint actions), safety and equipment issues, and appropriate cueing. You also need to know a large variety of exercises and stretches. A few common principles guide the muscle conditioning and flexibility segments of most group exercise classes. In this chapter, we discuss muscular conditioning first and then cover flexibility and cooling down. After that, we provide detailed descriptions and photographs of exercises and stretches; these make up the majority of this chapter. The descriptions begin with the upper-body muscles, move through the torso muscles, and conclude with the lower-body muscles. The main points on the Group Exercise Class Evaluation Form (found in appendix A) that apply to muscular conditioning and flexibility training are listed in "Group Exercise Class Evaluation Form Essentials."

Recommendations and Guidelines for Muscular Conditioning

Most group exercise instructors include some form of muscle strength and endurance training in their classes. To promote total fitness, you must include exercises for maintaining muscular strength, endurance, and tone as well as exercises for promoting flexibility and cardiorespiratory fitness. The American College of Sports Medicine (ACSM) (2014) has published the following guidelines regarding resistance training for the average healthy adult:

- Each major muscle group (chest, shoulders, abdomen, back, hips, legs, arms) should be trained with 2 to 4 sets. Multijoint exercises affecting more than one muscle group and targeting opposing muscles are recommended; single-joint exercises may also be included. Perform a variety of exercises using equipment and/or body weight. Perform 8 to 12 repetitions for most adults; 10 to 15 repetitions may be more appropriate for beginner middle-aged and older individuals.

- Intensity (the amount of weight lifted) can vary depending on one's goal and fitness level: for example, 60%-70% 1RM (moderate to vigorous intensity) for beginners and intermediates, 40%-50% 1RM (very light to light intensity) for sedentary and/or older people, and >80% 1RM (vigorous to very vigorous intensity) for experienced strength trainers to improve strength.

- Exercise each muscle group 2 to 3 nonconsecutive days per week, and if possible, perform a different exercise for each muscle group every 2 to 3 sessions.

- Maintain a normal breathing pattern; breath holding can cause increases in blood pressure.

Considerable debate continues regarding single-set versus multiple-set programs. The National Strength and Conditioning Association (NSCA) currently recommends performing multiple sets for optimal strength gains (2005), but some of the studies on which this recommendation is based have been discredited (Otto and Carpinelli 2006). In fact, the ACSM has reversed its position on this matter several times. We recommend staying up to date with the most current guidelines and remaining aware that they will most likely change based on future research. Note that the current (2014) ACSM guidelines state that a single set can be effective, particularly is the exerciser is a beginner or an older adult.

For example, in an earlier publication, Faigenbaum and Pollock (1999) stated that single-set programs performed a minimum of 2 times per week can be recommended over multiple-set programs because they are less time consuming, are more cost efficient, and still produce most of the health and fitness benefits of resistance training. Other studies, however, have reported that multiple-set programs provide superior results, especially for intermediate and advanced exercisers (Wolfe et al. 2004; Rhea et al. 2002). The NSCA adds that training should occur at least 3 days per week and that there should be a minimum of 24 hours rest between training sessions (Pearson et al. 2000). Even though controversy exists, the bottom line is that muscular training is an important health-related fitness component that needs to be included in group exercise instruction. The many benefits of muscular resistance training are listed in the sidebar. However, in the group exercise setting, teaching resistance training is not always easy to do according to the guidelines since you may not have access to heavier weights. The typical group exercise room stocks only 2-, 3-, 5-, 8-, and 10-pound (1, 1.4, 2.3, 3.6, 4.5 kg) dumbbells, making it difficult for most participants to reach muscle fatigue in one set of 8 to 12 repetitions or to adhere to the ACSM guidelines for intensity.

Group exercise class participants often ask the following question: "How many sit-ups (curl-ups, leg lifts, and so on) should I do?" The answer is, "It depends." Participants should do

Benefits of Resistance Training

- Easier performance of daily activities
- Increased lean body (muscle) mass
- Increased metabolism due to increased lean body mass
- Stronger muscles, tendons, and ligaments
- Stronger bones and reduced risk of osteoporosis
- Decreased risk of injury
- Decreased risk of low-back pain
- Enhanced feelings of well-being and self-confidence

as many as they can while maintaining good form and alignment and should stop when they reach the point of fatigue (not total muscle failure). The optimal number of repetitions varies from exercise to exercise and from person to person. Also, the more challenging the exercise, and the harder you push yourself during the exercise, the more quickly you'll reach the point of fatigue. For example, you will find that you are able to do more abdominal curl-ups when you hold your arms at your sides rather than overhead (holding them overhead creates a longer lever and thus is more biomechanically challenging). Participants who are performing more difficult variations may do fewer repetitions than participants who are performing an easier modification or participants who are not pushing themselves.

How do you increase participants' intensity when instructing muscular conditioning in the group exercise setting? There are at least three ways to increase intensity:

1. Have your students focus on consciously contracting the muscle with each repetition. Conscious muscle contractions create tension similar to that experienced during isometric muscle actions. Most people can squeeze their biceps while holding the elbow at a fixed angle. Continuing that squeeze while moving the elbow through its full range of motion (ROM) is what we mean by conscious muscle contraction, and it's a great technique to teach your students. In addition to increasing the exercise intensity, conscious muscle contractions promote increased body awareness and better alignment.

2. Use various resistance devices to increase intensity and provide overload. Commonly used devices include dumbbells, Body Bars, barbells, kettlebells, medicine balls, elastic tubing, and elastic bands. Steps can be inclined or declined to increase the resistance depending on the exercise. You can also use stability balls, BOSU balance trainers, foam rollers, and core boards to increase the potential for overload in a wide variety of exercises. Body leverage training, also known as suspension training, is increasingly popular in the group exercise setting; this type of muscular training requires suspension devices such as the TRX to be installed in the room.

Resistance in water exercise can be increased with aquatic gloves, dumbbells, barbells, paddles, fins, elastic bands and tubes, and buoyancy boots. Because it is impractical to supply a wide range of dumbbells or weight plates in the group setting, most facilities stop stocking large quantities of dumbbells at 8 or 10 pounds (3.6-4.5 kg). Therefore, creativity is needed in order to provide sufficient overload for more advanced participants.

3. Change the exercise mode (Yoke and Kennedy 2004). In group resistance training, this means using the functional training continuum (see chapter 3, figure 3.4) to progress from easier to more difficult (compound) exercises. To do this, you need a comprehensive knowledge of a wide variety of exercise choices for all major muscle groups and the ability to evaluate which exercises are appropriate for which participants. As a general rule, the more advanced a student becomes, the more he needs to emphasize multimuscle, multijoint exercises (Sorace and LaFontaine 2005). Many exercises have several variations that can move participants along the exercise continuum. For example, push-up modifications from easiest to hardest include: wall push-up, hands and knees (tabletop) push-up, knee push-up with hands on step, knee push-up with hands on floor, knee push-up with knees elevated on step, full-body push-up with hands on step, full-body push-up with hands on floor, full-body push-up with feet on step, full-body push-up with feet on stability ball, and full-body push-up using one arm. A competent instructor will be familiar with these progressions, regressions, and modifications and be able to help participants determine which one is right for them. See the section "Demonstrating Progressions, Regressions, Modifications, and Alternatives" later in this chapter for more information.

Another technique that instructors commonly use to increase exercise difficulty is to increase the duration of the strength training or to encourage more repetitions. Although this method may be appropriate in some classes, you must be cautious with this approach. It's hard to challenge 8 to 10 major muscle groups in a 1-hour class that also includes a cardio component if you are prescribing large numbers of repetitions for each exercise.

When it comes to monitoring intensity in the muscular fitness segment, be cautious using heart rate as a gauge because oxygen consumption does not increase proportionately to heart rate during most resistance exercises. A higher heart rate during a strength and endurance session is caused by sympathetic nervous system activation and doesn't necessarily mean you're getting a great workout (Beckham and Earnest 2000). Heart rate is more appropriately used as an intensity indicator during cardio activities such as step, high-low impact exercise, and stationary indoor cycling—all activities that repeatedly engage large muscle groups for a prolonged duration.

Key Definitions

Stress Adaptation

Gradually and progressively increase the intensity of the workout by increasing the number of repetitions or the amount of resistance. Sudden increases in intensity, such as abruptly doubling the repetitions or the resistance, can result in muscle damage and injury. On the other hand, staying at the same intensity will not allow musculoskeletal stress adaptation to occur. Instruct your participants to add 1 to 2 pounds (0.5-1 kg) or go to the next thickness of rubber band if they can perform 15 or more repetitions at their current level. The ACSM recommends that resistance be increased by 2% to 10%, depending on the muscle groups used, when the participant can complete 1 to 2 repetitions beyond the desired number and has done so for at least two consecutive sessions (American College of Sports Medicine [ACSM] 2002).

Rebuilding Time

When a muscle is stressed beyond its normal limitations, it needs time for repair, recovery, and positive physiological change. This time is known as *rebuilding time*. Generally, muscles require 1 to 2 days (24-48 hours) to rebuild, so resistance training should be performed every other day. If you are strength training daily, you should emphasize different muscle groups on each day, especially if your intensity is high.

Controlled Movement

Slow, smooth, and controlled movement speed ensures consistent application of force throughout the entire ROM. Keep in mind that music tempos of 130 beats per minute or faster increase momentum and the risk of injury. Slower music tempos ($\sim$ 116 beats per minute) demand control and strength. If you want to progress a class, use slower speeds and music tempos as the class session proceeds.

Full Range of Motion

Use the full range of motion of the muscle and joint structure to help preserve flexibility. Training the muscles and tendons through a greater ROM enables more muscle fibers to perform work. Pulsing (or performing a limited ROM) is discouraged unless limited range of motion is your goal, as it is in some abdominal work. Using limited ROM may be appropriate for rehabilitation or for injury avoidance. For example, performing partial ROM exercises during weight training can help an injured rotator cuff to heal.

Training Specificity

The principle of specificity states that specific adaptations occur in response to specific exercises, activities, or stretches. This means that the results of exercise training are specific to the part of the body being trained; for example, training the upper body has little effect on the lower body, and vice versa.

Cueing Muscular Conditioning Exercises

The type of cueing required for muscle conditioning is different from that required when leading cardio exercise to music. When you are leading a dance-based class, for example, good anticipatory cueing is essential so you can let your class know about upcoming moves before they actually happen, helping to ensure that your class moves safely together as a unit. During muscle conditioning, however, anticipatory cues are much less important than alignment, safety, and motivational cues.

Some instructors fall into the monotonous trap of counting every repetition of every strength exercise. There are so many other valuable things to say. We recommend that you save counting for the last set or the last few repetitions. For example, tell your class that they have 8 more biceps curls and that you want them to go to the point of fatigue, squeezing their biceps as hard as possible for the last 8 repetitions. Then, counting backward from 8, increase the intensity in your voice and add a motivational cue or two to encourage participants to achieve muscle overload by the last repetition. Motivational cues are used liberally by experienced instructors. You can do it!

Additionally, the muscular conditioning segment is an ideal time to face your class, because complex choreography is not an issue. Facing your class is more personal and more direct than facing the mirror and generally provides you with better visibility of your students' alignment. After demonstrating proper form and alignment for the first few repetitions of an exercise, walk around your class to check everyone's form and give personalized modifications when needed. This is an excellent time to address participants by name and give encouragement! The following sections discuss the basic types of cues for muscular conditioning.

Alignment Cues

Because 8 of 10 Americans will experience back problems during their lifetime (Frymoyer and Cats-Baril 1991), it is essential to give verbal cues on posture and spinal alignment in each segment of the class; giving appropriate postural and alignment cues is especially critical during the muscular conditioning and stretching segments. See figure 8.1 for points to remember when teaching correct posture in the standing position.

When giving alignment cues, focus on joints of the neck, spine, pelvis, scapulae, shoulders, wrists, elbows, hips, knees, and ankles. As a general rule, most conditioning exercises engage the stabilizer muscles. Give several posture cues *before* providing instruction on the specific muscle groups to be worked or stretched. For example, when leading the class in a latissimus dorsi strengthening exercise using elastic tubing, cue the participants to soften the knees, get a good base of support with the feet apart comfortably, and contract the abdominals while keeping the spine in a neutral position. In other words, clearly cue the exercise setup. After that, you may cue the movement itself, in this case a standing lat pull-down for the latissimus dorsi.

Here's an example of providing useful alignment cues during the squat: "Be sure your knees are behind your toes, and your weight is directed back toward your heels. Point your tailbone toward the back wall. Tighten up those abdominals and lift your chest!" Visual and tactile cues are also very useful for promoting proper alignment. When describing knee alignment in the squat, try visual cueing, as follows: point to your knees and use the wrong, right technique—first demonstrate incorrect knee alignment, drawing an imaginary line from the hyperflexed knee to the floor. Then reposition your knees to demonstrate correct alignment. You can also visually cue by placing your finger over your tailbone to show how it should point toward the back wall. Touch your abdominals to indicate abdominal support. Alignment can be thought of as joint alignment. If you are at a loss as to what to say or show, verbally and/or visually describe the alignment of all the joints. Even in a simple biceps curl, students need to be mindful of lower-body alignment. How should the knees be positioned? What about the pelvis or the spine, shoulders, neck, and wrists?

Safety Cues

A safety cue educates your participants on how to make the exercise safer and prevent injury.

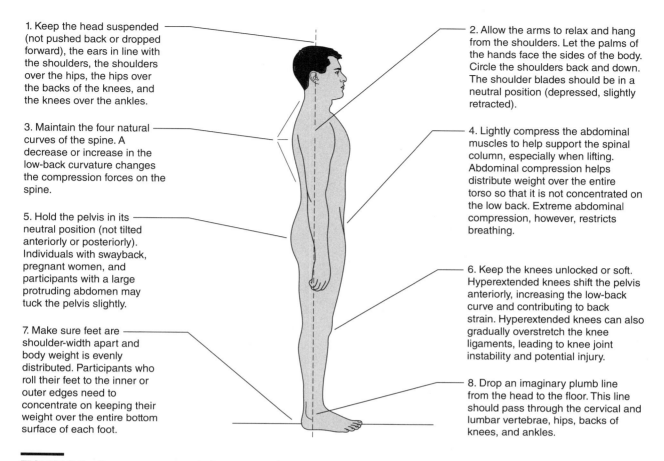

1. Keep the head suspended (not pushed back or dropped forward), the ears in line with the shoulders, the shoulders over the hips, the hips over the backs of the knees, and the knees over the ankles.

2. Allow the arms to relax and hang from the shoulders. Let the palms of the hands face the sides of the body. Circle the shoulders back and down. The shoulder blades should be in a neutral position (depressed, slightly retracted).

3. Maintain the four natural curves of the spine. A decrease or increase in the low-back curvature changes the compression forces on the spine.

4. Lightly compress the abdominal muscles to help support the spinal column, especially when lifting. Abdominal compression helps distribute weight over the entire torso so that it is not concentrated on the low back. Extreme abdominal compression, however, restricts breathing.

5. Hold the pelvis in its neutral position (not tilted anteriorly or posteriorly). Individuals with swayback, pregnant women, and participants with a large protruding abdomen may tuck the pelvis slightly.

6. Keep the knees unlocked or soft. Hyperextended knees shift the pelvis anteriorly, increasing the low-back curve and contributing to back strain. Hyperextended knees can also gradually overstretch the knee ligaments, leading to knee joint instability and potential injury.

7. Make sure feet are shoulder-width apart and body weight is evenly distributed. Participants who roll their feet to the inner or outer edges need to concentrate on keeping their weight over the entire bottom surface of each foot.

8. Drop an imaginary plumb line from the head to the floor. This line should pass through the cervical and lumbar vertebrae, hips, backs of knees, and ankles.

FIGURE 8.1 Proper posture and alignment in the standing position.

For example, during the squat you could say, "Keeping both hands on the thighs, or performing alternating front raises in which you keep one hand on the thigh, helps protect your low back. Maintaining an abdominal contraction while squatting also supports the low back and guards against injury."

Motivational Cues

Motivational cues can make the difference between a mediocre workout and a great workout. Tell your participants, "Great job!" "I really like how all of you are keeping your knees in good alignment!" "You people are terrific!" "All right!" Many instructors cue on every (or almost every) repetition of a muscle conditioning exercise. Here are additional cues you can use to offer encouragement: "Squeeze!" "Contract!" "Press." "Breathe!" "Oh yeah!" "Release." "Make it look like work!" "Consciously tighten that muscle!" "Go!" "You can do it!"

Educational Cues

The following list includes examples of cueing that can be used during strengthening segments to optimize educational opportunities:

- Perform this exercise slowly, smoothly, and with control.
- Breathe in, and as you begin the movement, perform the work, lift the weight, or pull against the resistance—exhale!
- The number of repetitions is not as important as tuning in to the area you are working.
- If you feel any pain, twinges, or joint discomfort, stop!
- Correct form is more important than the number of repetitions or the amount of weight.
- You can do one side until fatigued; then switch to the other side or alternate sides each time.

- If you are new to class, change sides or stop when you get tired, even if the rest of the class keeps going.
- Even though we are doing many repetitions, this type of exercise will not remove fat from this area. To remove fat, you need aerobic exercise. This exercise will help you tone and shape muscles and will allow you to tuck in, pull up, and contour your body.

Looking closer at verbal and physical cues will help you understand that there is more than one way to communicate and direct movement. Verbal cues include cueing movement with appropriate terminology and instruction as previously discussed. For example, when you are teaching a standing outer-thigh leg lift to strengthen the gluteus medius, you might do the following:

- Ask participants to contract the stabilizers (abdominals, gluteus maximus).
- Give appropriate alignment cues joint by joint.
- Remind participants that the range of motion of the movement is around 45°, so lifting with the side of the heel is important. If the participant's toe comes up, that means hip flexion is being performed, which works the quadriceps and hip flexors. Remind participants to keep the movements slow and controlled and alternate sides to promote greater comfort and better muscle balance.
- Always be encouraging when giving any cue; try to word all corrections in a positive way. Instead of saying, "Don't lock your knees" or "You're locking your knees," say, "Bend your knees slightly, OK?" or "Would you mind softening your knees a bit? That will help reduce both knee stress and back stress and keep you safe."

Physical, hands-on (tactile) cues are another way to give participants feedback on their form. When you give physical cues, walk around the room and observe participants from different angles. Gently placing your hands on a participant's shoulders to remind her to relax the shoulder blades is an example of a physical or tactile cue. Before touching, be sure to ask the participant's permission. Do not touch if the participant seems uncomfortable in any way.

Demonstrating Exercises With Proper Form and Alignment

Performing exercises and stretches correctly when giving verbal cues is important. If you say to keep a leg movement at a 45° ROM but at the same time lift your leg higher than that, you will confuse the participants. Whatever instructions you give need to be duplicated in your demonstration of the movement. Most participants are visual learners and will copy what they see you doing. Since many people are visual learners, it's very helpful to give visual alignment cues. For example, if you say, "Soften your knees," you might simultaneously point to your own flexed knees. If you say, "Pull your abdominal muscles in," you can point to your own abdominals while you pull them in in an exaggerated fashion. Practice is the key to becoming an effective visual demonstrator. Work constantly on your own form and alignment so that you can inspire your class and enhance safety and effectiveness by becoming a superior role model.

Demonstrating Progressions, Regressions, Modifications, and Alternatives

A big difference between the teacher-centered instructor and the student-centered instructor is that the student-centered instructor helps individual participants make their exercise safer and less painful or problematic. To help your participants, you must observe them and understand their problems and limitations.

In addition to knowing the basic exercises, skilled instructors are familiar with a wide variety of progressions, regressions, modifications, and alternatives they can use to suggest appropriate exercises for every person in their class. If a participant complains that the knee, shoulder, back, or any other body part hurts in an exercise, modify the exercise to make it more

Exercise Continuum Terminology

progression—Making a specific exercise harder by increasing the balance and/or coordination challenge, increasing the need for core stability, and/or making the exercise more multimuscle and multijoint. Progression can also be accomplished by choosing a different and harder exercise.

regression—Making a specific exercise easier by providing more stability or support, reducing the need for strong core stabilizers, and/or focusing on muscle isolation or single-joint moves. Regression can also be achieved by choosing a different and easier exercise.

modification—Adjusting a specific exercise to accommodate an issue such as joint pain. A modification may make an exercise easier (see regression criteria) or not. For example, performing a push-up on the knuckles is a modification for someone with wrist pain; however, it does not make the exercise itself easier—it just reduces the stress on the wrists.

alternative—Providing a completely different (but ideally at the same level) exercise for the same muscle group in order to accommodate a participant's issue.

comfortable or provide a completely different exercise that works the same muscle group. For example, imagine that a student tells you her wrists hurt when she does push-ups. You can suggest that she try the push-up on her fists or on her fingers or that she curl her hands around sturdy dumbbells; all of these modifications help keep the wrists in a straight line during the push-up movement and may alleviate the problem. Or you might suggest that the student try push-ups on the wall, where she has to lift less of her body weight (this would be a regression). If none of these options relieves the pain, suggest an alternative exercise that still targets the chest muscles, such as a bench press. If her wrists still hurt, you can recommend that she see her physician if she hasn't already done so.

The functional training exercise continuum (discussed in chapters 1, 3, 5, 8, 9, 13, and 15 and shown in figure 8.2) ranks the exercises for a particular muscle group according to their difficulty level (Yoke and Kennedy, 2004). As a participant gradually improves strength and

endurance, he will be able to progress, performing harder exercises and moving along the continuum to the right. Conversely, a participant who is having trouble performing an exercise from the more difficult end of the continuum can regress to an easier exercise that can be done safely with good form. An exercise modification can also be a regression, but not necessarily. An example of this could be moving a participant from the hands and knees (all fours) position for hip extension to an elbows-and-knees position. While this is a modification that can help a participant experiencing wrist or back pain, it is not significantly easier in terms of core stability or resistance. The ACSM (2002) recommends that novice exercisers start with simple exercises and progress to complex exercises as they become more advanced.

It's important to be out on the floor observing and assisting your participants. Demonstrate the exercise, perform a few repetitions, and then begin to move around the room, watching the participants. When you stay in one place,

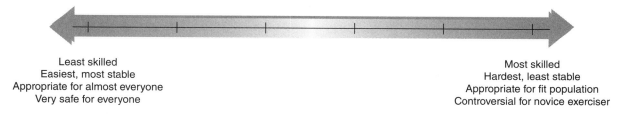

Least skilled
Easiest, most stable
Appropriate for almost everyone
Very safe for everyone

Most skilled
Hardest, least stable
Appropriate for fit population
Controversial for novice exerciser

FIGURE 8.2 Progressive functional training continuum.

you give your participants only one frame of reference. Plus, coaching participants is a large part of the group exercise experience, and when you are nearby and observing, participants will listen and perform more effectively. When you move around the room, you allow participants to see that you have empathy as well as the knowledge to modify exercises that are problematic for them.

 See online video 8.1 for muscle conditioning progression options and instructor cueing for the following exercises: squat, bent-over row, push-up, and abdominal exercises performed on a stability ball and a BOSU balance trainer.

Safety Issues in Muscular Conditioning

Safety is a major concern when you are leading a group fitness class. In general, group exercise instructors need to be more cautious and conservative than personal trainers when designing a muscular strength and conditioning program. Responsible personal trainers take thorough health histories on all their clients, require physicians' clearances when appropriate, and create individualized programs that account for each client's unique musculoskeletal needs. Group leaders usually don't have the luxury of individually assessing each participant in their class or tailoring the program to a specific participant. Ideally, each exercise that is given in a class is safe for everyone in that class, including beginners or deconditioned members. You may show progressions for participants who are in better shape, although after demonstrating an advanced move, you'll want to demonstrate the variation that best fits the majority of the people in your class. Most participants will try to copy whatever the instructor is demonstrating, even though that particular variation may be inappropriate for them. (Participants will also unconsciously copy your form and alignment, so always demonstrate all exercises using excellent alignment.)

Encourage your participants to listen to their bodies and note twinges or slight annoyances,

which can be warning signals of future injury. Most participants have heard the saying, "No pain, no gain" and think that if they don't hurt after an exercise session, it wasn't a good workout. No pain, no gain may be appropriate for competing athletes, but is completely inappropriate in a group health and fitness setting. Educate your students about the difference between muscle soreness and joint pain. Muscle soreness usually disappears after 24 to 48 hours and may be acceptable for students who want to challenge themselves. Joint pain, however, is never okay and is a sign that something is wrong. Teach your students to distinguish between the two and stop whatever activity is causing joint pain. Remember, if there is pain, there is little gain!

The major cause of exercise-related injury is doing too much, too soon. Students must progress gradually to harder, more intense exercises and longer duration. Your exercise choices must be appropriate for the students in your class. This means that you must be prepared to alter your class plan on a moment's notice, depending on the fitness levels and skills of the participants who have shown up for the session. Experienced instructors have a large repertoire of exercises and exercise modifications that they can use to reformat or even individualize a class on the spot.

When teaching your class, follow the tenets of good technique and correct alignment. Avoid the following:

- Hyperextended knees or elbows
- Excessive momentum
- Inappropriate torque (a rotational twisting force applied to a joint, as in the hurdler's stretch)
- Hyperflexed knees (knees bent past 90°) in a weight-bearing position such as a squat or lunge

Avoid risky moves and follow industry guidelines on high-risk exercises to protect your students and yourself. Moves that are considered higher risk include

- ballistic stretches,
- deep squats (in which the hips drop below the knees),

- extreme or ballistic lumbar hyperextension,
- cervical spinal hyperextension,
- unsupported forward flexion of the lumbar spine (avoid toe touches without back support; place hands on a block, the floor, ankles, shins, or thighs),
- unsupported forward flexion of the lumbar spine with rotation (e.g., windmills),
- unsupported lateral spinal flexion,
- hurdler's stretch,
- full sit-ups,
- full straight-leg sit-ups,
- double straight-leg raises,
- deadlifts,
- good mornings,
- plow (yoga),
- full cobra (yoga), and
- V-sits.

For the average class participant interested in health-related fitness, the risks of performing these exercises can outweigh the potential benefits (Yoke 2010). For example, although the deep squat is an essential skill for Olympic lifting, and is found in yoga, ballet, and baseball, the majority of researchers agree that it's a risky move that increases the risk of knee pain and injury (Anderson 2003; Kreighbaum and Barthels 1996). As such, we do not recommend including it in your group exercise classes—unless, of course, you're teaching Olympic weightlifting athletes, professional baseball catchers, ballet dancers, or advanced yoga participants. Always consider the risk-to-benefit ratio and the issue of appropriateness when choosing exercises for your class.

Being able to analyze an exercise in terms of its effectiveness and safety is an important skill for all fitness professionals. One way to do this has been devised by the Aerobics and Fitness Association of America (2010). Here are five key questions with added comments:

1. What is the purpose of the exercise? (And is it important for activities of daily living or for a specific sport?)

2. Is the exercise effective for the stated purpose? (For a resistance exercise, look at the resistance applied against the primary movers.)
3. Does the exercise create any safety concerns? (Look at the major joints.)
4. Is the participant able to perform the exercise in proper alignment for the duration of the set?
5. For whom is the exercise appropriate or inappropriate?

Follow-up questions might address the risk-to-benefit ratio and whether there are any modifications that would make the exercise safer or more appropriate.

Equipment for Muscle Conditioning

A wide variety of equipment can be used in group exercise muscle conditioning. Dumbbells, elastic tubes, and resistance bands are standard in most fitness facilities, and many clubs also stock weighted bars, barbells with plates, stability balls, BOSU balance trainers, medicine balls, kettlebells, foam rollers, core boards, wobble boards, TRX, fitness circles, and more. See Figure 8.3 for some of the many equipment options and "Equipment Resources" for a list of websites. The following sections discuss the use of various types of equipment.

Dumbbells

Most health clubs and fitness centers supply several sets of dumbbells ranging from 1 to 10 pounds (0.5-4.5 kg) for use during group exercise

Equipment Resources

- www.power-systems.com
- www.gymsource.com
- www.thera-band.com
- www.optp.com
- www.spri.com
- www.amazon.com

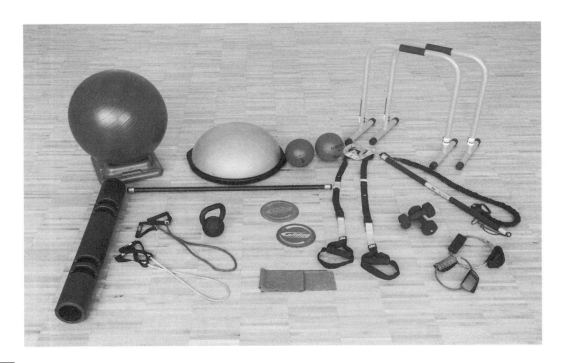

FIGURE 8.3 Some types of equipment that may be used for muscle conditioning in group exercise.

class. Dumbbells provide a practical, convenient way to overload the musculoskeletal system and can be used in a wide variety of exercises. Here are recommendations for the safe and effective use of dumbbells:

1. Do not let participants use weights until they can perform muscle conditioning exercises with proper form and technique against gravity alone; this includes being able to consciously contract the targeted muscle throughout its entire ROM. The eccentric, or lengthening, phase of the muscle action (when the weight is lowered) should be performed with awareness and care. An uncontrolled eccentric action is a primary mechanism of musculoskeletal injury (see "Common Mistakes in Weight Training").

2. Teach participants to hold the weights with a relaxed grip because lifting with tight fists may inadvertently raise blood pressure. Many participants also hold their breath and strain when clenching their fists. This action, called the Valsalva maneuver, can be potentially dangerous for people with heart disease, people with high blood pressure, and women who are pregnant. The Valsalva maneuver also increases the possibility of fainting, light-headedness, and

irregular heart rhythms. Consistently remind your students to breathe!

3. Make sure participants maintain a neutral wrist throughout all exercises, especially when holding hand weights, tubes, or bands. Repeatedly flexing or extending the wrists while holding weights or tubes increases the likelihood of developing carpal tunnel syndrome or tennis elbow.

4. Encourage participants to select a weight load that allows them to move with proper form yet still fatigues the targeted muscle group after several repetitions.

Use caution when adding hand weights to the cardio segment of class. Studies have shown that adding 1- to 2-pound (0.5-1 kg) weights to the cardio routine does not significantly increase the caloric expenditure or oxygen uptake (Blessing et al. 1987; Kravitz et al. 1997; Stanforth et al. 1993; Yoke et al. 1988). Although adding weight to cardio sessions may improve local muscle endurance, the risk-to-benefit ratio must be considered: Rapidly moving 1- to 2-pound (0.5-1 kg) hand weights while performing complex lower-body patterns offers questionable benefit while increasing the risk of injury, especially to the vulnerable shoulder joint. Upper-body

Common Mistakes in Weight Training

- Using weights that are too heavy for maintaining good form
- Failing to stabilize the core (pelvis, spine, and scapulae)
- Holding the breath (Valsalva maneuver)
- Using excessive speed or momentum, especially during the eccentric phase
- Using too much or too little range of motion

form may be compromised when the attention and focus are on footwork. We encourage you to reserve the use of weights for the time when they can provide the greatest benefit—the muscular conditioning portion of your class.

Technique and Safety Check

Teach participants how to pick up and put down their weights correctly without jeopardizing their low backs:

- Face the dumbbells with the feet shoulder-width apart. Placing one hand on the front of the thigh for support; use the other hand to reach for a dumbbell.
- Pick up the dumbbell and transfer it to the hand that is resting on the thigh. Hold the dumbbell against the thigh, continuing to lean on the thigh for support.
- Pick up the other dumbbell with your free hand. Hold this dumbbell against the other thigh and press up to standing.
- Reverse this process to put the dumbbells back on the floor.
- The idea is to always keep one hand on the thigh for support and perform a one-handed lift. This is a great method for protecting the spine when picking up objects; whenever possible, use one hand to lift the object while supporting your back by keeping the other hand on the thigh.

Barbells, Weighted Bars, and Portable Cable Column Systems

Some facilities invest in sets of barbells and weight plates for group exercise; a few facilities even invest in portable cable column systems, such as the one manufactured by Free Motion. Barbells can provide an excellent option for participants who are more advanced. However, barbells may be troublesome in a mixed-level class that includes beginners and intermediates since many of the exercises that are performed bilaterally with a barbell are more challenging because of the increased need for core stabilization. It's important that instructors provide several alternatives and modifications and be wary of continually demonstrating and exercising with barbells while in front of the group. Even when the instructor gives an easier variation, if she continues to demonstrate the more advanced version, participants are likely to copy whatever is being demonstrated even if it goes beyond their level. Examples of barbell exercises that may not be appropriate for many group exercise participants are the weight room–style back or front squat, bent-over bilateral lat row, bent-over bilateral high (horizontal) row, upright row, and deadlift. All these exercises require a high degree of core stability and body awareness for safe execution.

Additionally, participants need to be able to perform a proper weight room–style squat to safely pick up the barbell from the floor. We encourage you to reserve group barbell work for classes clearly labeled as advanced. Weighted bars, such as Body Bars, can be a good option for use in a group exercise class. Even better are portable cable columns, which some facilities have used in a controlled group exercise environment. Old racquetball courts are sometimes used for portable cable classes. Each participant has a cable column and can change weight easily and effectively in order to work at his own pace.

Elastic Resistance

Elastic bands and tubes are another option for overloading the muscular system. Many facilities stock tubing and bands in different strengths and thicknesses, allowing participants to progressively overload their exercises. Elastic resistance is different from most weighted exercise in that the tension is less at the starting position and the greatest at the end of the range of motion For instance, when participants perform a biceps curl with the tubing anchored under the foot, the tension is greatest at the top of the curl—the end range of motion (Miller et al. 2001; Stoppani 2005). In contrast, when participants perform a biceps curl with a dumbbell, the tension is greatest at the sticking point, the point where the elbow is at approximately 90° of flexion and the force

needed to overcome gravity is at its greatest. Providing a variety of exercises with both free weights and elastic resistance is an optimal way to provide overload and stimulate improvement throughout a muscle's entire ROM. Note that even more exercises can be created by combining elastic resistance with dumbbells or barbells. Figure 8.4 shows a group setup for the RIP Trainer, a type of resistance equipment that combines elastic resistance with a barbell, creating an asymmetrical pull and a multiplanar core challenge.

The following are recommendations for safe, effective band and tubing use:

1. For safety and reduced joint stress, match the line of pull with the direction of the tubing or bands. In other words, position the elastic resistance so it's in the same plane as the muscle

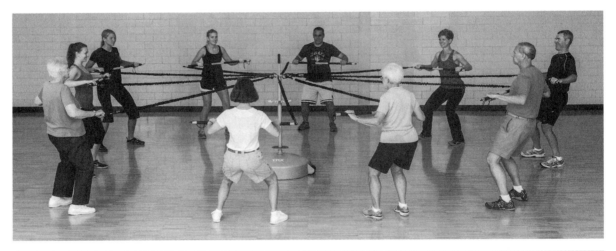

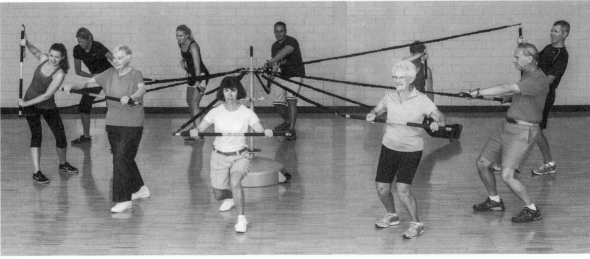

FIGURE 8.4   This RIP Trainer station can accommodate 10 exercisers at once.

action of the exercise. In a biceps curl, for example, the tubing would fall straight down from the forearm; the anchor point should be directly below, behind, or even in front of the moving arm. If the anchor point is off to the side (not in the same plane), the exercise tends to be less safe; in this case, a rotary force, or torque, is applied to the moving joints and ligaments and may lead to injury (Page and Ellenbecker 2003). However, some experts recommend multiplanar training, in which joints and muscles are challenged in more than one plane (Cressey et al. 2007). The new TRX Rip Trainer, for example, is designed to integrate rotational movements with traditional exercises, such as a squat (an exercise in the sagittal plane) performed while holding a bar attached on one end to an elastic tube. Because the pull of the tube is not symmetrical and is only on one side of the bar, a rotational or horizontal plane force is applied. As a result, significantly more core stabilization is required. Since many Rip Trainers can be attached to a central anchoring device, this type of resistance can be used in group exercise. However, we recommend this format for intermediate and advanced exercisers only, due to the skill and core stability required.

2. Adjust elastic resistance by choosing different thicknesses of bands or tubing or by having participants choke up on the tubing to shorten it. Multiple pieces of thin tubing may also be used to increase the resistance. This method has the advantage of allowing for multiple lines of pull within the plane of motion. For example, tubing can be anchored both anteriorly and posteriorly to the elbow joint in a standing biceps curl.

3. Make certain participants maintain a neutral wrist when holding tubes or bands. Have participants who have carpal tunnel syndrome check with a physician before using elastic resistance.

4. Remind participants to maintain a relaxed grip whenever possible so as not to elevate blood pressure. Using tubing with handles makes it easier to avoid a clenched fist and keep the hands relaxed.

5. Teach participants to control the eccentric (negative) phase of the exercise. Avoid the rebound effect and joint stress that occur when participants abruptly stop the contraction and let the elastic yank the joint back to its starting point.

6. Regularly inspect the tubing or bands for cracks and tears.

7. When placing tubing under a step, use tubing designed for that purpose (usually there is a nylon strip that prevents excessive rubbing and deterioration of the tubing as it contacts the step).

8. Place tubes and bands over clothing whenever possible to avoid pinching or rubbing the skin and pulling body hair.

9. Look away from the band (especially in upper-body resistance work) to protect the face in the event that the band might break.

Steps

Steps, or benches, can be used to increase or decrease the amount of resistance in a given exercise and to change the muscle-group focus. If you place the steps on risers only at one end, participants can be inclined or declined, and the exercise can be gravity assisted or gravity resisted. For example, if participants are inclined (head is higher than the hips) when performing an abdominal curl-up, the exercise becomes easier than if they were lying flat (supine). The exercise is gravity assisted. If participants are declined (head is lower than the hips), the curl-up is harder than if they were supine, and the gravitational resistance is greater (gravity resisted).

The muscle-group focus can also be altered by inclining or declining an exercise. A classic example is the bench press, an exercise that in the supine position targets the majority of the pectoralis major muscle fibers as well as the anterior deltoid. If the bench press is performed in an inclined position, anterior deltoid and clavicular pectoral involvement increases, and sternal pectoral involvement decreases. When the bench press is performed in a declined position, the reverse is true: There is increased sternal pectoral and latissimus dorsi involvement and less anterior deltoid and clavicular pectoral recruitment.

Steps are also useful props for lower-body conditioning. The lunge, squat, and single-leg step-up are all exercises that can be performed with a step. The use of a step adds variety to your muscular conditioning segment and increases the potential for individualizing your conditioning sessions and appropriately overloading your students.

Stability Balls and BOSU Balance Trainers

Large, resilient stability balls (also known as *Swiss balls* or physioballs) have been used for years by physical therapists for both strength and flexibility training. The BOSU balance trainer (*BOSU* stands for *both sides up*), on the other hand, is a relatively new device for muscle training. Stability balls are an extremely effective prop for training the core muscles (abdominals and low back) to stabilize the trunk and spine (Hahn et al. 1998; Willardson 2004). Other muscle groups can also be strengthened effectively on the stability ball and BOSU balance trainer. Studies show that core muscles are recruited to a greater extent when exercises targeting other muscle groups (e.g., the bench press for the chest and triceps) are performed on the stability ball (Marshall and Murphy 2006). In general, exercises performed using stability balls and BOSU balance trainers are more advanced than those performed without these devices because they require greater balance and thus greater recruitment of the stabilizer muscles (Cosio-Lima et al. 2001). The ball, of course, provides an unstable surface and improves balance by improving muscle reflex, proprioception, and small-muscle involvement. Depending on how the BOSU is used (dome side up or flat side up), it can also significantly challenge balance and coordination (see figure 8.5). We recommend that participants develop basic muscle strength and endurance before progressing to stability ball and BOSU exercises. Stability balls should be sized according to the participant's height or leg length and should always be inflated to the designated size (see table 8.1). Exercises using the stability ball and the BOSU are included later in this chapter.

TABLE 8.1 Stability Ball Size Recommendations

Participant height	Ball size
<60 in (<152 cm)	18 in (45 cm)
60-67 in (152-170 cm)	22 in (55 cm)
68-74 in (173-188 cm)	26 in (65 cm)
>74 in (>188 cm)	30 in (75 cm)

The knees and hips should both form 90° angles when the participant sits on the ball.

Recommendations and Guidelines for Flexibility Training

Stretching a muscle group immediately after it's been strengthened can promote a relative balance between flexibility and strength for that group. Note that, contrary to popular misconceptions, resistance training alone does not improve flexibility (Nobrega et al. 2005). Coupling a strengthening exercise with a stretching exercise ensures that you have included both aspects in your class format and optimizes the benefits of each.

Flexibility training is an integral part of any exercise session; it helps release tight muscles and can reduce the risk of injury by correcting muscle imbalances (see "Benefits of Flexibility Training"). There are several points during a group exercise class when stretching is appropriate. These include the warm-up, the cool-down after the cardio segment, the end of a resistance training exercise for a specific muscle or muscle group, and the end of class. Alternatively, learning to teach an entire class devoted to flexibility and relaxation can expand your opportunities as a group leader. If you teach your class how to release and relax each muscle, as well as how to breathe deeply and slowly to release excess tension, you'll have many grateful students!

Remember to focus on stretching the muscle groups that are relied on the most in the class you

Benefits of Flexibility Training

- Enhanced performance of daily activities
- Decreased risk of low-back pain
- Increased motor performance
- Decreased risk of injury
- Reduced muscle tension
- Increased relaxation
- Increased range of motion (ROM)
- Decreased stress and tension
- Increased mind–body connection
- Improved posture

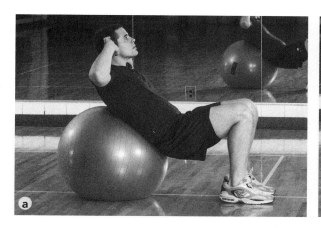
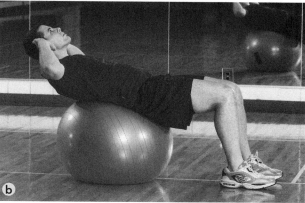
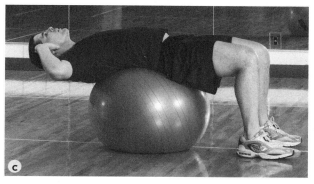
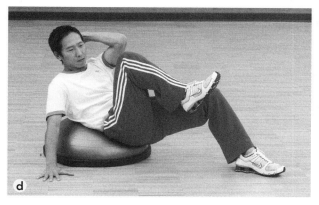
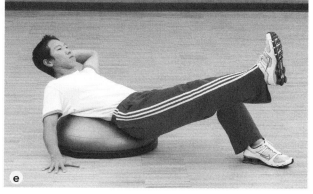

FIGURE 8.5 Curl-ups performed on a stability ball can be (*a*) inclined (gravity assisted), (*b*) parallel to the floor, and (*c*) declined (gravity resisted); they can also be done (*d-e*) with a diagonal-twist crunch (with added leg movement) for obliques on the BOSU.

teach. For instance, after teaching a stationary indoor cycling class, stretching the quadriceps, calves, and hamstrings makes sense because they are the major muscles used for cycling. After a kickboxing class, lead the participants in stretching the muscles that surround the hip and are used in kicking; it is also important to work on stretching the anterior chest muscles, which are used in punching.

Following are the ACSM (2014) guidelines for flexibility:

- Precede stretching with a warm-up to elevate muscle temperature.

- Static stretches should be held for 10 to 30 seconds for most people, with 30- to 60-second holds recommended for older adults. Stretch a minimum of 2 to 3 days per week, although daily stretching has been found to be most effective. Stretch to the point of muscle tightness without inducing discomfort. Repeat each stretch 2 to 4 times, with a total of approximately 60 seconds per muscle group.

- Deep stretching is best performed at the end of class, particularly if the class includes competitive-type exercises for strength or power.

Other stretching recommendations include the following:

- Encourage your participants to tune in and listen to their bodies. Stretching should feel good!
- Encourage muscle balance (see chapter 3).
- Encourage participants with extreme flexibility around a joint to focus on strengthening the muscles around the joint instead of working toward more mobility. Flexibility without strength can lead to injury.

The previous guidelines are for the improvement of flexibility; stretching 2 or 3 days per week has been shown to be sufficient to maintain flexibility (Rancour, Holmes, and Cipriani 2009). Note that stretches do not need to be held long in the warm-up segment; the goal of the warm-up is not to make flexibility gains but to move joints and muscles through their full ROM before vigorous activity. Studies show that static stretching during the warm-up does not necessarily reduce the risk of injury (Thacker et al. 2004).

Stretching should be comfortable. Encourage proper form by giving cues such as, "Move to the position where you can feel the muscle stretch slightly and then hold that position. You should feel the sensation of stretch but no pain. If you are shaking, reduce the intensity of your stretch." A student-centered teacher will provide options for stretching and will model average flexibility so that participants do not imitate a form they cannot safely match. As with any other fitness activity, it is important to move participants ahead appropriately and progressively. Yoga (see chapter 15) has long been touted as an activity that enhances flexibility. Be careful, however, when incorporating challenging yoga postures into your general fitness classes; these postures are meant to be practiced by advanced yoga students in a mindful setting such as an actual yoga class.

A relatively new way to elongate and relax muscles has become popular; this method involves self-myofascial release and is usually performed on foam rollers or special supple balls. Fascia is connective tissue located within and around muscles; it forms a connective web throughout the body and is thought to be a primary factor in whether or not a person is flexible (Myers 2008; Alter 2004). In self-myofascial release, flexibility is promoted by applying pressure (by lying on or over a foam roller or ball) perpendicular to the muscle fibers—this helps release any tightness in the connective tissue (see figure 8.6). Usually, when a tight spot is found while rolling, the recommendation is to hold the position for approximately 20 to 60 seconds, giving the muscles and connective tissue time to let go and relax. Some facilities provide enough foam rollers for use in group exercise, so you may want to become familiar with self-myofascial release techniques through courses or tutorials

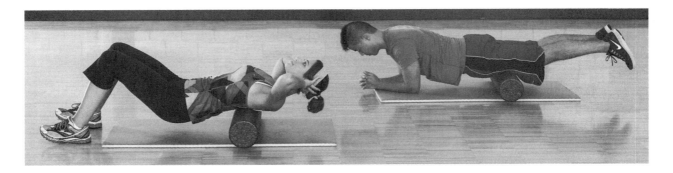

FIGURE 8.6   Use of a foam roller to provide self-massage for the erector spinae and quadriceps muscles.

(e.g., "Myofascial Release in Sports Medicine," offered through ACSM via Human Kinetics).

Cueing Flexibility Exercises and Ending a Class Appropriately

When teaching flexibility exercises, remind participants of proper alignment so you can promote overall body awareness and enhance the effectiveness of the stretching experience. Give at least 2 or 3 verbal cues for every stretch to make sure body positioning is effective. For example, when you are leading a class in the standing hamstring stretch (see figure 8.7), cue the participants to tilt the pelvis anteriorly to lengthen the hamstring muscle. Sullivan, Dejulia, and Worrell (1992) studied anterior and posterior pelvic tilt using two types of stretching techniques and found that the anterior pelvic position was the most important variable for enhancing hamstring flexibility.

The final flexibility segment of a class is the time when stretching for long-term improvement is optimal. Students are warm and psychologically ready to relax and hold a given stretch. During this segment, the focus is on providing a variety of stretches held for longer durations (15- 60 seconds each). Studies show that flexibility improvement relates to both the frequency and duration of a stretch (Bandy and Irion 1994; Feland 2000). We have found that one of the best techniques for promoting comfortable stretching that helps reduce stress is to have your students count their breaths while holding a position; have them count 3 to 5 deep, slow breaths per stretch. Suggest that they imagine that all their stress and tension (both muscular and otherwise) is draining out of their bodies with each prolonged exhalation, leaving them progressively more relaxed and refreshed. At the very end of class, it's important to end on a positive note. Remind participants of what they've accomplished and ask them how they feel. This gives them a moment to integrate and acknowledge the good feelings you and they have created; it also provides a graceful transition back to the outside world. And finishing with a sincere "thank-you for your participation today" will make them want to return!

Figuring out how to stretch a muscle is easy if you know your kinesiology (joint actions). To stretch a muscle, simply move it into the opposite position of its concentric joint action. For example, if you have just led your class members in shoulder abduction exercises such as lateral raises and overhead presses for the deltoids, you can now lead them in a stretch involving shoulder adduction, which is the opposite position from the concentric muscle-shortening action of the deltoid exercises. Once you understand this principle, you can come up with your own stretches for any muscle group (keeping in mind safety guidelines). Later in this chapter you will review standing stretches (appropriate for both the warm-up and the final flexibility segment of class) and floor stretches (generally not used during the warm-up) for each major muscle group.

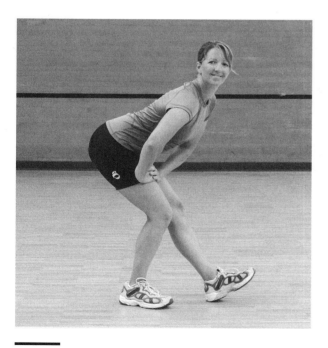

 See online video 8.2 for an example of a flexibility segment that covers the inner and outer thigh, low back, hamstrings, abdominals, quadriceps, hip flexors, upper back, neck, deltoids, triceps, and pectorals as well as breathing, relaxation, and visualization.

FIGURE 8.7 Standing hamstring stretch with anterior pelvic tilt. Instructors must always keep in mind the tenets of good alignment and use injury-prevention strategies to protect the major joints.

Safety Issues in Flexibility Training

Just as with resistance exercises, we want to consider the risk-to-benefit ratio and the issue of appropriateness when choosing stretches for our classes. For example, the hurdler's stretch is appropriate for hurdlers who are training to run hurdles in competition, but for all other groups, the benefits of the hurdler's stretch are outweighed by the risk to the medial collateral ligaments of the knee (overstretching these ligaments can lead to knee instability, which can lead to serious knee injury). Instead of using the hurdler's stretch, teach a modified version (much safer for the knees) or present a completely different hamstring stretch (see figure 8.8).

Additionally, it's important that participants take precautions when stretching. Both passive overstretching and ballistic stretching can initiate the stretch reflex. Whenever you suddenly stretch or put excessive tension on your muscle, special receptors (muscle spindles) within the muscle fibers detect the action. There is a complicated and continual interplay between opposing muscle groups that leads to precise, controlled, and coordinated movement; if a muscle is activated by a sudden stretch or is continually overstretched, then the system stimulates the muscle to contract rather than lengthen and maintains the contraction to oppose the excessive length-ening force. Simply put, if you overstretch or bounce and stretch, then the muscle shortens to protect itself. Keep pulling on a shortened muscle, and it will either cramp up or tear—but it will not lengthen. This process is often referred to as the *myotatic stretch reflex* (figure 8.9). It is an involuntary reflex that happens at the spinal cord level; we cannot mentally override it no matter how hard we try. Therefore, for most exercisers, static stretching is recommended.

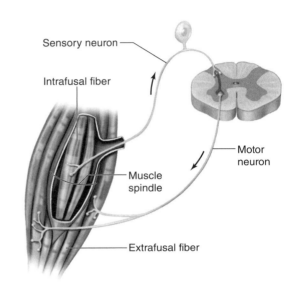

FIGURE 8.9 Special receptors are active during a strong contraction or stretch. They inhibit or facilitate contraction in order to protect the muscle.

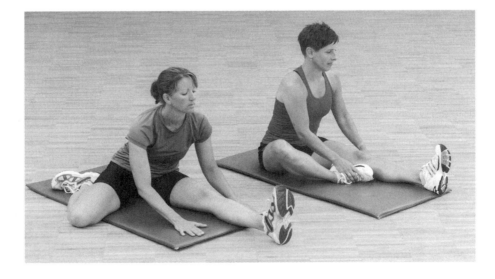

FIGURE 8.8 Avoid the hurdler's stretch (left) due to increased risk of knee injury. Instead, perform the modified version (right) that is shown here.

MUSCULAR CONDITIONING AND FLEXIBILITY EXERCISES

In this section we examine the major muscles, joint by joint. For each joint we show anatomical illustrations of each major muscle, list joint actions, and include appropriate strengthening and then stretching exercises—all with corresponding verbal cues.

Shoulder Joint and Shoulder Girdle

Figures 8.10 and 8.11 illustrate the major muscles of the shoulder joint and shoulder girdle. Tables 8.2 and 8.3 list common activities using these muscles as well as basic strengthening exercises appropriate for the group setting. Tables 8.4 and 8.5 list the shoulder joint and shoulder girdle muscles and their joint actions. Table 8.6 gives the ROM of select shoulder joint actions. The photos and descriptions that follow demonstrate muscular conditioning exercises and stretches for the shoulder joint and shoulder girdle muscles. Remember that keeping the shoulder girdle (scapular) muscles strong is very important for good posture and injury-free shoulders.

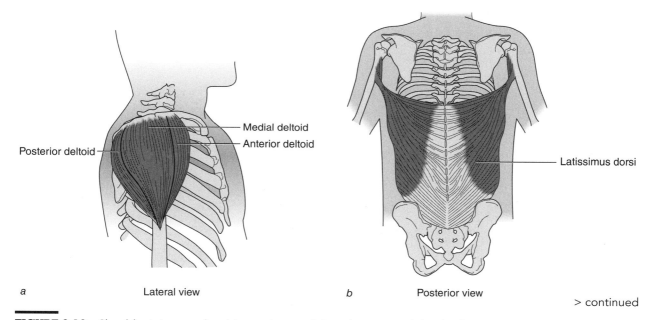

a Lateral view

b Posterior view

> continued

FIGURE 8.10 Shoulder joint muscles: (*a*) anterior, medial, and posterior deltoids; (*b*) latissimus dorsi;

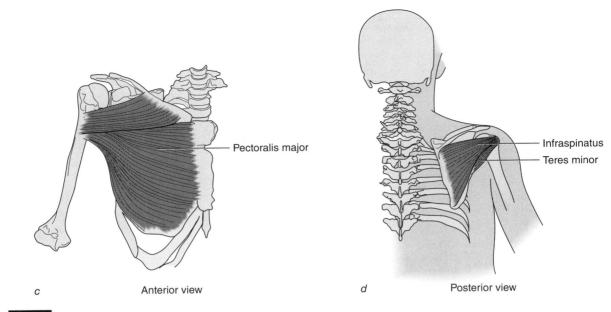

c   Anterior view   *d*   Posterior view

FIGURE 8.10 > continued   (*c*) pectoralis major; and (*d*) external rotator cuff (infraspinatus and teres minor).

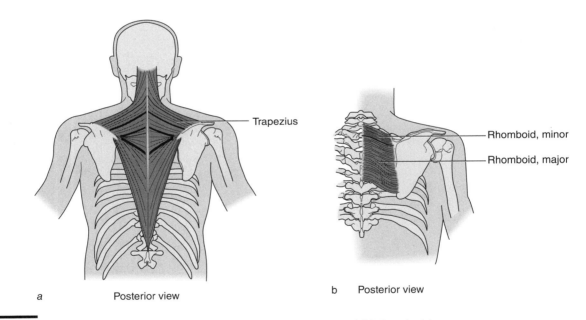

a   Posterior view   *b*   Posterior view

FIGURE 8.11   Important shoulder girdle muscles: (*a*) trapezius, and (*b*) rhomboids.

TABLE 8.2 Shoulder Joint Muscles

Muscle	Daily activities	Exercises for groups
Anterior and medial deltoid	Lifting and carrying, pushing items up overhead	Front raise, lateral raise, overhead press, upright row
Latissimus dorsi	Pulling items toward the body, lifting	Bent-over low row, bent-over shoulder extension, seated low row, unilateral adduction with tube
Pectoralis major	Pushing items in front of the body, lifting, throwing	Push-up, bench press, dumbbell fly, standing chest press with tube
Posterior deltoid (works with scapular retractors)	Pulling items toward the body, lifting	Bent-over high row, reverse fly, prone dorsal lifting, seated high row
Rotator cuff muscles (supraspinatus, subscapularis, infraspinatus, teres minor)	Opening and closing doors, stabilizing the shoulder joint	Side-lying external shoulder rotation, supine internal rotation, standing rotation with tube

TABLE 8.3 Shoulder Girdle (Scapulothoracic) Joint Muscles

Muscle	Daily activities	Exercises
Trapezius I and II	Holding phone to ear	Shrug
Trapezius III and rhomboids	Posture stabilizer	High row, reverse fly, prone dorsal lift, seated high row
Trapezius IV	Stabilizer when pushing out of a chair	Resisted depression in a dip position

TABLE 8.4 Shoulder Joint Muscles and Their Actions

Muscle	Actions
Anterior deltoid	Prime mover for shoulder flexion and shoulder horizontal adduction; assistor for shoulder abduction and internal rotation
Medial deltoid	Prime mover for shoulder abduction and shoulder horizontal abduction
Posterior deltoid	Prime mover for shoulder horizontal abduction; assistor for shoulder extension and external rotation
Latissimus dorsi	Prime mover for shoulder extension and shoulder adduction; assistor for internal rotation and horizontal abduction
Teres major	Prime mover for shoulder extension, shoulder adduction, and shoulder internal rotation; assistor for horizontal abduction
Pectoralis major, clavicular	Prime mover for shoulder horizontal adduction and shoulder flexion; assistor for shoulder internal rotation
Pectoralis major, sternal	Prime mover for shoulder horizontal adduction, shoulder adduction, and shoulder extension; assistor for internal rotation
Supraspinatus	Prime mover for shoulder abduction
Infraspinatus	Prime mover for shoulder external rotation and shoulder horizontal abduction
Teres minor	Prime mover for shoulder external rotation and shoulder horizontal abduction
Subscapularis	Prime mover for shoulder internal rotation; assistor for flexion, abduction, adduction, and horizontal adduction
Biceps and Triceps	Assistors for shoulder flexion and shoulder extension, respectively

TABLE 8.5   Shoulder Girdle (Scapulothoracic) Muscles and Their Actions

Muscle	Actions
Trapezius I	Prime mover for scapular elevation
Trapezius II	Prime mover for scapular elevation and upward rotation; assistor for retraction
Trapezius III	Prime mover for scapular retraction
Trapezius IV	Prime mover for scapular depression and upward rotation; assistor for retraction
Rhomboids	Prime mover for scapular retraction, elevation, and downward rotation
Levator scapulae	Prime mover for scapular elevation
Pectoralis minor	Prime mover for scapular depression, protraction, and downward rotation
Serratus anterior	Prime mover for scapular protraction and upward rotation

TABLE 8.6   ROM of Select Shoulder Joint Movements

Joint movement	ROM
Flexion	90°-120 °
Extension	20°-60°
Abduction	80°-100°
Horizontal abduction	30°-45°
Horizontal adduction	90°-135°
Internal rotation	70°-90°
External rotation	70°-90°

Exercises for the Deltoids

FRONT RAISE

Anterior deltoid, clavicular pectoralis major (shoulder flexion)

CUES   Stand (or sit on a step or stability ball) with feet shoulder-width apart; knees slightly bent; and neck, spine, and pelvis in neutral. Elbows are straight but not hyperextended. Shoulder blades are down and slightly retracted (neutral position). Wrists are straight throughout. Palms are down (pronated). Keep torso stable while flexing shoulders to about shoulder height (90°). Avoid momentum.

FYI   Consider limiting the use of this exercise when leading a group. The reason is that everyday activities (and high-low and step classes) challenge the anterior muscles much more frequently than they challenge the posterior muscles. Dumbbells, barbell, or tubing may be used for resistance. This exercise may be performed bilaterally or unilaterally; the unilateral version is safer for the back.

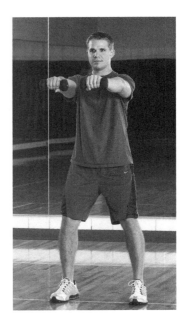

LATERAL RAISE

Medial deltoid, supraspinatus (shoulder abduction)

CUES Stand (or sit on a step or stability ball) with the feet shoulder-width apart and the knees slightly flexed. Maintain the neck, spine, and pelvis in neutral. In addition, keep the scapulae neutral (down and slightly retracted). Wrists should also be neutral (neither flexed nor extended). Elbows may be bent at 90° for a short-lever variation or flexed at about 15° (so that arms are nearly straight) for the more traditional long-lever version (using the long lever is more difficult). Palms face the sides (midpronated position) at the start of the exercise and maintain this position throughout, thumbs facing straight ahead. As the shoulders abduct, they stay in partial internal rotation, lifting to no more than 90°. At the end of the movement, the shoulders are slightly higher than the elbows, which are slightly higher than the wrists.

FYI During this exercise it is particularly important to avoid momentum and bringing the arms higher than the shoulders (they should not abduct any higher than 90°). Both of these actions can cause shoulder impingement. Lateral raises can be performed with dumbbells or tubing for added resistance.

OVERHEAD PRESS

Medial and anterior deltoids, supraspinatus, triceps (shoulder abduction, elbow extension)

CUES Stand (or sit on bench or stability ball) with feet shoulder-width apart for stability. Knees are soft; spine, neck, and pelvis are in neutral. The shoulder girdle is down and slightly retracted (neutral). Start in the down position, holding the dumbbells at shoulder level with the palms facing forward (pronated) and the hands slightly wider than the shoulders. When pressing up, straighten but do not lock (hyperextend) the elbows. Keep the chest lifted and avoid leaning backward.

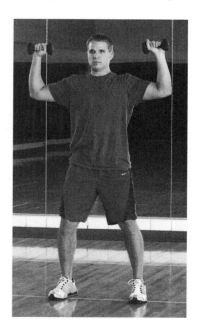

FYI This exercise can be performed with dumbbells, barbell, or tubing for added resistance. The press should be performed in front of the head to minimize injury to the shoulder joint; the behind-the-neck press has become controversial because of the vulnerable shoulder position and the increased risk of injury from external rotation behind the frontal plane. This exercise may be performed unilaterally or bilaterally.

UPRIGHT ROW

Medial and anterior deltoids, supraspinatus, biceps brachii (shoulder abduction, elbow flexion)
Optional: upper trapezius, rhomboids, and levator scapulae (scapular elevation)

CUES (*a*) Stand with feet shoulder-width apart, knees flexed, and spine, neck, and pelvis in neutral. Hands are pronated (overhand grip) and 6 to 8 inches (15-20 cm) apart. (*b*) Lead with the elbows (not the wrists) and do not lift the elbows above the shoulders. Keep wrists as neutral as possible (watch for the tendency to flex the wrists, which increases the risk of wrist and elbow injuries). Avoid momentum.

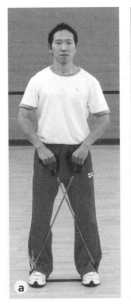
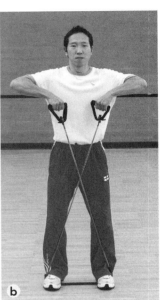

FYI The upright row has become somewhat controversial due to concerns about shoulder joint injury. Because the exercise is performed while the shoulders are internally rotated, it is very important that the elbows do not come higher than the shoulders (no more than 90° of abduction) because of the risk of shoulder joint impingement. Even though the traditional variation of the upright row includes shoulder girdle elevation, we do not recommend this for the general public or for group exercise. From a functional training perspective, most fitness and health exercisers need to strengthen the muscles required to keep the scapulae down, not up. Therefore, scapular elevation can be considered an optional movement in an upright row. This exercise may be performed with dumbbells, barbell, or tubing for added resistance.

DELTOID STRETCHES

Anterior, medial, and posterior deltoids

CUES

Variation 1

(*a*) To stretch the medial and anterior deltoids, stand in ideal standing alignment and bend one elbow behind your body. Gently press your arm across and toward the back of your body. Try tilting your head to the opposite side for a great stretch of the side of your neck (upper trapezius).

Variation 2

(*b*) To stretch the medial and posterior deltoids, stand with your feet shoulder-width apart; knees slightly flexed; and pelvis, spine, and neck in neutral. Keep your shoulder blades down and maintain a large space between shoulders and ears. Gently press your arm across the body and in toward the torso.

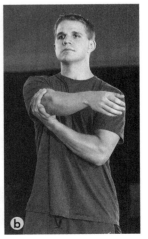

FYI These stretches may also be performed in a seated position.

Exercises for the Latissimus Dorsi

BENT-OVER ROW

**Latissimus dorsi, teres major, posterior deltoid, biceps brachii
(shoulder extension, elbow flexion)**

NOTE The middle trapezius and rhomboids are strong stabilizers for this exercise because of their antigravity position. If the exercise is performed bilaterally, the erector spinae and abdominals are also important stabilizers of the spine.

CUES (a) Stand with the feet staggered, front knee bent, and the nonworking hand placed on the front thigh for support. All joints face the same direction, with the hips and shoulders evenly squared and level. Ideally, one long line is created from the back heel to the top of the head. The spine is in neutral, with no rounding or hunching of the upper back. The neck continues the line of the spine with no ducking toward the weight. (b) During the lift, keep scapulae stabilized in neutral; do not protract or retract with the exercise. The only moving joints are the working-side shoulder and elbow; keep all else still. The moving arm brushes against the rib cage. Avoid rotating the spine when lifting the weight. Keep shoulders level throughout.

FYI This exercise is one of the best choices for working the latissimus dorsi in group exercise; we recommend performing it unilaterally when in a group. Although the bilateral version is excellent, it is quite unlikely that every student in a group class will be able to correctly stabilize the spine and maintain proper alignment for the bilateral version. This exercise may be performed with dumbbells or tubing or, for advanced participants, both. Another variation is long-lever shoulder extension with the elbow held straight.

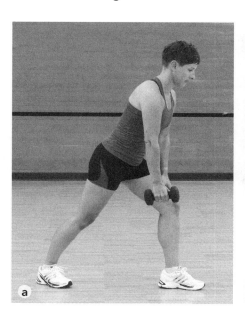
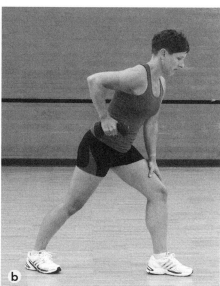

SEATED LOW ROW

Latissimus dorsi, teres major, sternal pectoralis major, posterior deltoid, biceps brachii
(shoulder extension, elbow flexion)

CUES (a) Sit on the floor (or step) and bend knees slightly to ensure that the pelvis and spine are aligned directly over the sitting bones (ischial tuberosities). Hold the spine erect and tall, maintaining neutral alignment throughout. Keep the neck in line with the spine and the scapulae down and away from the ears. (b) Move the arms through the sagittal plane, keeping the upper arms close to the rib cage. Hold the handles of the tubing in a midpronated position (palms face each other). Move only the shoulders and elbows; keep the low back still.

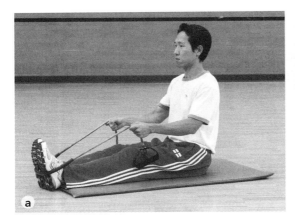 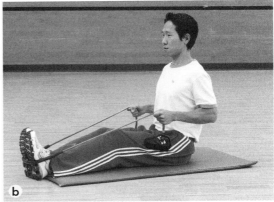

UNILATERAL LAT PULL-DOWN

Latissimus dorsi, teres major, sternal pectoralis major, biceps brachii
(shoulder adduction, elbow flexion)

CUES (a) Stand with feet shoulder-width apart for stability. Spine, neck, and pelvis are in neutral. Grasp the elastic tubing or band with one hand, keeping it anchored overhead. (b) Perform the pull-down with the other hand, keeping the shoulder blades down and the head high. Release the tubing or band upward slowly, with control.

FYI Without a high pulley (found in most weight rooms), the only way to make this exercise effective in the group setting is to use elastic resistance. Although some instructors try to duplicate the pull-down exercise with dumbbells, the muscles actually resisting gravity's pull when holding free weights are the deltoids, not the latissimi dorsi.

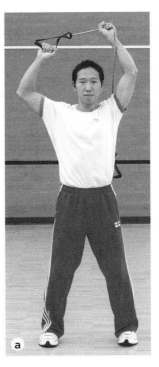 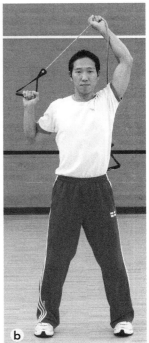

LATISSIMUS DORSI STRETCHES

CUES

Variation 1
(a) Stand with feet shoulder-width apart, knees bent, and pelvis tucked under (posterior pelvic tilt). Curve (flex) the spine, pull the abdominals in, and reach one arm up and out in front, allowing the upper back to round and curve slightly to one side to increase the lengthened feeling through the latissimus dorsi. Keep the opposite hand on the thigh to support the low back.

Variation 2
(b) Stand with feet shoulder-width apart; knees slightly bent; and pelvis, spine, and neck in neutral. Place one hand on the outer thigh and reach the other hand overhead. Lengthen along your side as you lift up your hand, separating the ribs from the hip; perform a comfortable, gradual side bend, allowing the neck to continue the line of the spine. Leave the opposite hand on the thigh to help support the low back.

FYI These stretches may be performed in a seated position.

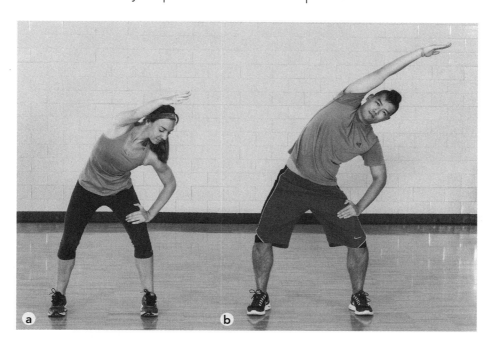

Exercises for the Pectoralis Major

CHEST FLY

Pectoralis major, anterior deltoid (shoulder horizontal adduction)

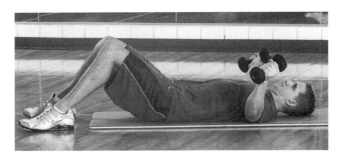

CUES   Lie supine, with the feet flat on the floor or bench and the knees bent. Keep the neck, spine, and pelvis in neutral alignment. Start in the up position with the elbows just slightly flexed. Palms can be pronated or midpronated (facing each other). Moving only the shoulder joints, stabilize the elbows, wrists, scapulae, spine, and pelvis. Lower the arms out to the sides until the upper arms are parallel with the chest, being especially careful not to exceed the appropriate end ROM, which can lead to shoulder injury.

FYI   This exercise is performed with dumbbells and can be inclined or declined on a step. Another variation is the short-lever fly, or pec dec, in which the elbows are flexed at a 90° angle.

BENCH OR CHEST PRESS

**Pectoralis major, anterior deltoid, triceps
(shoulder horizontal adduction, elbow extension)**

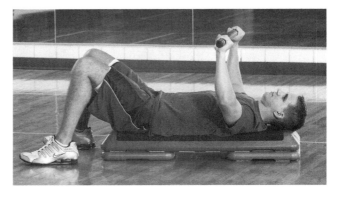

CUES   Lie supine on the floor or bench with the knees bent and the feet on the floor. Keep the spine, neck, and pelvis in neutral and the abdominals engaged. Use a wide, pronated grip. Stabilize all joints, including the scapulae, wrists, and spine, while the shoulders and elbows move. Angle the upper arm 80° to 90° out from the torso; forearms are perpendicular to the floor. Keep the movement slow and controlled, avoiding a sudden descent. If on a step avoid letting the elbows drop too far below the bench, as doing so increases the shoulder joint stress. Avoid rolling the wrist, arching the back, and hyperextending the elbows.

FYI   The narrower the grip, the more the triceps are involved and the less the chest is involved. This exercise can be performed with dumbbells or a bar and may be inclined or declined on a step. Performing this exercise while lying supine on the floor hinders the ROM—the floor gets in the way of the movement.

PUSH-UP

Pectoralis major, anterior deltoid, triceps
(shoulder horizontal adduction, elbow extension)

NOTE There are several important stabilizers used for this exercise—the abdominals, erector spinae, gluteus maximus, trapezius, rhomboids, serratus anterior, and pectoralis minor.

CUES Keep the head, neck, spine, and pelvis in neutral. The head and neck continue the line of the spine. In all positions except tabletop, the hips are in neutral as well (in the tabletop position, the hips are flexed at 90°). The fingers point straight ahead to minimize wrist stress; the hands are slightly wider than the shoulders, and the upper arms are perpendicular to the torso (in the horizontal plane). The only moving joints are the shoulders and elbows; all other joints are stabilized, which is important for injury prevention. Avoid sagging through the back, hyperextending the elbows, or hyperextending the cervical vertebrae. Exhale on the way up.

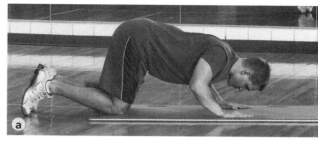

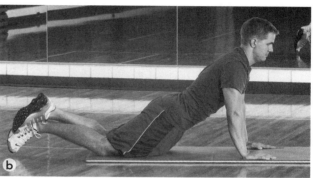

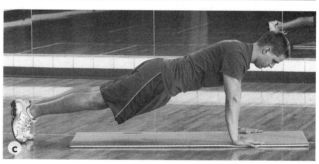

Variations
There are many pushup variations. Here are a few, listed from easiest to hardest wall push-up, (*a*) tabletop push-up, knee (intermediate) push-up with hands on step, (*b*) knee push-up with hands on floor, knee push-up with knees on step and hands on floor (decline), full-body push-up with hands on step, (*c*) full-body push-up with hands on floor, full-body push-up with feet on step, and full-body push-up on one leg.

FYI Push-ups are a good option for chest work in the group setting. Always show at least three variations to accommodate varying ability levels. The closer the elbows are to the ribs, the more the exercise becomes a triceps push-up and the less it challenges the chest muscles.

STANDING CHEST PRESS

Pectoralis major, anterior deltoid, triceps
(shoulder horizontal adduction, elbow extension)

CUES   (a) Stand with feet parallel and shoulder-width apart or staggered and hip-width apart. Loop elastic tube or band around a ballet barre or hook (or use a partner) and face away from the barre, grasping the ends of the tube or band in the hands with the elastic under the arms. Place spine, neck, pelvis, scapulae, and wrists in neutral; contract abdominals. (b) Moving only the shoulders and elbows, exhale and press directly away from the anchor point of the tubing. Stabilize the entire torso throughout the movement.

FYI   For an ideal line of pull and optimal muscle recruitment, anchor the tube or band on a stationary object behind the body; wrapping the elastic behind the back instead of anchoring it reduces the exercise effectiveness. (Alternatively, loop two bands around each other as in the partner exercise shown) Traditional standing chest exercises with dumbbells are not effective choices because gravity does not directly oppose the muscle action. The muscles holding the arms up against gravity are the deltoids; the chest muscles actually do very little work.

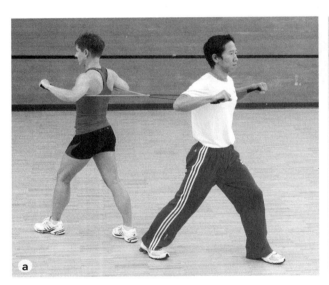
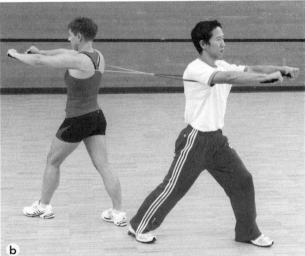

PECTORALIS MAJOR STRETCHES

CUES

Variation 1

(*a*) Stand with the feet hip-width or shoulder-width apart; knees soft; and pelvis, spine, and neck in neutral. Bring your arms behind your body, clasping the hands together if possible (although this is not essential). Keep the shoulders down and abdominals contracted; avoid arching the low back. Hold a towel or strap if desired to help increase the stretch.

Variation 2

(*b*) Stand with the feet shoulder-width apart; knees soft; and pelvis, spine, and neck in neutral alignment. Place the hands behind the ears with the elbows high and shoulders down, and gently open the elbows toward the back while lifting and opening the chest. Feel the shoulder blades scrunch together in the back as the chest muscles stretch.

FYI These stretches may be performed in the seated position.

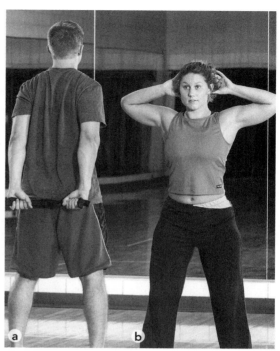

Exercises for the Middle Trapezius, Rhomboids, and Posterior Deltoids

PRONE SCAPULAR RETRACTION (PRONE DORSAL LIFT)

**Middle trapezius, rhomboids, posterior deltoids
(scapular retraction, shoulder horizontal abduction)**

CUES Lie prone on the floor (or on a step) with the forehead down and the neck in line with the spine. Place arms on the floor with the upper arms at a 90° angle to the torso and the elbows flexed at 90°. Place palms down on the floor. Retract the scapulae, pulling the shoulder blades toward each other. Keep your forehead on the floor and your neck and spine in neutral. Be sure to lift the elbows up toward the ceiling, not back toward the hips.

FYI This exercise requires no equipment other than a mat and can make a great superset when alternated with sets of push-ups. Most participants will have a small ROM in this position and will be unable to lift much more than the weight of their arms. Even so, prone scapular retraction is an excellent exercise for posture correction and education.

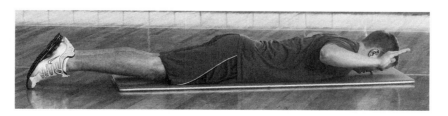

SEATED HIGH (HORIZONTAL) ROW

**Middle trapezius, rhomboids, posterior deltoids, biceps brachii
(scapular retraction, shoulder horizontal abduction, elbow flexion)**

CUES (a) Sit on the floor with the hips flexed at 90° and the spine and neck in neutral. Keep the knees slightly bent to help keep the torso aligned over the sitting bones. Wrap the elastic tubing around the feet and grasp the handles with palms down (pronated). Start with the elbows extended and the arms in the horizontal plane in front of the chest. (b) Row the elbows back (keeping them in the horizontal plane, parallel to the floor) and consciously retract the shoulder blades. Keep the wrists straight and avoid rocking the lower spine.

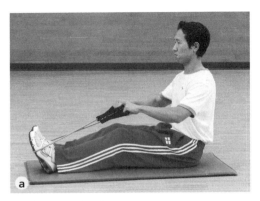

FYI Do not confuse this exercise with a low row, which targets the latissimus dorsi. In a high row, the arms are held up in the horizontal plane just slightly below the shoulders. Perform a standard row, or, for variety, try a 4-count row: pull back on 1, retract the shoulder blades on 2, release the shoulder blades on 3, and release the row on 4.

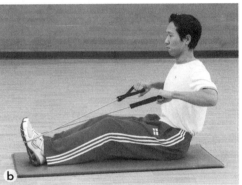

UNILATERAL REVERSE FLY

**Middle trapezius, rhomboids, posterior deltoid
(scapular retraction, shoulder horizontal abduction)**

CUES Choose whichever standing bent-over position feels the most comfortable: feet shoulder-width apart and parallel with one hand on the thigh or feet staggered with one hand on the front thigh. Square the hips and shoulders and place the spine and neck in neutral alignment. Press the shoulders and shoulder girdle down, away from the ears. With the working arm perpendicular to the torso, lift that arm backward toward the ceiling, finishing the move with the scapula moving toward the spine (retraction). Only the scapula and shoulder joint move; the spine, neck, hips, elbow, and wrist remain perfectly still. Consciously contract the rear deltoid, middle trapezius, and rhomboids.

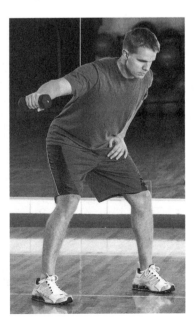

FYI This exercise may be performed with dumbbells, band, or tube for resistance. Bilateral bent-over reverse flys are not recommended for most group exercise classes. Most participants are unable to properly stabilize the torso and maintain strongly contracted abdominal and erector spinae muscles when working bilaterally. Bent-over movements performed unilaterally with one hand on the thigh to support the spine are much less risky. This exercise may also be performed in the half-kneeling position or prone on a step.

UNILATERAL BENT-OVER HIGH ROW

Middle trapezius, rhomboids, posterior deltoid, biceps brachii
(scapular retraction, shoulder horizontal abduction, elbow flexion)

CUES   Choose whichever standing bent-over position feels the most comfortable: feet shoulder-width apart and parallel with one hand on thigh or feet staggered with one hand on the front thigh. Square the hips and shoulders and place the spine and neck in neutral alignment. Press the shoulders and shoulder girdle down, away from the ears. With the working arm perpendicular to the torso, lift the elbow of that arm backward toward ceiling, finishing the move with the scapula moving toward the spine (retraction). Only the scapula, shoulder joint, and elbow move; the spine, neck, hips, and wrist remain perfectly still. Consciously contract the rear deltoid, middle trapezius, and rhomboids.

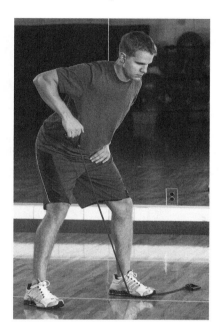

FYI   This exercise may be performed with dumbbells, barbell, band, or tubing for resistance. Do not confuse this exercise with a low row, which targets the latissimus dorsi. In a high row, the arms are held in the horizontal plane just slightly below the shoulders. For variety, try a 4-count row: Pull back on 1, retract the shoulder blade on 2, release the shoulder blade on 3, and release the row and return to start on 4. Again, be very cautious with bilateral bent-over high rows in the group setting; most participants have difficulty stabilizing the torso when moving bilaterally in the bent-over position.

TRAPEZIUS STRETCHES

CUES

Variation 1

(*a*) To stretch the upper trapezius, stand in ideal standing alignment and gently tip the head forward (cervical spinal flexion), moving the chin toward the chest. Do not allow the upper back to round forward; this stretch is only for the neck. If desired, the hands can rest lightly on the top of the head; do not pull. Experiment with slightly and carefully tipping your head diagonally (in the direction of your left little toe and then your right little toe) to release neck and shoulder tension.

Variation 2

(*b*) To stretch the upper trapezius, stand with feet shoulder-width apart, knees soft, and pelvis and spine in neutral. Consciously press the shoulder blades down. Tilt the head sideways (lateral flexion) to the left and feel a comfortable stretch on the right side of your neck. If you like, gently rest your left hand on your head to increase the stretch sensation (do not pull). Repeat on the other side.

Variation 3

(*c*) To stretch the middle trapezius and rhomboids, stand with the knees flexed, pelvis slightly tucked under (posterior pelvic tilt), back rounded and flexed, and hands clasped together directly in front of your chest. Allow the shoulder blades to come apart as far as possible. Contract the abdominals, bringing navel to spine, and allow your head to gently continue the line of the spine. Maintain your upper body over your hips (avoid unsupported forward spinal flexion).

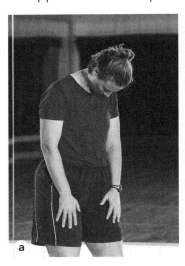 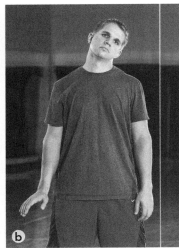 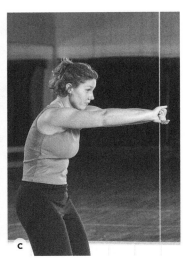

a b c

Exercises for the External Rotators

STANDING SHOULDER EXTERNAL ROTATION

Infraspinatus, teres minor (shoulder external rotation)

CUES Stand with the feet shoulder-width apart and the spine, neck, and pelvis in neutral. Keep the shoulder blades down and slightly retracted (neutral scapulae). Anchor the tube by holding it on the opposite hip with the nonworking hand. On the working side, flex the elbow to 90° and grasp the tube or band. Hold the upper arm close to the side of the body and move the forearm to the side, externally rotating the shoulder joint (as if you were opening a door). Keep your forearm parallel to the floor and maintain a neutral wrist. Move slowly and with control.

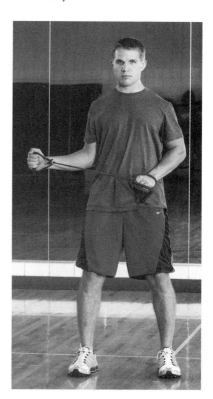

FYI Strengthening the external rotator cuff is important to counteract the large forces generated by the powerful internal rotator muscles of the shoulder. These muscles include the subscapularis, teres major, pectoralis major, anterior deltoids, latissimus dorsi, and biceps brachii. Strong external rotator muscles help maintain proper function of the shoulder joint and decrease the risk of injury. We recommend occasionally incorporating this exercise into your class.

Shoulder Joint and Shoulder Girdle

Elbow Joint

The major muscles of the elbow joint are illustrated in figure 8.12. Table 8.7 lists the common activities that use these muscles as well as basic strengthening exercises for these muscles. Table 8.8 lists the elbow and radioulnar joint muscles and their joint actions. Table 8.9 lists the ROM of the elbow and radioulnar joints. The photos and descriptions that follow demonstrate exercises and stretches for the elbow joint.

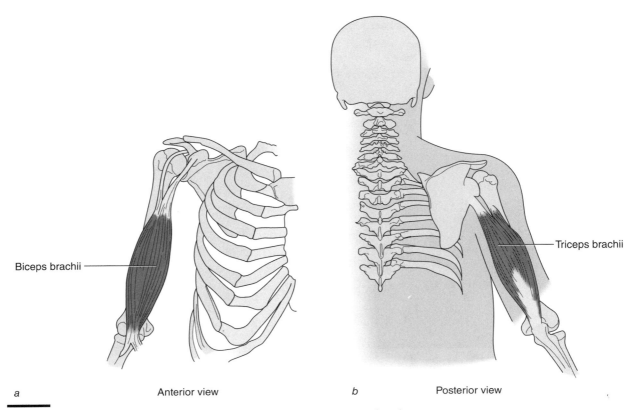

Biceps brachii

Triceps brachii

a   Anterior view   *b*   Posterior view

FIGURE 8.12 Elbow joint muscles: (*a*) biceps brachii and (*b*) triceps brachii.

TABLE 8.7   Elbow Joint Muscles

Muscle	Daily activities	Exercises
Biceps brachii, brachialis, brachioradialis	Carrying, lifting	Biceps curl, concentration curl, hammer curl, reverse curl
Triceps brachii	Getting in and out of chairs, throwing balls	Dip, kickback, press-down with tube, supine elbow extension

TABLE 8.8 Elbow and Radioulnar Joint Muscles and Their Actions

Muscle	Actions
Biceps brachii	Prime mover for elbow flexion; assistor for radioulnar supination
Brachialis	Prime mover for elbow flexion
Brachioradialis	Prime mover for elbow flexion; assistor for both radioulnar pronation and supination
Pronator teres	Assistor for elbow flexion and radioulnar pronation
Pronator quadratus	Prime mover for radioulnar pronation
Triceps brachii	Prime mover for elbow extension
Anconeus	Assistor mover for elbow extension
Supinator	Prime mover for radioulnar supination
Flexor carpi radialis	Assistor for elbow flexion and radioulnar pronation
Flexor carpi ulnaris	Assistor for elbow flexion
Extensor carpi radialis longus	Assistor for elbow extension and radioulnar supination
Extensor carpi ulnaris	Assistor for elbow extension

TABLE 8.9 ROM of Elbow and Radioulnar Joint Movements

Joint movement	ROM
Flexion	135°-160°
Supination	75°-90°
Pronation	75°-90°

Exercises for the Biceps Brachii

ALTERNATING DUMBBELL BICEPS CURL

Biceps brachii, brachialis, brachioradialis (elbow flexion)
Optional: supinator (radioulnar joint supination)

CUES Stand with the feet shoulder-width apart; the knees flexed; and the spine, neck, and pelvis in neutral. Press the shoulders down and slightly back (neutral scapulae). Hold the upper arms close to the ribs (shoulder joints are neutral), palms facing the outer thighs. Curl one arm and then the other, smoothly supinating the palms (turning the palms face up) at the end ROM. Keep hands as relaxed as possible, maintaining tension in the biceps. Wrists stay completely neutral (no active wrist flexion or extension). Control the movement on the way down, avoiding elbow hyperextension. Return the palms to the midpronated position (facing the thighs) on the way down.

FYI This exercise may be performed while standing or while seated on a step. Barbell, dumbbells, or tubing may be used for resistance. Supinating the wrist (turning the palms face up) at the end of the lift is optional. Other variations include maintaining supination throughout and performing the exercise bilaterally, without alternation.

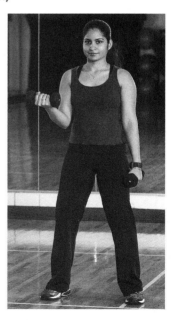

The hammer curl (palms stay in midpronated position throughout the movement) and reverse curl (palms are pronated and facing down throughout the movement) are additional exercises that challenge the biceps, brachialis, and brachioradialis.

CONCENTRATION CURL

Biceps brachii, brachialis, brachioradialis (elbow flexion)

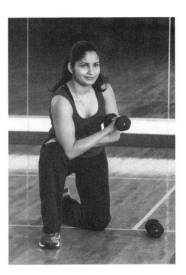

CUES   Kneel, placing one knee on the floor. Rest the opposite foot on the floor so that knee is bent at 90°. Place the elbow of the working arm slightly inside the thigh of the bent leg and place the opposite hand behind the elbow for support. Hinge forward from the hips, maintaining a neutral spine and neck and keeping the shoulders down. Flex the elbow, lifting the weight diagonally across the body; keep the wrist neutral. Slowly return to the starting position, keeping the elbow from locking (hyperextending).

FYI   This exercise may also be performed while seated on a step.

BICEPS STRETCHES

CUES

Variation 1

(*a*) Stand with the feet shoulder-width apart; the knees soft; and the pelvis, spine, neck, and scapulae in neutral. Hold one arm out in front of your body (shoulder flexion), elbow straight, and use your other hand to gently support the wrist, extending your wrist if desired.

Variation 2

(*b*) Stand in the same alignment; reach your arms behind your body with your elbows extended

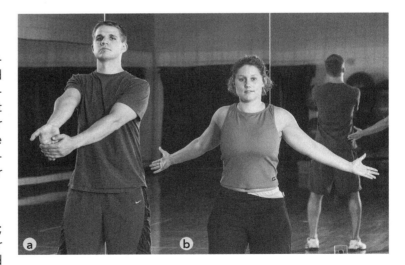

and shoulders externally rotated; your palms should face forward and up (thumbs up). Allow the biceps muscles to lengthen.

 See online video 8.3 for muscular conditioning exercises and progression options for the biceps.

Exercises for the Triceps Brachii

SUPINE TRICEPS EXTENSION

Triceps brachii (elbow extension)

CUES   Lie supine on the floor or on a step. Keep the knees bent, the spine and neck in neutral, and the abdominals contracted. Flexing the shoulder of the working arm, point the elbow straight up toward the ceiling; your hand should be near the side of your head. Smoothly extend the elbow to lift the dumbbell, contracting the triceps. Without flaring the elbow, carefully lower the dumbbell back to the starting position. Keep the upper arm still throughout the movement.

FYI   This exercise may be performed unilaterally, which is the easiest variation. It may also be performed bilaterally by holding a dumbbell in each hand, by holding a single dumbbell in both hands, or by holding a barbell (this last variation is the most challenging).

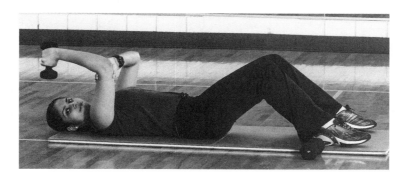

TRICEPS PRESS-DOWN WITH TUBE

Triceps brachii (elbow extension)

CUES   Stand with the feet shoulder-width apart and the spine, pelvis, and neck in neutral. Contract the abdominals and press the shoulders down. Holding one end of the tube or band in the working-side hand, use the other hand to anchor the tube or band to the working-side shoulder. Extend the elbow so that the working arm presses straight down. Straighten the elbow without hyperextending it and keep the wrists as neutral as possible. Control the motion on the way up (eccentric phase), maintaining a conscious muscle contraction.

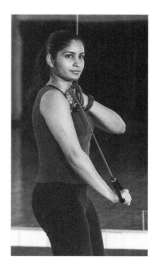

TRICEPS KICKBACK

Triceps brachii (elbow extension)

CUES (*a*) Stand in a bent-over position with the feet staggered and all joints pointing in the same direction; keep the hips and shoulders squared. Place the nonworking hand on the same-side thigh for low-back support. Place the spine and neck in neutral and pull the abdominals in; be sure the shoulders are pressed down, and the scapulae are neutral. Bring the working arm up so that the upper arm is parallel to the floor (shoulder stays down). (*b*) With control and conscious muscle contraction, straighten the elbow without hyperextending it. Maintain a neutral wrist.

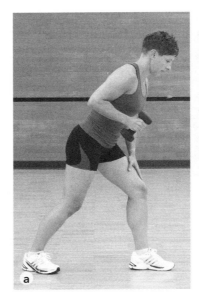

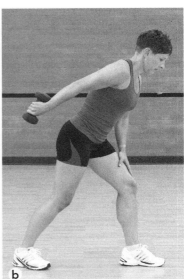

FYI Although this exercise may be performed bilaterally, we don't recommend doing so in the average group fitness class. Most students are unable to assume the proper bent-over position with a neutral spine and correct alignment; in addition, sufficient core stability is critical for low-back protection. Performing the exercise unilaterally is a fine modification for almost everyone. Kickbacks can also be performed in the half-kneeling position. Common mistakes when performing the kickback include rotating the spine, hunching the shoulders, locking the elbow, and using momentum.

FRENCH PRESS (OVERHEAD PRESS FOR TRICEPS)

Triceps brachii (elbow extension)

CUES Stand (or sit on a step) with the knees soft; the pelvis, spine, and neck in neutral; and the abdominals contracted. Point the working elbow straight up to the ceiling; the working forearm should be behind the head. Support the upper arm with the opposite hand. Smoothly, maintaining careful control, move the weight straight up toward the ceiling and carefully lower it back behind the head. Hold your head high and maintain a perfectly neutral neck throughout the exercise, keeping your elbow next to your head.

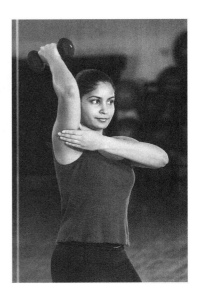

FYI This exercise is difficult for participants with tight shoulder muscles or excessive kyphosis. If proper alignment is difficult or impossible, suggest a different triceps exercise (such as a press-down or kickback) that participants can perform more safely. The French press may be performed bilaterally, but doing so is especially inappropriate for those with poor upper-body flexibility.

TRICEPS DIP

Triceps brachii (elbow extension)

CUES Place your hands on the floor or step with the fingers pointing forward. Suspend your buttocks off the floor or step, supporting your body weight on your hands. Press the shoulder blades down and away from the ears, lengthening the neck. Stabilize the lower body and avoid moving the legs and hips. The elbow joint should be the only moving joint. Straighten and flex the elbows, keeping them close to the sides of the body. Avoid hyperextending the elbows as you straighten them.

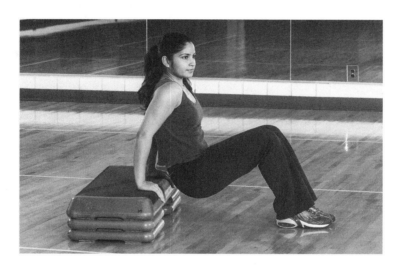

FYI This is an advanced exercise. Even the beginner version (seated with the hands behind the buttocks) demands heightened body awareness. Avoid flexing the elbows more than 90° and extending the shoulder joints too far back (avoid dips that are too deep) as doing so increases the risk of shoulder joint injury. A dip progression, listed from easiest to hardest, is as follows: dip while seated on the floor, dip on floor with buttocks lifted, dip with hands on step, dip with hands on step and feet on another step, and dip with hands on a stability ball.

TRICEPS STRETCHES

CUES

Variation 1

(*a*) Stand with feet shoulder-width apart, knees flexed, tailbone pointing straight down, abdominals in, and spine in neutral. Point one elbow toward the ceiling and reach that hand down your back. Gently support the stretch by placing your other hand on either your upper arm or elbow. Keep the head and neck in alignment; avoid hunching the shoulders or hanging the head forward. Keep the shoulders down and away from the ears.

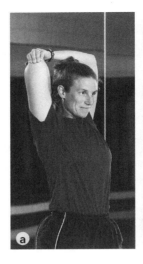
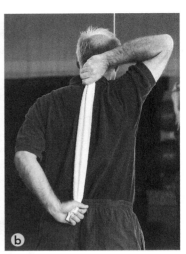

Variation 2

(*b*) For a more intense triceps stretch that also stretches the anterior deltoids and the external rotators on the opposite side, stand in the same ideal alignment, again pointing one elbow toward the ceiling so that hand reaches down the back. Reach the opposite hand behind the back, bringing it up along the spine so that it is reaching toward the other hand. Use a towel or strap to help move the hands toward each other and deepen the stretch.

FYI

This stretch can identify dramatic muscle imbalances between the right and the left sides. Many people will have one side that is noticeably tighter than the other—keep stretching! Try not to force this stretch, particularly on the side with the elbow pointing down toward the floor; the weaker external rotator cuff muscles are already in a strong stretch on this side, and injuries may easily occur when trying to force the stretch deeper. Release from the stretch gradually.

 See online video 8.4 for muscular conditioning exercises and progression options for the triceps.

Spinal Joints and Torso Muscles

The major muscles of the torso are illustrated in figure 8.13. Table 8.10 lists muscles of the spinal joints, activities that use these muscles, and basic strengthening exercises for these muscles. Table 8.11 lists the spinal joint muscles and their joint actions. Table 8.12 gives the ROM of various spinal movements. The photos and descriptions that follow show muscular conditioning exercises and stretches for the spinal joint muscles.

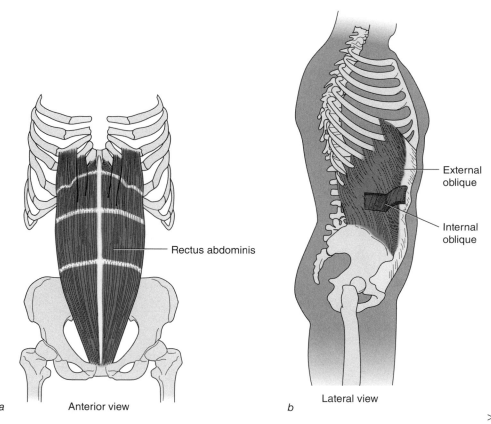

a Anterior view

Rectus abdominis

External oblique

Internal oblique

b Lateral view

> continued

FIGURE 8.13 Spinal muscles: (*a*) rectus abdominis, (*b*) internal and external obliques,

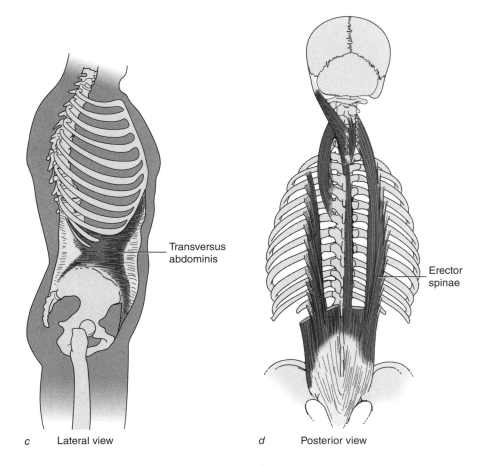

c   Lateral view   d   Posterior view

FIGURE 8.13 > continued   (c) transverse abdominis, and (d) erector spinae.

TABLE 8.10 Spinal Joint Muscles

Muscle	Daily activities	Exercises
Rectus abdominis	Getting out of bed, posture maintenance	Crunch, pelvic tilt, hip lift
Internal and external obliques	Bending sideways to pick something up, maintaining posture	Diagonal twist crunch
Transverse abdominis	Laughing, coughing, maintaining posture	Hollowing in plank, crunch, Pilates exercises, quadruped
Erector spinae	Bending forward to pick something up, maintaining posture	Prone extension, quadruped

TABLE 8.11   Spinal Joint Muscles and Their Actions

Muscle	Flexion	Extension	Lateral flexion	Rotation to same side	Rotation to opposite side
Sternocleidomastoid	PM		PM		
Erector spinae group (iliocostalis, longissimus, spinalis)		PM	PM	PM	
Multifidus		PM	PM		PM
Rectus abdominis	PM		Asst		
Internal obliques	PM		PM	PM	
External obliques	PM		PM		PM
Quadratus lumborum			PM		

PM = prime mover; Asst = assistant mover. Transverse abdominis performs no joint actions but is responsible for abdominal compression, vigorous exhalation, and expulsion.

TABLE 8.12   Spinal ROM

Spinal movement	ROM
Flexion	30°-45°
Extension	20°-45°
Lateral flexion	10°-35°
Rotation	20°-45°

Exercises for the Abdominals

PELVIC TILT FOR ABDOMINALS

**Rectus abdominis, transverse abdominis
(spinal flexion and posterior pelvic tilt, abdominal compression)**

CUES   Lie supine with the knees bent, the upper body relaxed on the floor, and the spine in neutral. Using a diaphragmatic or abdominal breath, exhale and firmly contract the abdominals, allowing them to tilt the pelvis posteriorly. Because this exercise is focusing on the abdominals, avoid allowing the buttocks muscles to participate. Work to isolate the abdominals, feeling a tug on the pubic bone attachment. Keep the movement small; more is not better. Avoid arching the low back on the return; simply go back to the neutral spine.

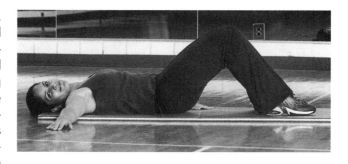

FYI   This is an excellent exercise to teach abdominal awareness and proper diaphragmatic breathing. Here is a progression for the pelvic tilt (modifications are listed in order from easiest to hardest): feet flat on floor with knees bent, legs somewhat straight with heels on floor, supine on a slanted bench with pelvis below head, and pelvis hanging off a stability ball. In all variations, try to perform lumbar spinal flexion and posterior pelvic tilt by using the abdominals but not the buttocks.

BASIC CURL-UP (CRUNCH)

Rectus abdominis (spinal flexion and posterior pelvic tilt)

CUES Lie supine with the knees bent and the spine and neck in neutral. Perform a diaphragmatic breath, exhale, and flex the spine, pulling the ribs toward the hips. Keep the neck in neutral; it has no independent movement of its own (it just goes along for the ride). Avoid performing neck-ups or hyperextending the neck. Bring the shoulder blades off the floor; avoid arching the low back on the descent, returning only to neutral.

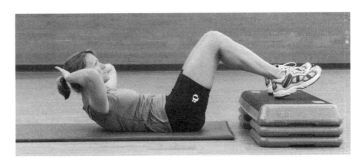

FYI There are many variations of this exercise. Arm variations (listed from easiest to hardest) include arms at sides, arms crossed on chest, hands behind ears, hands on forehead, arms crossed behind head, and arms extended overhead. Lower-body variations (again listed from easiest to hardest) include feet supported on a wall or bench (great for participants with low-back problems), supine on an inclined step (hips below head) with knees bent, supine with feet on floor and knees bent, supine with legs elevated and knees bent, supine with legs elevated and knees straight, supine on declined step (head below hips), supine on a stability ball (may be inclined, flat, or declined), and supine with a medicine ball toss. For variety and increased difficulty, combine the upper-body curl-up with a hip lift and pelvic tilt.

ABDOMINAL HIP LIFT

Rectus abdominis (spinal flexion and posterior pelvic tilt)

CUES Lie supine and elevate the legs with the knees slightly bent. Stabilize the knees and the hips at one joint angle. Keep this angle (or position) constant, exhale, and contract the abdominals firmly, posteriorly tilting the pelvis. The movement will be small. Avoid active hip flexion or swinging and rocking the legs.

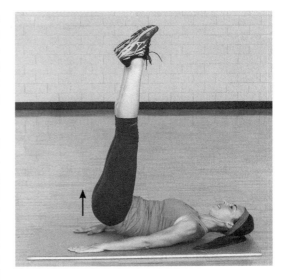

FYI This exercise is the more difficult version of the pelvic tilt described earlier. Before progressing to the hip lift, make certain your participants can perform a correct pelvic tilt with coordinated abdominal breathing. The knees may be bent or straight during the hip lift, depending on hamstring flexibility and low-back status. Using an inclined step with the hips below the head increases the difficulty, as does adding an upper-body crunch (full spinal flexion). For variety, try this 4-count variation: Tilt the pelvis (legs are in the air) on 1, curl the upper body up on 2, curl the upper body down on 3, and lower the pelvis on 4.

RECTUS ABDOMINIS STRETCHES

CUES

Variation 1

(a) Lie prone and prop yourself up onto your elbows, stretching the spine up and away from your hips. Lengthen the neck and allow it to continue as a natural extension of the spine (avoid cervical spinal hyperextension). Press down against the floor with your forearms to lower the shoulders away from the ears; slide your shoulder blades down your back.

Variation 2

If variation 1 is uncomfortable, modify it (b) by reaching your arms out in front and lifting your upper torso just slightly off the floor, lengthening the abdominals. Keep the neck in alignment.

FYI The full cobra pose, used in yoga, is an advanced version of this stretch. Since the cobra pose has a greater tendency to overstretch the long ligaments of the spine, we do not recommend including it in a group exercise class.

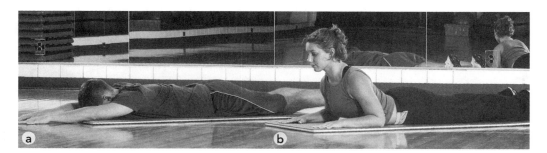

Exercises for the Obliques

DIAGONAL TWIST CRUNCH

External and internal obliques (spinal flexion and rotation)

CUES Lie supine with one knee bent, foot on the floor. Place your other foot on the thigh of your bent leg. Place one hand on the floor and the other hand behind your head. Exhaling, crunch diagonally, moving the ribs toward the opposite hip. Keep your neck in neutral (apple-sized space between chin and chest) and bring the shoulder blade off the floor. Keep the movement slow and controlled, avoiding momentum. Change legs and repeat the set on the opposite side.

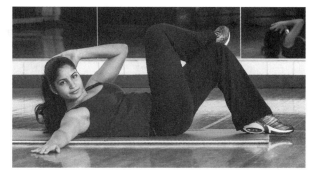

FYI Many variations exist for this exercise. Upper-body arm variations may be performed unilaterally and bilaterally and include (from easiest to hardest) arms at sides, arms crossed on chest, hands behind ears, arms crossed behind head, and arms stretched overhead. Lower-body variations include (again from easiest to hardest) both feet on floor (knees bent), both legs in the air (knees bent or straight), and one foot on the floor with the other leg extended in the air. In addition, a slanted step or a stability ball may be used for additional overload.

OBLIQUE STRETCHES

CUES

Variation 1

(a) Sit with your knees bent, one hip externally rotated (open) and the other hip internally rotated. Walk your hands around to the externally rotated side as far as is comfortable, stretching the obliques as well as the latissimus dorsi. Allow your arm to reach up and over in this position if desired.

Variation 2

(b) Lie supine with both knees bent in toward the torso. Allow the knees to slowly drop toward the floor. Reach the opposite arm to the other side, turning your head in that direction. Breathe deeply, relax, and enjoy this multiple-muscle stretch (the obliques, pectorals, hip abductors, erector spinae, and rectus abdominis are all being stretched).

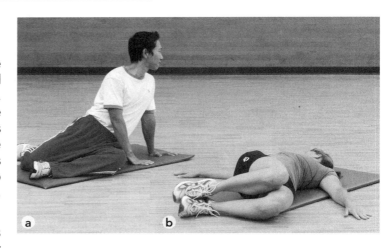

Exercises for Training the Core

The purpose of the next three exercises is to train the core muscles to stabilize the spine in neutral. The first exercise, the single-leg circle, is easiest since it is performed in the supine position; the quadruped that follows requires greater balance and core stability. The plank is even more difficult as increased core stability is required to maintain good alignment.

SINGLE-LEG CIRCLE

Iliopsoas, rectus femoris, transverse abdominis
(hip circumduction, abdominal compression)

CUES Lie supine with one leg extended along the floor and the other leg extended toward the ceiling, toes pointed. Firmly anchor the torso by hollowing the abdominals and pulling the navel toward the spine, all the while staying in neutral spinal alignment that maintains the four natural curves of the spine. Press both hips and shoulders evenly into the floor. Make small circles in the air with the perpendicular leg, moving first clockwise and then counterclockwise. Increase the size of the circles only as long as the pelvis can be kept level and absolutely still. Repeat on the other side.

FYI In this Pilates exercise, the hip flexors act as the prime movers; the rectus abdominis, obliques, transverse abdominis, and erector spinae muscles stabilize the spine. Adequate hamstring flexibility is required to perform the exercise as described; keeping the bottom knee bent is an acceptable modification.

QUADRUPED

Erector spinae, transverse abdominis, gluteus maximus, hamstrings, deltoids, serratus anterior (maintenance of neutral spine and scapulae, abdominal compression, hip extension, shoulder flexion)

CUES   Kneel on all fours with the hands directly under the shoulders and the knees directly under the hips. Place the pelvis, spine, neck, and scapulae securely in neutral alignment. Slowly reach one arm forward and extend the opposite leg back, maintaining level hips and shoulders and the neutral spine and neck. Hold. Return slowly to all fours without disturbing your alignment and repeat on the other side.

FYI   This exercise may be performed statically (holding 5-30 seconds per side) or dynamically (smoothly alternating back and forth between sides). The purpose of both variations is to promote torso stability and challenge both the erector spinae and the abdominals as stabilizers.

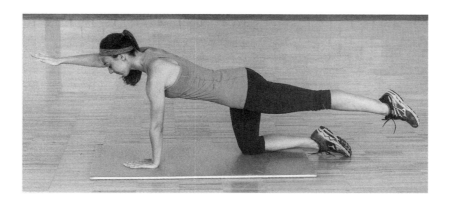

PLANK

Erector spinae, transverse abdominis, gluteus maximus, hamstrings, quadriceps, deltoids, serratus anterior (maintenance of neutral spine and scapulae, abdominal compression, hip extension, knee extension, shoulder flexion)

CUES   On hands and toes, align the body to make a straight line from the crown of the head all the way to the heels. Pelvis, spine, neck, and scapulae are all held in neutral alignment. Lift abdominals up toward the spine. Hold and breathe.

FYI   There are many plank variations— from easiest to hardest: plank on knees, plank on forearms, basic plank shown in photo, plank with one leg lifted, plank with

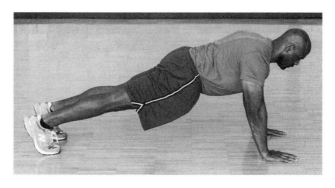

one leg abducting and adducting in frontal plane, plank rotating to side plank and back again, and more.

Exercises for the Erector Spinae

PRONE SPINAL EXTENSION

Erector spinae (spinal extension)

CUES Lie prone with your forehead on the mat and your neck in neutral. Press your hips into the floor and keep your arms at your sides. Lengthen the spine and slowly lift the upper body, maintaining a neutral neck (chin will remain slightly tucked). Lower smoothly and repeat.

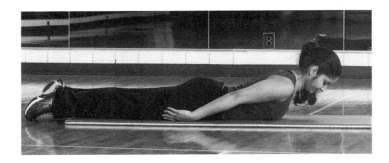

FYI Active lumbar extension or hyperextension can be problematic for some participants. Always ask your participants how they feel and provide modifications when needed. Tell participants to stop if they feel any pain. The most conservative approach to strengthening the low back is to perform isometric extension only (simply lift the chest an inch or so off the floor and hold) and encourage students to work with their physicians. Other variations of this exercise, moving from easiest to hardest, include extension with arms at 90°, extension with arms overhead, extension with opposite arm and leg, and extension performed on a stability ball.

ERECTOR SPINAE STRETCHES

CUES

Variation 1

(a) Stand with the feet shoulder-width apart and the knees bent. Place your hands on your thighs, tuck your pelvis (posterior pelvic tilt), and round (flex) your spine, pulling your navel in. Allow your head and neck to be a natural extension of the spine and your hands to support your back as you press your waist backward, lengthening the muscles of the low back.

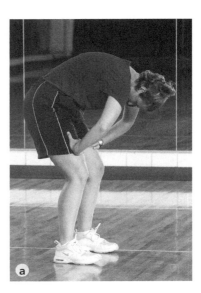

Variation 2

(*b*) Kneel on all fours and perform the angry cat stretch, flexing your spine upward and contracting your abdominals up and in. Keep your pelvis tucked under and tailbone pointing down. Allow your head and neck to flex gently, following the line of the spine. Press your waist back and up to increase the low-back stretch.

Variation 3

(*c*) Lie supine and hug both knees to your chest, placing your hands behind the knees. Allow your spine to flex and your tailbone to curve upward. If comfortable, gently rock side to side, back and forth, or in a circular pattern, massaging the low-back muscles. Allow the head and neck to rest in neutral alignment on the floor.

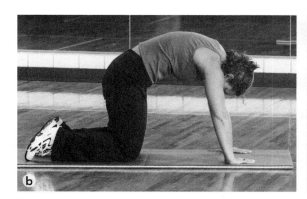 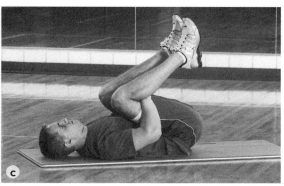

FYI   Encourage your participants to find low-back and abdominal stretches that make their backs feel good. Provide them with several options and let them discover their preferences.

Hip and Knee Joints

Since so many lower-body exercises use the hip and knee joints simultaneously, we combine the information for these two joints. Figures 8.14 and 8.15 show the muscles of the hip and knee joints. Tables 8.13 and 8.16 list the major muscles of each joint, activities of

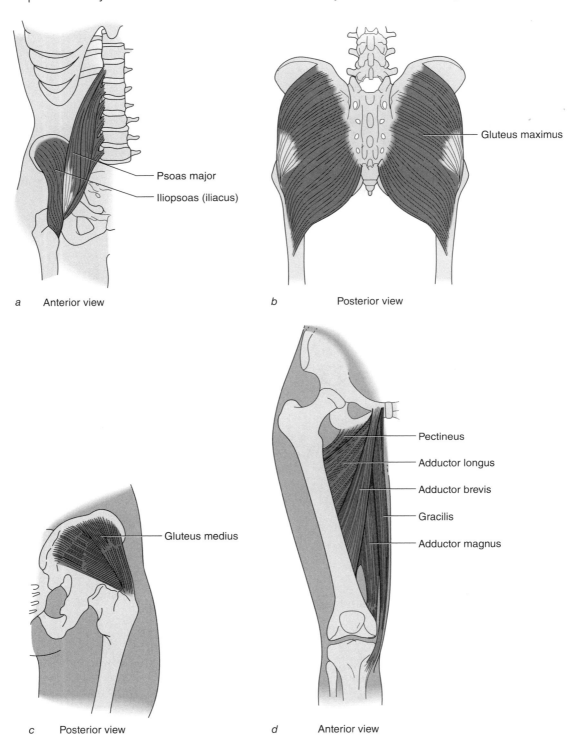

a   Anterior view

Psoas major

Iliopsoas (iliacus)

b   Posterior view

Gluteus maximus

c   Posterior view

Gluteus medius

d   Anterior view

Pectineus

Adductor longus

Adductor brevis

Gracilis

Adductor magnus

FIGURE 8.14   Hip joint muscles: (*a*) anterior view of the psoas major and iliopsoas, (*b*) gluteus maximus, (*c*) posterior view of the gluteus medius, and (*d*) anterior view of the hip adductors.

daily living that use each joint, and basic strengthening exercises for each joint. Tables 8.14 and 8.17 list the muscles and joint actions of the hip and knee. Tables 8.15 and 8.18 give the ROM of selected hip and knee movements. The photos and descriptions that follow demonstrate muscular conditioning exercises and stretches for the hip and knee joint muscles.

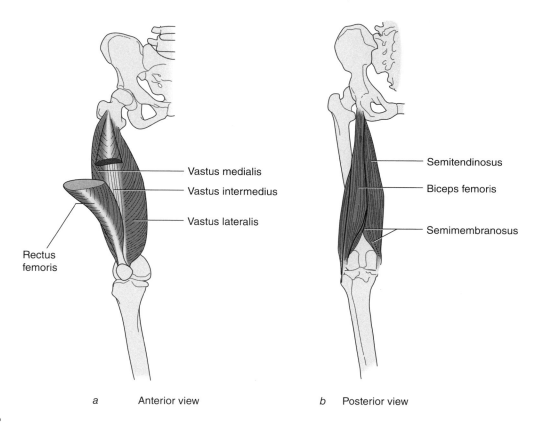

a   Anterior view   b   Posterior view

FIGURE 8.15   Knee joint muscles: (a) quadriceps and (b) hamstrings.

TABLE 8.13   Hip Joint Muscles

Muscle	Daily activities	Exercises
Psoas and rectus femoris	Climbing stairs, walking, getting in a car, kicking a ball	Standing and supine leg lift (hip flexion)
Gluteus maximus, hamstrings	Climbing stairs, running, walking uphill	Squat, lunge, leg lift in all-fours position, pelvic tilt
Gluteus medius	Stabilizing hip when walking, balancing	Side-lying leg lift, standing abduction
Hip adductors	Stabilizing hip when walking, horseback riding	Side-lying leg lift, supine adduction

TABLE 8.14   Hip Joint Muscles and Their Actions

Muscle	Actions
Psoas	Prime mover for hip flexion; assistor for hip abduction and outward rotation
Iliacus	Prime mover for hip flexion; assistor for hip abduction and outward rotation
Rectus femoris	Prime mover for hip flexion; assistor for hip abduction
Sartorius	Assistor for hip flexion, abduction, and outward rotation
Gluteus maximus	Prime mover for hip extension and outward rotation; assistor for abduction and adduction (select fibers recruited for each)
Bicpes femoris	Prime mover for hip extension; assistor for outward rotation
Semitendinosus	Prime mover for hip extension; assistor for inward rotation
Semimembranosus	Prime mover for hip extension; assistor for inward rotation
Gluteus medius	Prime mover for hip abduction; assistor for hip flexion, extension (select fibers recruited for each), inward and outward rotation
Gluteus minimus	Prime mover for inward rotation; assistor for hip flexion, extension, abduction, and outward rotation
Tensor Fasciae latae	Assistor for hip flexion, abduction and inward rotation
Pectineus	Prime mover for hip adduction and flexion; assistor for inward rotation
Gracilis	Prime mover for hip adduction; assistor for hip flexion and inward rotation
Adductor longus	Prime mover for hip adduction; assistor for hip flexion and inward rotation
Adductor brevis	Prime mover for hip adduction; assistor for hip flexion and inward rotation
Adductor magnus	Prime mover for hip adduction; assistor for hip flexion, extension, and inward rotation
Six outward rotatos: piriformis, obturator internus, obturator externus, quadratus femoris, gemellus superior, gemellus inferior	Prime movers for hip outward rotation

TABLE 8.15 ROM of Select Hip Joint Movements

Joint movement	ROM
Flexion	90°-135°
Extension	10°-30°
Abduction	30°-50°
Adduction	10°-30°
Internal rotation	30°-45°
External rotation	45°-60°

TABLE 8.16 Knee Joint Muscles

Muscle	Daily activities	Exercises
Quadriceps (rectus femoris, vastus medialis, vastus intermedius, vastus lateralis)	Walking, cycling, stair climbing, sitting down, standing up	Squat, lunge, knee extension, plié
Hamstrings (biceps femoris, semitendinosus, semimembranosus)	Swimming, running	Prone knee-curl, knee-curl on all fours

TABLE 8.17 Knee and Joint Muscles and Their Actions

Muscle	Actions
Biceps femoris	Prime mover for knee flexion and knee inward rotation
Semitendinosus	Prime mover for knee flexion and inward rotation
Semimembranosus	Prime mover for knee flexion and outward rotation
Rectus femoris	Prime mover for knee extension
Vastus lateralis	Prime mover for knee extension
Vastus intermedius	Prime mover for knee extension
Vastus medialis	Prime mover for knee extension
Sartorius	Assistor for knee flexion and inward rotation
Gracilis	Assistor for knee flexion and inward rotation
Popliteus	Prime mover for knee inward rotation; assistor for knee flexion
Gastrocnemius	Assistor for knee flexion
Plantaris	Assistor for knee flexion

TABLE 8.18 ROM of Knee Joint Movements

Joint movement	ROM
Flexion	130°-140°
Extension	5°-10°

Exercises for the Quadriceps, Gluteus Maximus, and Hamstrings

SUPINE LEG LIFT AND KNEE EXTENSION

Iliopsoas, quadriceps (hip flexion, knee extension)

CUES   Lie supine with the spine in neutral and the abdominals firmly anchored. Place one foot on the floor with the knee bent. Straighten the other knee and raise it to a 45° angle off the floor. Using a controlled, smooth motion, bend and straighten the elevated knee (a). Alternate with hip flexion (b), if desired, lifting and lowering the leg while keeping the knee straight.

FYI   Knee extension and hip flexion can be performed supine, supine propped up on the elbows, or standing. Supine is the easiest position. In addition, the knee extension can include a quad set (isometric-type contraction of the quadriceps that tighten the patella) and terminal knee extensions (moving the knee joint only through the last few degrees of motion). These variations help to correct potential muscle imbalances around the knee joint. Bands or ankle weights can be added for additional overload.

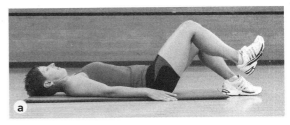

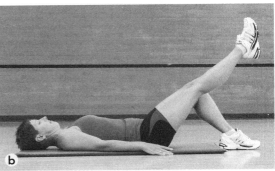

SQUAT

Quadriceps, gluteus maximus, hamstrings (knee extension, hip extension)

CUES   Stand with the feet shoulder-width apart and the toes straight ahead or slightly rotated outward (in the same direction as the knees). The spine, neck, and pelvis are in neutral, and the abdominals are pulled up and in. Bending the knees, press the tailbone and the middle third of the body back. Keeping the torso erect, the chest lifted, and the head in line with the spine, lower the body until the thighs are almost parallel to the floor or until the lumbar curve becomes excessive. Do not allow your hips to drop below your knees; keep the knees behind the toes (avoid overshooting the toes) and keep the heels on the floor. Keep the abdominals contracted and the spine stable throughout the movement. Keep one hand on your thigh for low-back safety and allow the other arm to flex forward, providing a counterbalance.

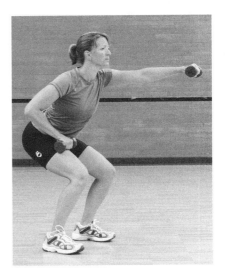

FYI   Almost everyone can benefit from learning to squat properly. This functional exercise helps participants have better mechanics in lifting, getting in and out of chairs, and completing other daily activities. Variations, listed in order from easiest to hardest, include a sit-back squat while holding onto a ballet barre or a partner's hands, a squat while holding onto a Body Bar placed vertically in front of the body, a squat with hands on thighs, a squat with one hand on one thigh, a squat with dumbbells held at the sides, a back squat with a barbell, and a front squat with a barbell (the last three variations pose a greater risk for the low back).

PLIÉ

Quadriceps, gluteus maximus, hamstrings, adductors (knee extension, hip extension, hip adduction)

CUES Stand with the feet wide apart and the toes angled away from the midline of the body. Turn out from the hips, making sure that the knees are aligned in the same direction as the toes (if this isn't possible, adjust the feet so that the toes and knees are in the same line). The pelvis is in neutral with the tailbone pointing straight down, and the spine is in neutral with the shoulders level and chest lifted. Maintaining this lifted, turned-out alignment, bend the knees to no more than a 90° angle (thighs will be parallel to the floor). Straighten the knees and return to the starting position, consciously contracting the buttocks and inner thighs.

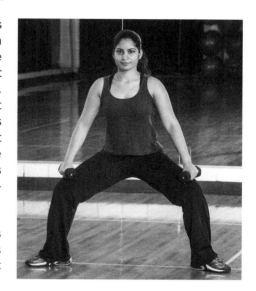

FYI This exercise may be performed with dumbbells or a barbell for added resistance; upper-body exercises can be combined with the plié once good alignment has been mastered. A plié is really just a modified squat. Some students may find it easier than a squat because the pelvis is kept neutral and the spine is kept upright. Other students may find it more difficult because of the amount of turnout required. Although the quadriceps is the prime mover of this exercise, the gluteus maximus isometrically contracts to maintain external hip rotation, and the adductors can be recruited during the lifting phase of the movement (although there is no resistance against gravity).

LUNGE

Quadriceps, gluteus maximus, hamstrings, hip abductors, hip adductors (knee extension, hip extension, hip stabilization)

CUES For a stationary lunge, stand with the feet staggered at least 3 feet (1 m) apart; participants with long legs should stand with their feet even farther apart. Lift up onto the ball of the back foot. Place the pelvis in neutral, the tailbone down, and the spine and neck in neutral; contract the abdominals. The hips and shoulders are level. Bend both knees and slowly lower your body. Go only low enough that the front knee bends to a right angle (90°) and the front thigh is parallel to the floor Avoid dropping the hips below the knee or letting the back knee touch the floor. Keep the pelvis and spine upright; avoid leaning forward. Return to the starting position, keeping the back heel elevated. To perform a front lunge, start in a standing position with the feet shoulder-width apart and the spine, pelvis, and neck in neutral. Step forward and

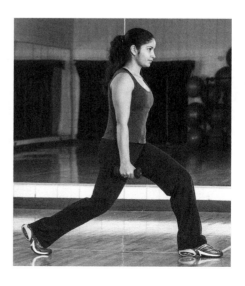

land on the heel, ball, and then toe. Slowly lower the body and bend the front knee to no more than 90°. Keep the front knee behind the toes (avoid overshooting). The torso remains completely upright (requiring hip flexor flexibility), and the heel of the back foot is off the floor. Push off with the front foot and return to standing. When performing a long lunge with the back leg straight, it may be necessary to stutter-step back with the front foot—this more advanced move uses two or three smaller steps.

FYI In general, lunges are a more advanced exercise. To perform a proper lunge, students need lower-body strength, flexible hip flexors, stable torsos, balance, and coordination. There are many variations of the lunge, including the front, back, side, and crane lunges. All of these can be performed with stationary, dynamic, or traveling variations. Front, back, and crane lunges can be performed with the back leg bent or straight (using the straight leg is more difficult and requires much more flexibility). The lunge can be an excellent lower-body strengthener but care must be taken to maintain strict form (especially with regard to the knees) to avoid injury.

ALL-FOURS BUTTOCK AND HAMSTRINGS EXERCISE

Gluteus maximus, hamstrings (hip extension, knee flexion)

CUES Assume the all-fours position; place the hands directly under the shoulders (or rest on the forearms) and the knees directly under the hips, forming a tabletop with the spine, neck, and head. Lift the abdominals, placing the spine in neutral with the head and making the neck a natural extension of the spine. The hips and shoulders are level. Keeping the torso absolutely still, slowly raise one leg straight behind you on 1, flex the knee on 2, straighten the

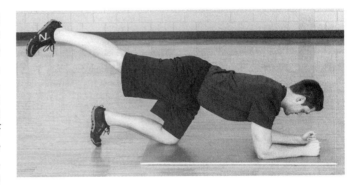

knee on 3, and lower the leg back to the starting position on 4. Consciously squeeze the buttocks and hamstring muscles as you perform this exercise.

FYI The hip extension and knee-curl can be performed prone, on all fours, or even standing. Hip extension and knee flexion can each be performed alone, or the two moves can be combined, as described previously. The prone position is the most stable and appropriate for beginners, although ROM at the hip joint is small. Both the all-fours and standing positions are more difficult to stabilize, and both isometrically challenge the abdominal and low-back muscles. Avoid momentum in this position because performing the movements too quickly can lead to back hyperextension and potential injury. Performing the exercise on elbows and knees is an excellent alternative to hands and knees; ROM may be increased without as much risk of back hyperextension.

 See online video 8.5 for muscular conditioning exercises and progression options for the hamstrings.

ILIOPSOAS (HIP FLEXOR) STRETCHES

CUES

Variation 1

(*a*) Stand with the feet staggered, as pictured. Your feet should be far enough apart to prevent your front knee from bending excessively (the front knee should be directly over the heel, with the lower leg perpendicular to the floor). Turn all the joints in the same direction: The toes, knees, hips, and shoulders should all face the same way. Firmly squeeze the buttocks and press the pelvis into a posterior pelvic tilt (tailbone tips slightly forward and under). Hold the abdominals securely in and the torso upright with neutral spine, scapulae, and neck. Feel the hip flexor muscles lengthen and stretch across the front of the right hip. If necessary, stand by a wall for balance.

Variation 2

(*b*) For a more intense version of this stretch, move into a runner's lunge, bringing the back foot even farther back. The front knee will now make a right angle; the shin will be perpendicular and the thigh will be parallel to the floor. Keep the torso as upright as possible, place your hands on the floor or balance them on your thighs. The back knee may be placed on the floor, if desired (although avoid placing it directly on a wood floor—use a mat for cushioning). If you choose to show the runner's lunge first, always show the easier version as well since many participants will be uncomfortable in the runner's lunge. Pay special attention to the front (bent) knee as overbending is a common mistake and can lead to knee problems. The rectus femoris is also stretched in these first two stretching examples.

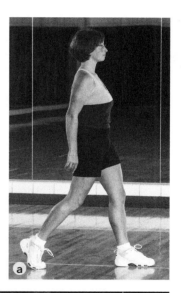

Variation 3

(*c*) Lie supine on the floor with one knee pulled into the chest (hands on the knee or behind the thigh) and the other leg stretched out straight on the floor. Lie with the spine and neck in neutral and the abdominals contracted. Gently attempt to press the back of the straight knee toward the floor while maintaining the bent knee pressed into the chest. Feel the hip flexor stretch on the top of the extended hip.

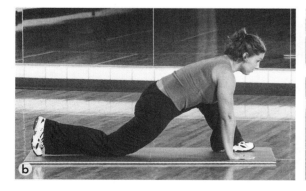

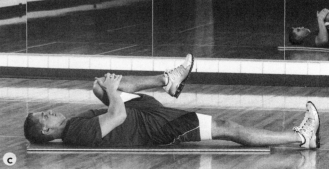

QUADRICEPS STRETCHES

CUES

Variation 1

(*a*) Stand on one foot and keep the knee soft; the abdominals contracted; and the pelvis, spine, neck, and scapulae in neutral. Grasp the other foot with your hand (usually the same-side hand, although either hand is acceptable as long as it feels comfortable) and gently pull the heel into your buttocks, making certain that the hip, knee, and ankle joints are all in a line (no torque), and the knee is pointing toward the floor. Check to see that your hips and shoulders are level and even. If balance is a problem, stand near the wall for support. If you cannot comfortably reach your foot or ankle, try holding onto your pant leg or sock, or place your foot on a bench or chair and then squeeze your buttocks, tucking your pelvis posteriorly.

Variation 2

(*b*) Lie on your side and grasp your top foot with your top hand, flexing the knee and gently pulling it toward your buttocks. Keep your hips stacked, abdominals in, and spine and neck in neutral, with your bottom arm bent under your head (do not place your head on your hand because this takes your neck out of alignment).

FYI Another excellent position for quadriceps stretching is the prone position. Simply place one hand under the forehead (avoiding cervical hyperextension) and reach back with the other, grasping the same-side ankle and gently pulling it in toward the buttocks.

GLUTEUS MAXIMUS AND HAMSTRING STRETCHES

CUES

Variation 1

(*a*) Stand with the feet hip-width apart, with one foot forward just far enough that the heel is in line with the toes of the other foot. Press the tailbone backward as if preparing to sit or squat; keep the hips and shoulders square. Hinging at the hips (no spinal flexion), fold the torso forward while maintaining a long, neutral spine. Contract the abdominals and place both hands on the thigh of the bent knee (this helps protect the low back). The leg with the bent knee is the support leg, and the other leg is the stretching leg. The knee of the stretching leg is straight but not hyperextended. Your foot may be dorsiflexed or plantar flexed. Keep the hips square and hinge in the direction of the straight leg so you are stretching along the longitudinal line of the hamstring muscle.

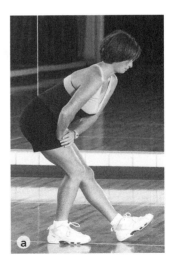

Variation 2

(b) Lie supine with one knee bent, that foot on the floor, and the spine, neck, and scapulae in neutral. With the other knee straight (but not hyperextended), gently pull the straight leg in toward your torso (your foot may be pointed or flexed).

Variation 3

(c) Sit perfectly upright on the sitting bones (ischial tuberosities) so that your pelvis, spine, and neck are in neutral alignment. If you find it difficult to sit upright without slumping, wedge a towel slightly under the tailbone or use a stretch strap (or towel) around the foot, enabling you to pull yourself upright. (It is harmful to your spine to slouch in this position.) Extend one leg. Keeping the hips square and the opposite knee bent out to the side, hinge at the hip as much as possible in the direction of your extended leg. Keep your spine long and straight, your chest lifted, and your head and neck in a natural extension of the spine.

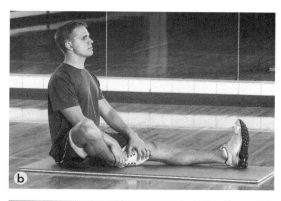

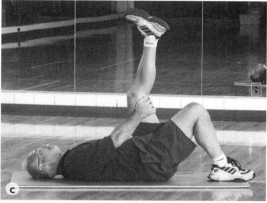

FYI Be familiar with the modifications for the seated hamstring stretches: Many participants won't be able to perform them with acceptable alignment and will risk hurting their backs. Have participants use props (a wedge or towel under the edge of the buttocks and a strap around the feet), place their hands behind the body for support (instead of reaching forward), or choose an alternative hamstring stretch. The seated stretch can be performed either unilaterally or bilaterally (both legs in front), although the bilateral position is potentially more stressful to the low back.

Exercises for the Gluteus Medius

HIP ABDUCTION

Gluteus medius

CUES

Variation 1

To perform side-lying hip abduction (a), lie on your side with your head resting on your arm. Maintain a neutral neck and spine (do not place your head on your hand; doing so can place undue stress on the neck) and keep your hips stacked. Make sure both kneecaps face

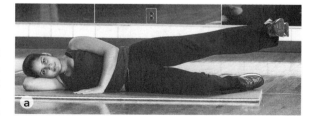

forward (to avoid external hip rotation and flexion and the subsequent use of muscles other than the hip abductors) if the goal is to isolate the outer-thigh muscles. Consciously contract the abductors and slowly raise and lower the leg.

Variation 2

If you are performing this exercise while standing (*b*), make certain that the standing knee is bent slightly, allowing the pelvis and spine to maintain a neutral position. Keep the hips level, keep the moving kneecap facing forward, and maintain a stable torso as the leg abducts and returns.

FYI Effective isolation-type exercises for the abductors may be achieved in either the side-lying or the standing position. The side-lying position is the safest and arguably the most effective choice because of its stability and direct resistance against gravity. There are several variations of this exercise, including top leg straight, top leg bent, top leg in line with the body, and top leg at 45° of hip flexion. There are also numerous rhythm variations. Bands or ankle weights may be added for additional overload.

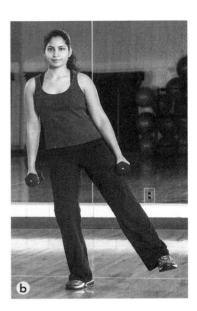

GLUTEUS MEDIUS STRETCHES

CUES

Variation 1

(*a*) Lie on your side with your arm comfortably under your head, hips stacked, and spine in neutral. Flex the bottom hip so that your bottom leg is in front of your body (knee can be bent). Place your top leg in a straight line with your torso and bend the knee. Gently lower the bent top knee toward the floor, maintaining level, stacked hips and avoiding any lateral spinal flexion. Do not let your top leg move in front of or in back of the torso; it needs to be in exactly the same plane for the most effective outer-thigh stretch.

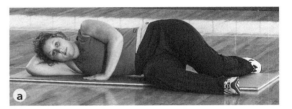

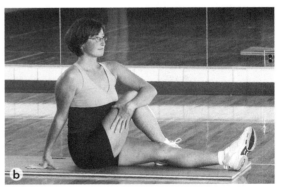

Variation 2

(*b*) Sit in good alignment, up on the sitting bones, with the spine, neck, and scapulae in neutral and one leg extended out in front. Bring the opposite knee diagonally across the torso, attempting to press the knee into the opposite shoulder. Feel the stretch in the right outer-thigh and buttock muscles.

Exercises for the Hip Adductors

HIP ADDUCTION

Adductor longus, adductor brevis, adductor magnus, gracilis, pectineus

CUES

Variation 1

To perform hip adduction from the side-lying position (*a*), lie on your side with your head resting on your arm. Keep your hips stacked and your spine and neck in neutral (do not place your head in your hand because this takes the neck out of alignment). The bottom (moving) leg is in line with the body, and the top leg is in front of the body with the inside edge of the foot resting on the floor. (Unless students have long thigh bones and narrow hips, they should hold the top knee in a slightly elevated position to ensure that the hips remain stacked—unstacking the hips leads to greater reliance on muscles other than the hip adductors and can stress the back.) Consciously contract the muscles and slowly raise and lower the bottom leg.

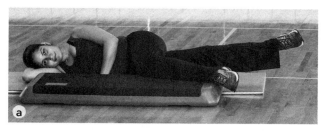

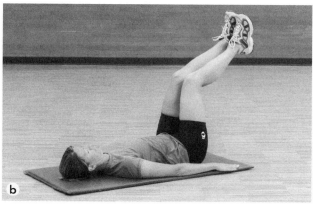

Variation 2

To perform hip adduction from the supine position, lie supine with the legs elevated in the air (*b*). Participants with tight hamstrings should bend their knees to ensure that the weight of the legs is over the torso and not over the floor. Anchor the abdominals to help maintain torso stability. (*c*) Open and close the legs, consciously tightening the inner thigh muscles.

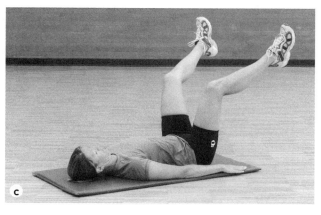

FYI Isolation of the adductors can be performed in the side-lying or the supine position; the side-lying position is more effective because it optimizes resistance against gravity's pull. Hip adduction exercises may be varied by using short or long levers, adding rhythmic variations, and using bands or weights. To help maintain the slight elevation of the top knee in the side-lying position, use a step, towel, or small ball.

Hip and Knee Joints

HIP ADDUCTOR STRETCHES

CUES

Variation 1

(a) Sit on the floor in the straddle position, legs wide apart, weight securely on sitting bones (ischial tuberosities). If necessary, place the hands on the floor behind the body to help place the pelvis, spine, scapulae, and neck in a neutral alignment directly in line with the sitting bones. Rotate the hips open so that the kneecaps face the ceiling; the feet may be pointed or flexed. Hinging at the hips, not the waist (no spinal flexion), point the tailbone backward and bring the torso forward, maintaining neutral alignment. The farther you are able to hinge at the hips and bring the torso forward, the more you'll need to place your hands in front for support.

Variation 2

(b) Lie supine with the knees bent; the feet on the floor; and the pelvis, spine, scapulae, and neck in neutral. Allow the legs to fall open (abduct) until you feel a comfortable inner thigh stretch; keep the feet together on the floor and the knees bent.

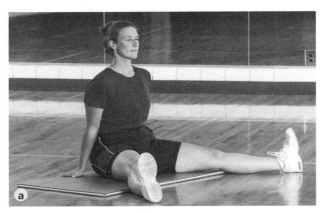

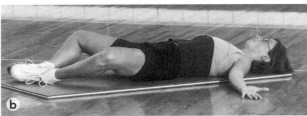

Ankle Joint

Figure 8.16 shows the major muscles of the ankle joint. Table 8.19 lists the ankle joint muscles, activities that use these muscles, and basic strengthening exercises for these muscles. Table 8.20 lists the ankle joint muscles and their joint actions. Table 8.21 gives the ROM of ankle joint movements. The photos and descriptions that follow demonstrate exercises and stretches for the ankle joint muscles.

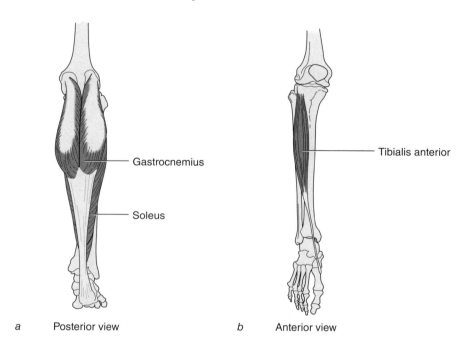

Gastrocnemius

Soleus

Tibialis anterior

a   Posterior view   *b*   Anterior view

FIGURE 8.16   Ankle joint muscles: (*a*) gastrocnemius and soleus and (*b*) tibialis anterior.

TABLE 8.19   Ankle Joint Muscles

Muscle	Daily activities	Exercises
Tibialis anterior	Walking uphill, toe tapping	Toe lift
Gastrocnemius, soleus	Walking, running, jumping	Heel raise

TABLE 8.20   Ankle Joint Muscles and Their Actions

Muscle	Actions
Tibialis anterior	Anterior: prime mover for ankle dorsiflexion and inversion
Extensor digitorum longus	Prime mover for ankle dorsiflexion and eversion
Peroneus tertius	Prime mover for ankle dorsiflexion and eversion
Gastrocnemius	Prime mover for ankle plantarflexion
Soleus	Prime mover for ankle plantarflexion
Peroneus longus	Prime mover for ankle eversion; assistor for plantarflexion
Peroneus brevis	Prime mover for ankle eversion; assistor for plantarflexion
Flexor digitorum longus	Assistor for ankle plantarflexion and inversion
Tibialis posterior	Prime mover for ankle inversion; assistor for plantarflexion

Ankle Joint

TABLE 8.21 ROM of Ankle Joint Movements

Joint movement	ROM
Dorsiflexion	15°-20°
Plantar flexion	30°-50°
Inversion	10°-30°
Eversion	10°-20°

Exercises for the Shin Muscles

SHIN EXERCISE

Anterior tibialis (ankle dorsiflexion)

CUES Sit in good alignment, with your weight over your sitting bones and your spine and neck in neutral alignment. Keeping the knees slightly bent, point and flex each foot one at a time. Move through the full ROM, allowing each foot to point fully and then bringing the toes as far toward the shin as possible. Consciously contract the shin muscles.

FYI This exercise may be combined with basic abdominal crunches. As you curl up, simultaneously dorsiflex one ankle, releasing as the spine returns to neutral. Alternate ankles with each curl-up.

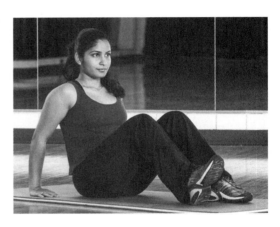

SHIN STRETCHES

CUES

Variation 1

(a) Stand with the feet staggered, one foot behind the body. While maintaining one long line from the back foot to the head, contract the abdominals as you balance on the front leg and point the back foot (ankle plantar flexion). Keep all joints in line and avoid letting the ankle collapse to the right or left side. Feel the stretch through the shin and along the top (front) of the foot.

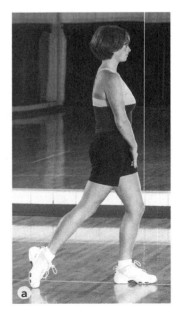

Variation 2

(b) Lie in the prone position for the quadriceps stretch, one hand under your forehead and the other hand holding your foot. Point your foot as you gently bring the heel toward the buttocks, feeling the stretch not only in the quadriceps but also in the shin (anterior tibialis) and the top (front) of the foot.

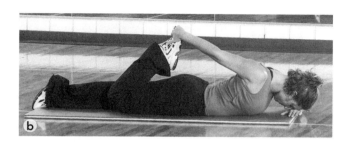

Exercises for the Calves

CALF EXERCISE

Gastrocnemius and soleus (ankle plantar flexion)

CUES Stand with the knees soft; the pelvis, spine, and neck in neutral; the abdominals tight; and the feet hip-width apart. Lift both heels off the floor, rising onto the balls of the feet as far as possible. Return to the floor.

FYI To achieve full ROM for the calf muscles, stand on the edge of a step, lowering the heels as far off the step as possible and then returning to normal standing, using a bar or railing for balance as necessary.

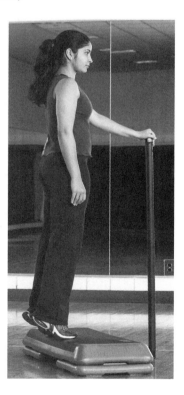

CALF STRETCHES

CUES

Variation 1

(*a*) Stand with the feet staggered, one foot behind the body. Adjust the distance between your feet so that your back heel comfortably reaches the floor yet your front knee is still directly over the heel and the front lower leg is perpendicular to floor. Turn all joints in the same direction: The toes, knees, hips, and shoulders should all face the same way. Place both hands on your front thigh and check to see that your body forms one long line from heel to head; the spine should be neutral. Contract the abdominals, keep the chest slightly lifted, and keep the shoulders back and down. This stretch may also be performed with the hands on a wall.

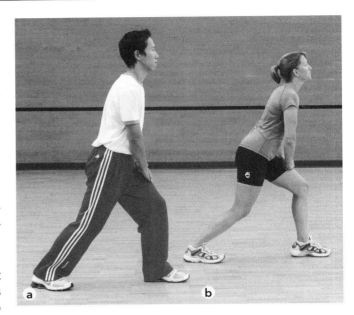

Variation 2

(*b*) Stand in the position just described and let your back knee bend as far as feels comfortable; your back heel should remain down, and your joints should remain in alignment—pointing in the same direction. Bending the knee provides a deeper stretch for the soleus muscle and helps lengthen the Achilles tendon (which is often too tight).

Practice Drill

Practice each of the preceding exercises and stretches with a partner, taking turns performing each movement. Study the pictures, cues, and other information; practice giving cues as your partner performs the exercise. Make sure to perform each exercise and stretch with excellent form and alignment. Write down two cues for every exercise and stretch in this chapter.

Exercises Using the Stability Ball

Many exercises can be performed using a stability ball or BOSU. Several of the exercises described next incorporate multiple joints and muscles in one move. Performing multijoint and multimuscle exercises is more difficult, so adapt these moves to your class accordingly.

SEATED KNEE EXTENSION WITH BAND AND SEATED OVERHEAD PRESS

Quadriceps; Deltoids and triceps

CUES

Knee Extension
Sit with good posture on the ball; with the band around both ankles, smoothly extend one knee (a). Maintain level hips and shoulders; keep the abdominals contracted.

Overhead Press
Sit on the ball with good alignment and a neutral spine; contract the abdominals. Press the arms overhead, keeping the scapulae down (b).

FYI For an additional challenge, lift one leg.

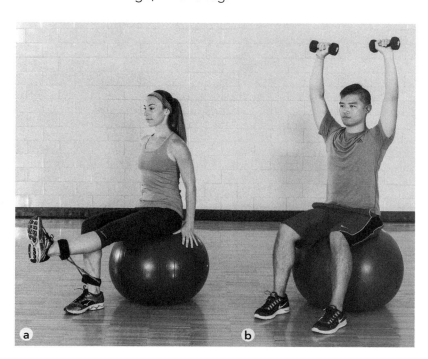

Exercises Using the Stability Ball

SUPINE BUTTOCKS SQUEEZE AND SQUAT

Buttocks and hamstrings; quadriceps, buttocks, and hamstrings

CUES

Supine Buttocks Squeeze
Lying supine with your feet on the ball (*a*); contract the buttocks and smoothly press up into a planklike position, abdominals contracted.

Supine Buttocks Squat
Execute the standing wall squat by standing with the ball against the wall and pressed into the low back (*b*). Place the feet far enough away from the wall so that when you squat your knees will form a 90° angle and your shins will be vertical. Toes, knees, hips, and shoulders should all face the same direction.

FYI   A standing squat may also be performed on a BOSU for more difficulty.

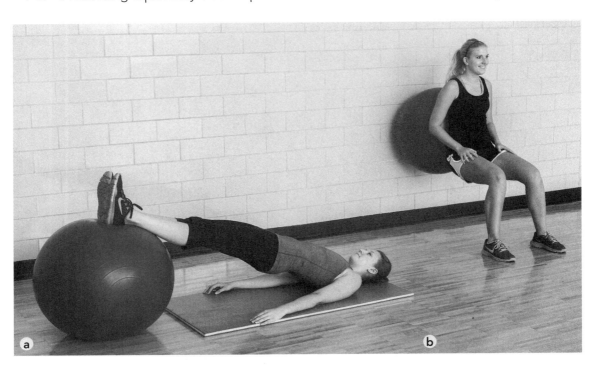

SIDE-LYING HIP ABDUCTION

Gluteus medius

CUES   Lying on one side over the ball, maintain proper alignment with the hips and shoulders stacked and the neck continuing the line of the spine. Perform hip abduction with the top leg.

FYI   You may let the bottom knee rest against the floor or, for greater challenge, keep the knee straight and stack the feet on top of each other as shown.

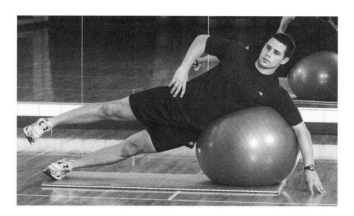

SIDE-LYING HIP ADDUCTION

Hip adductors, gracilis, pectineus

CUES   Lie on your side with the top leg resting on the ball and the ball resting on the bottom leg. The hips are stacked, and the spine and neck are in neutral. Moving both legs and the ball upward, adduct the bottom leg.

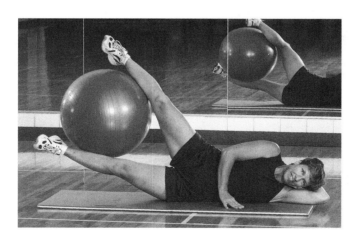

PUSH-UP WITH STABILITY CHALLENGE

Pectoralis major, anterior deltoids, triceps

CUES

Variation 1
Lie prone on the ball; then walk your hands away from the ball, maintaining a plank position with the abdominals securely contracted and the neck in line with the spine. Begin the push-ups (a).

Variation 2
Push-ups may also be performed with the flat side of the BOSU facing up (b-c).

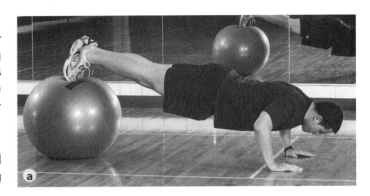

FYI The closer the ball is to your feet, the more difficult the push-ups will be. Try balancing on one leg for a difficult challenge!

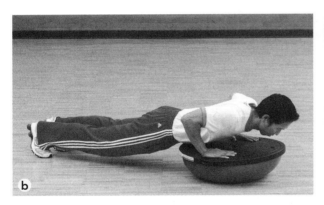 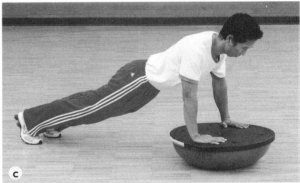

PRONE REVERSE FLY

Middle trapezius, rhomboids, posterior deltoids

CUES Lie prone with the ball under the lower ribs and the arms perpendicular to the torso. Keep the elbows slightly flexed, the wrists neutral, and the neck in line with the spine. Horizontally abduct the arms toward the ceiling, retracting the scapulae.

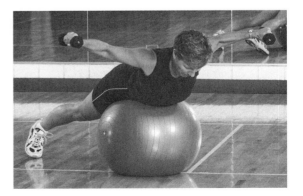

PRONE SHOULDER EXTENSION

Latissimus dorsi, posterior deltoids

CUES   Lie prone with the ball under the lower ribs and the arms at the sides, elbows straight, wrists neutral, and neck in line with the spine. Lift straight arms up toward the ceiling.

FYI   For additional challenge, lift one leg.

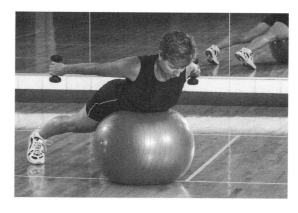

PRONE BACK EXTENSION

Erector spinae

CUES   Lie prone with the hands behind the ears, either with the spine flexed slightly forward over the ball or with the back flat. Smoothly extend the spine.

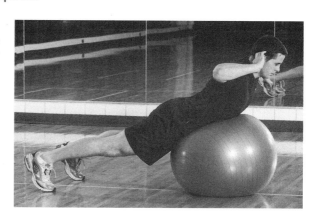

SUPINE ABDOMINAL CRUNCH

Rectus abdominis

CUES   Lie supine on the ball and perform abdominal curl-ups. Decrease the difficulty by moving into an inclined position; increase the difficulty by moving into a declined position or by lifting one leg.

FYI   Challenge the obliques by performing crunches with rotation.

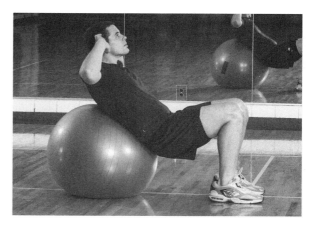

Exercises Using the Stability Ball

Chapter Wrap-Up

This chapter has outlined the variables that are common to most muscular conditioning and flexibility segments of group exercise. Knowing muscle anatomy and joint actions, selecting exercises and equipment, and demonstrating and cueing specific exercises and stretches with good alignment are all important when teaching classes. The information, skills, and exercises discussed in this chapter are fundamental for a skilled group exercise leader. Muscle conditioning and flexibility are key components of fitness, and we highly recommend that all group instructors become adept at leading these important class segments.

ASSIGNMENTS

1. Prepare in writing a stretch and strengthening exercise for each major muscle group (calves, shins, abductors, adductors, quadriceps, hamstrings, gluteus maximus, anterior and medial deltoids, latissimus dorsi, pectorals, middle trapezius and rhomboids, posterior deltoids, abdominals, erector spinae, biceps, and triceps). List ROM, joint action, muscles involved (use proper terminology), and at least three cues for each exercise. You may put these on note cards or any format that will help you study.

2. Pick five muscle groups from the following list of major muscle groups covered in this chapter: calves, shins, abductors, adductors, quadriceps, hamstrings, gluteus maximus, anterior and medial deltoids, latissimus dorsi, pectorals, middle trapezius and rhomboids, posterior deltoids, abdominals, erector spinae, biceps, and triceps. Give a regression and progression example for an exercise you select that uses each of the five groups you've picked.

Neuromotor and Functional Training

Chapter Objectives

By the end of this chapter, you will be able to

- understand neuromotor training principles and recommendations,
- understand functional training principles,
- ensure safety in a balance or functional training class,
- use equipment for balance and/or functional training classes,
- teach a balance class, and
- teach a functional training class.

This chapter addresses two emerging concepts in movement training: neuromotor fitness and functional exercise. Both types of activities fit well into the group exercise setting, as you will see. Neuromotor and functional training have a number of potential health benefits—see "Benefits of Neuromotor and Functional Training" for a partial list. Increase your ability to teach these modalities and help to further improve your participants' fitness and well-being!

Benefits of Neuromotor and Functional Training

- Reduced risk of falling
- Reduced risk of injury
- Improved gait
- Improved coordination and agility
- Improved reaction time and ability to move quickly
- Stronger core muscles
- Improved posture
- Improved ability to perform activities of daily living

Neuromotor Training Principles and Recommendations

Neuromotor training is a relatively new component of fitness officially identified by the American College of Sports Medicine in their 2011 position stand (Garber et al. 2011) as well as in the 2014 Guidelines (ACSM 2014). Neuromotor training involves training skills such as balance, coordination, gait, agility, and proprioception. It is important for everyone but has been shown to be especially important for older adults as an effective way to decrease the risk of falls (Bird et al. 2010; Nelson et al. 2007). Of the neuromotor activities, balance and agility training seem to have the most benefits (Karinkanta, Heinonen, and Sievanen 2007; Liu-Ambrose et al. 2004). Also, numerous studies have identified tai chi (tai ji) as an effective modality for improving balance, agility, motor control, proprioception,

and quality of life (Chin et al. 2008; Gatts 2008; Jahnke et al. 2010). You can learn more about tai chi in Chapter 17 (see "Mind–Body Classes" in that chapter). Additionally, some researchers have found that balance and agility training may reduce the risk of injuries, most notably anterior cruciate ligament injuries and ankle sprains in athletes (Hewett, Meyer, and Ford 2005; Hrysomallis 2007).

The ACSM 2014 guidelines recommend > 2 to 3 days per week (frequency) and sessions of > 20 to 30 minutes (duration) for a total of more than 60 minutes of neuromotor exercise per week. The ideal level of intensity and the optimal number of sets or reps has not yet been identified.

In this chapter, we'll focus primarily on exercises for balance, as well as those for functional training. Many functional training exercises incorporate both balance and agility skills. Balance is defined as the ability to adapt the body's center of mass with respect to its base of support. Having the ability to maintain balance, of course, is important both when standing still (static balance) and when moving the body through space (dynamic balance). Good posture, discussed in Chapter 8, is key for good balance. When moving, there are two types of postural control: anticipatory postural control and reactive postural control (Rose 2010). When you avoid an object that you can see or plan for, that is considered anticipatory control; when you must react quickly to an object that you did *not* plan for (e.g., tripping over a rock on a pathway), that is called reactive postural control. Both types of postural control are essential for full functioning in activities of daily living.

Several body systems are involved in balance and other neuromotor activities. These include the sensory systems (visual, auditory, etc.), the motor system, cognitive system, the somatosensory system (senses, touch, movement, body position, pain, etc.), and the vestibular system (located in the inner ear). Ideally, all of these systems work together to promote optimal balance in all situations. Unfortunately, in some individuals, and particularly with older adults, one or more of these systems may be impaired, thus compromising the ability to balance. It's important to note that studies show older adults pay more attention to maintaining balance in daily activities than younger adults; this is partly due to declining function in one or more of the body systems just listed (Shumway-Cook and Woollacott 2000). Fortunately, we now have increasing evidence that age-related changes in balance can be reversed—or at least slowed (Morrison et al. 2010).

Functional Training Principles

Per Olof Astrand coined the term *functional training* in a landmark article titled "Why Exercise?" He stated, "If animals are built reasonably, they should build and maintain just enough, but not more structure than they need to meet functional requirements" (1992, p. 154). Dr. Astrand was ahead of his time in predicting that people would soon be focusing more on why they should exercise, rather than on how exercise changes their physique. In a recent article on trends in fitness and wellness, Archer (2007) suggested that people need more of a sense of purpose for why they exercise and predicted that soon there will be a blending of fitness and wellness. Rather than exercising for aesthetics and to improve how we look, we will be exercising to improve our lives. The term *functional training* is often used to explain this movement from aesthetics to purposeful exercise.

The great majority of functional training literature has focused on the older adult population due to the link between physical activity or exercise, physical function, and risk for disability. For example, Anders (2007) took a group of fit older adults aged 58 to 78 years who engaged in traditional exercise training and had them focus on functional fitness movements for 4 weeks. The subjects were pre- and posttested using the Rikli and Jones (1999) Functional Fitness Test for older adults. Anders (2007) found that the focus on functional movements versus traditional fitness movements over a 4-week timeframe improved changes in functional fitness test scores even in exercise-trained individuals. Another example is found in the study by deVreede, Samson, and VanMeeteren (2005), who randomized older adults into two groups: a functional task–specific group (using sit-to-stand exercises and functional training) and

another group that performed a strength circuit using variable resistance machines. Although both groups improved in strength overall, the functional task–specific group reported that their quality of daily living improved. Quality of life indexes have been shown to improve in both types of muscle conditioning (Fiatarone, O'Neill, and Ryan 1994); however, due to the principle of muscle specificity, we can assume that a functionally based program will have the most significant effect on daily function. Unfortunately, few studies exist in the literature that evaluate functional fitness outcomes in younger adults and non-physically disabled individuals.

In functional fitness training, the muscles are trained and developed in such a way as to make the performance of everyday activities easier, smoother, safer, and more efficient. Functional exercises aim to improve the ability to function independently in the real world. In short, functional training is fitness training for life. Of course, everyone leads different lives; some spend their days lifting and carrying, others work in factories, many others sit all day long at their desks or driving in their cars. Almost everyone performs routine and familiar movements such as walking, standing up, sitting down, and bending over to retrieve something from the floor. The goal of functional training is to train the body to handle these and other real-life situations easily and safely.

Another hallmark of functional training is that exercises and movements are given that train the muscles to work together in a coordinated, whole-body way. Of course, that's what happens when you perform daily activities. Imagine how the muscles coordinate when you pick up a heavy laundry basket or a full trash can. Leg muscles work when you bend and straighten the hips, knees, and ankles, while the upper body muscles work to grasp and lift the heavy object. Meanwhile, the torso muscles are busy trying to maintain a stable spine. In real life, you hardly ever work just one muscle at a time. The idea of many muscles working all at once to perform smooth and efficient real-world movements is the idea behind functional exercise.

Traditionally, exercise scientists and fitness professionals have focused on standard weight room–type exercises for muscle conditioning, often performed on machines. While these exercises certainly have merit, they have tended to isolate specific muscles; in other words, only a single joint may have been used, while all other joints were kept still. A good example of this is a biceps exercise performed on a standard biceps curl machine. Here, the only moving joints are the elbows; all other joints are stabilized against the chair or strategically placed pads. Although such an exercise can be an excellent way to strengthen the biceps muscles, most of us do not use our biceps in this isolated way in real life.

Functional exercises tend to be multijoint, multimuscle exercises. Instead of only moving the elbow, as in the biceps exercise example described previously, a truly functional exercise might involve the elbows, shoulders, spine, hips, knees, and ankles. Instead of isolating the biceps muscles, a functional exercise may simultaneously strengthen the quadriceps, hamstrings, gluteals, abdominals, and back muscles; an example could be squatting to pick up dumbbells and then performing a standing biceps curl. Such an exercise duplicates the action of bending to pick up bags (with handles) full of groceries and then placing the bags on the kitchen counter. It is worth noting that most truly functional exercises are performed in a standing, or at least an upright, position since this more closely resembles our real-life daily positioning. Another hallmark of a functional exercise is that it tends to be multiplanar, moving the body through the sagittal, frontal, and horizontal planes. Traditional exercises are typically uniplanar; the standard biceps curl, for example, is only in the sagittal

plane. In real life we constantly move through a multitude of planes, so it doesn't make a lot of sense to repeatedly train in only one plane.

Functional training also has roots in the area of sport-specific training. This form of functional training was created by fitness professionals who desired to enhance the performance of athletes. Wolfe, Lemura, and Cole (2004) describe functional training as the art of training movements and not muscles. They believe this paradigm shift is what is needed to make a difference in the performance of athletes as well as in the performance of activities of daily living. According to Wolfe, Lemur, and Cole, when exercise programs exclusively use machines or isolated, repetitive movements, your client's functional needs are not being trained. You have to incorporate balance and speed and work the body through the various planes of movement (sagittal, frontal, transverse) rather than focus on single-plane movements that strengthen the body in only one direction. As a reminder, we are not suggesting that you avoid all isolated muscle actions for all participants. Single-joint and isolated-muscle exercises definitely have value, particularly for beginners, frail older adults, those with poor body awareness, and those with muscle imbalances. At the other end of the continuum, just because an exercise is challenging, it doesn't necessarily mean it is functional. For example, some kettlebell exercises, such as Turkish get-ups, are touted as functional, but we need to ask, for whom? Getting up off the ground is a good exercise to include for functional purposes; however, lifting a heavy weight with one hand overhead while getting up may not be necessary for life.

Santana (2002) has defined functional training by describing the various movement patterns that people use in their daily lives. His theory on functional training states that because in our daily lives we stand and move about, raise and lower the centers of our bodies, push and pull, and rotate with many movements, our exercise movements ought to mimic these basic daily patterns. Similarly, the American Council on Exercise (ACE), in their *Personal Trainer Manual* (2010), identified five primary movements that encompass all activities of daily living: bend-and-lift movements (e.g., squatting), single-leg

Hallmarks of a Functional Exercise

- Multijoint
- Multimuscle
- Multiplanar
- Occurs in a functional position (needed for activities of daily living)
- Incorporates balance
- Requires core stability

ACSM Guidelines for Elderly Adults

Older people are now the fastest growing segment of the population in the United States and the ACSM has created guidelines specifically for older adults and exercise (ACSM 2014) The increasing numbers of older adults in the population present a unique challenge as well as a vital opportunity for group exercise instructors. Old age is perhaps the most important time in a person's life for exercise and physical activity. What is the antidote for the tendency toward physical decline with aging and the eventual loss of independence that occurs with severely diminished physical function? The old adage, "If you don't use it, you lose it," holds true. Group exercise instructors can serve a valuable role in helping older adults stay vital and independent.

ACSM FITT Recommendations for Older Adults

Aerobic Exercise

Frequency: A minimum of 5 days/week for moderate intensity activities or 3 days/week for vigorous intensity activities

Intensity: RPE [rating of perceived exertion] is the preferred method for assessing intensity—5-6 for moderate intensity and 7-8 for vigorous intensity on a 0-10 scale

Time: For moderate-intensity activities—30-60 minutes in bouts of at least 10 minutes to total 150-300 minutes/week; for vigorous-intensity activities—20-30 minutes/day to total 75-100 minutes/week

Type: Any modality that does not impose excessive orthopedic stress; walking is highly recommended. Aquatic exercise and stationary cycle exercise may be preferred for those having trouble with weight-bearing activities

Muscle Strengthening and Endurance Exercise

Frequency: At least 2 days/week

Intensity: Between moderate (5-6) and vigorous (7-8) intensity on a scale of 0-10

Type: Progressive weight-training program or weight-bearing exercises (8-10 exercises involving major muscle groups; at least 1 set of 10-15 repetitions each)

Flexibility Exercise

Frequency: At least 2 days/week

Intensity: Stretch to the point of feeling tightness or slight discomfort

Time: Hold the stretch for 30-60 seconds

Type: Sustained stretches for each major muscle group; static rather than ballistic movements

Neuromotor (Balance) Exercises

Frequency: 2-3 days/week

Type: Postures that gradually reduce the base of support, dynamic movements that perturb the center of gravity, exercises with reduced sensory input (e.g., standing with eyes closed), and tai chi

movements (e.g., lunging), pushing movements, pulling movements, and rotational movements.

Underscoring the movement toward functional fitness, Cook (2010), a physical therapist working with professional athletes, created a series of tests to measure functional human movement. These assessments are used in some fitness and strength and conditioning programs and are called Functional Movement Screening Tests. Like the Rikli and Jones (1999) test for senior functional movement, Cook's tests were designed to measure functional movement for athletes. We have seen that using the functional movement screening protocols in an active-duty military population can enhance training outcomes (Kennedy-Armbruster et al. 2012). Our hope is that functional movement tests that focus on a larger segment of the population will eventually be designed.

Functional training assessments, theories, and recommendations are in line with the idea that participants need to take the benefits of the group exercise experience out of the fitness facility and into their lives. If we provide movements that relate to real life and even name movements after functional daily activities, we will help participants integrate fitness into their real world. For example, an overhead deltoid press exercise may be referred to as an exercise that assists with putting away things in a cupboard. A squat exercise with a bilateral deltoid raise may be a dryer exercise, simulating getting clothes out of a dryer. The more we integrate the importance of training for daily living activities into our conversation during group exercise, the more we teach participants about the relationship between movement and well-being.

Safety Issues in Balance and Functional Training

Functional training exercises for the average population are safe and easy to include in a group exercise class. Changing a traditional standing bilateral overhead press to a more complex move by adding standing unilateral hip abduction to the exercise is an example of an easy way to incorporate more functional movement into your class.

As always, though, safety is key whenever balance exercises are introduced. When teaching frail older adults or those with balance challenges, avoid progressing to harder exercises until participants can stand on their own comfortably and securely. Make certain they are within arm's reach of a chair or handrail unless you are able to stay at their side and provide appropriate spotting. Teach participants the options and progressions for hand support (see "Hand Support Progression for Balance Exercises") and encourage them to decide for themselves which option is best on any given day.

What about exercise safety and functional training? While an important benefit of exercise is reduced risk of injury, performing a difficult exercise before the body is sufficiently conditioned may actually cause an injury. Some functional exercises, such as a bent-over row performed bilaterally (with both arms at the same time), are considered riskier because of the core muscle endurance required to keep the back safe and stable while lifting heavy weights. It is recommended for beginners just starting an exercise program or new to resistance training that they start with more stable positions (e.g., supine or seated) or perform muscle-isolation exercises. After strength, endurance, flexibility, balance, coordination, core stability, and body awareness have improved, participants may progress toward more functional exercises where muscular integration is the focus. Figure

Hand Support Progression for Balance Exercises

Level 1: Securely hold on to support with both hands.

Level 2: Securely hold on with one hand.

Level 3: Lightly touch support with fingertips.

Level 4: Play piano (lift fingers off and then move them as if playing a piano) on the support.

Level 5: Float hands a few inches above the support.

Level 6: Balance with hands at sides or with shoulders abducted at 90°.

Level 7: Progress by performing Level 6 while looking around the room.

Level 8: Progress by performing Level 6 with eyes closed.

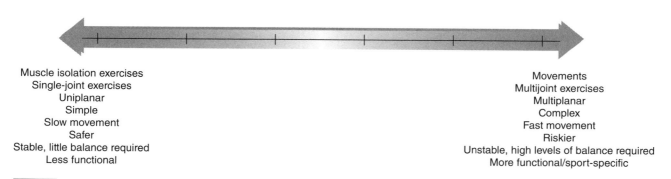

FIGURE 9.1 The progressive functional training continuum for functional and balance training.

9.1 adapts the progressive functional training continuum to note the factors that should be considered when choosing balance and functional exercises.

In summary, functional fitness is an important goal of exercise since participants are training for improved function in everyday activities. Muscle-isolation exercises are excellent for those new to resistance training, but over time, they will want to move toward functional exercises that use the body as an integrated whole, duplicating actions needed for life. This type of training, properly applied, can help reduce the risk of injuries, make everyday activities easier, and improve the quality of life.

Equipment for Balance and Functional Training

Although both balance and functional training classes can be readily taught with no equipment, several devices are available that can help provide overload and make your class more fun and interesting for participants (see figure 9.2).

- Stability balls are discussed in chapter 8; please review the information regarding proper sizing. These lightweight, large balls can be used to challenge balance in seated, side-lying, supine, or prone positions; a stability ball can also act as a bench for lying on, or as a chair.

- BOSU balance trainers are perfect for challenging balance in almost all positions: standing, seated, side lying, prone, supine, and on all fours. The BOSU can be used with either the domed side or the flat side up. Although some studies have shown that the BOSU does not increase core muscle activity (Willardson, Fontana, and Bressel 2009), no research has yet adequately studied its effects on balance.

- Foam rollers are often used for rolling and myofascial release techniques. However, they can make a great, inexpensive tool for core stability work and balance challenges, especially in the supine and prone positions.

- Core Boards and wobble boards are available in some facilities; these boards pivot on an axis and can provide a high-level balance challenge.

- Balance cushions (e.g., Dyna-disc) can be used in a variety of positions. Since these air-filled plastic cushions are low to the ground, they may help some participants feel safer in prone, supine, and seated exercises.

- Foam cushions (e.g., Airex) are great for providing balance overload in the standing position. After a participant has mastered single-leg balance exercises while standing on the floor, have him or her stand on a foam cushion for additional challenge.

- Agility dots, also known as balance pads, usually come in brightly colored sets of six. You can purchase perfectly flat dots or small pads that are domed, squishy, and can be used with either the flat or the domed side up. All are perfect for rock hopping or other balance and agility drills.

- Beams (e.g., Beamfit, Airex beams) are low, narrow, squishy beams (2.5 in high, 5 ft long [6.4 cm high, 1.5 m long]) on which a large variety of exercises can be performed. Some facilities offer Beamfit classes.

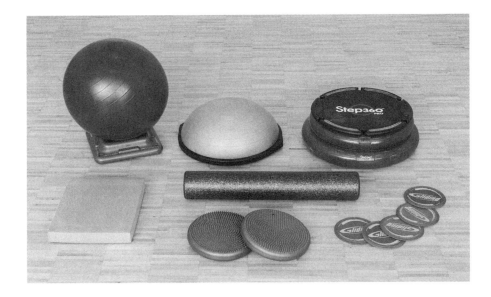

FIGURE 9.2   Equipment for balance training classes.

Teaching a Balance Class

As with other formats of group exercise instruction, all balance classes should begin with a warm-up and end with an appropriate cooldown. A formatting technique that works well is to organize all the exercises by position and then by equipment. For example, you might start with standing exercises, incorporating both static and dynamic balance challenges. You could have participants start with balance exercises that require no equipment, then move to exercises on the BOSU, then move to standing exercises on the foam roller, and so on. Follow these with traveling or dynamic balance challenges. All-fours or plank positions could be formatted next, followed by supine exercises. This type of formatting helps your class to flow more smoothly. Remember that you can use the Group Exercise Class Evaluation Form in appendix A as a template for this type of class.

 See online video 9.1 for a demonstration of exercises that can bring balance and neuromotor training into a group exercise class.

Balance Exercises

How many balance exercises do you know? Let's explore some of the many options available in a typical group exercise class.

Standing

The following exercises are probably what most people think of when they think about static balance.

BASIC SINGLE-LEG BALANCE

This exercise is sometimes known as the tree pose in yoga. Stand on one leg with the other knee bent; the bent knee can face forward (sagittal plane) or to the side (frontal plane). Shoulders can be abducted at 90°, arms can reach overhead, or hands can press together in front of the chest (prayer position). Lift the crown of the head upward even as the support foot presses downward. Hold for 30 seconds.

Regress
Hold onto a chair, handrail or Bodybar; stand against a wall.

Progress
Stand on a foam cushion; stand on a BOSU; stand on a foam roller. Raising the arms and/ or turning the head increases the challenge.

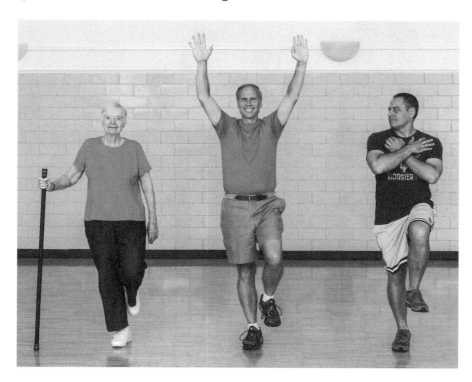

SINGLE-LEG BALANCE WITH LEG SWINGS

This exercise can be done with hip flexion and extension (*a, b*, sagittal plane) or with hip abduction and adduction (*c, d*, frontal plane). Stand on one leg in good alignment while swinging the opposite leg through hip flexion and hip extension. Keep the core stable and spine long. Perform 8 to 12 repetitions per side. Repeat the exercise while swinging the leg sideways through hip abduction and hip adduction. Regress or progress as shown in the photos or as suggested for the basic single-leg balance.

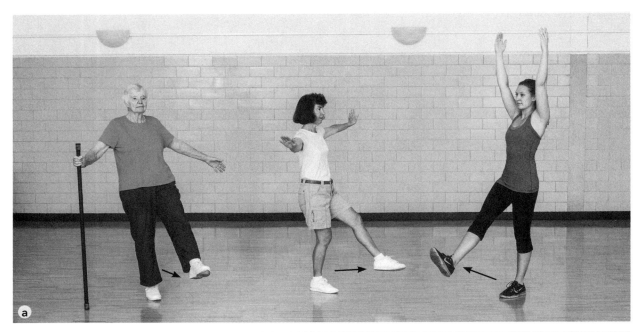

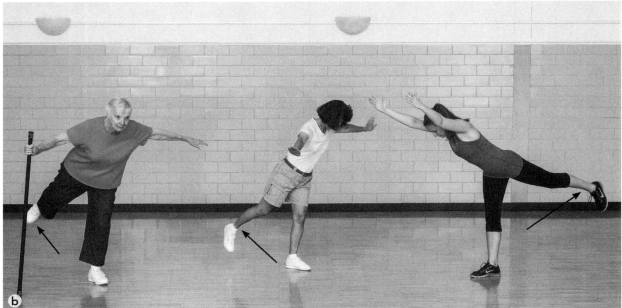

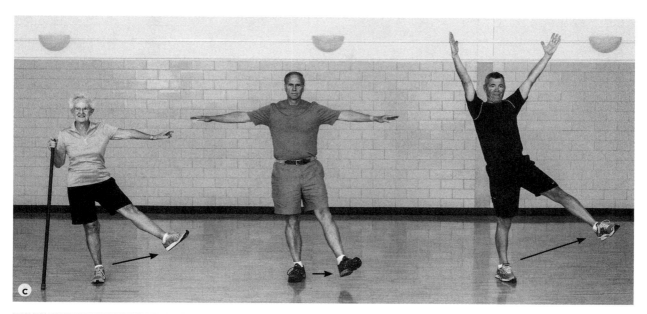

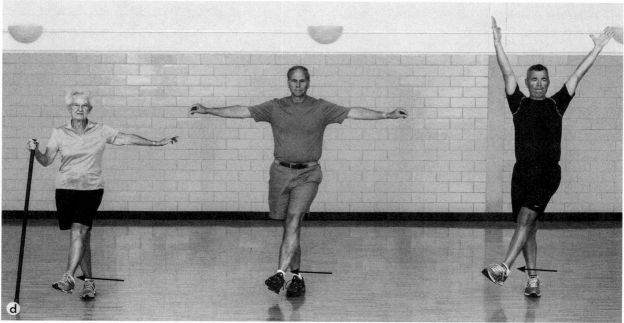

SINGLE-LEG BALANCE WITH CIRCUMDUCTION

Maintain single-leg balance while performing hip circumduction with opposite leg, or use other moves such as pedaling with the opposite leg, kicking with the opposite leg, heel-toe-heel-together pattern with the opposite leg, and so on. Regress or progress as shown in the photo or as suggested for the basic single-leg balance.

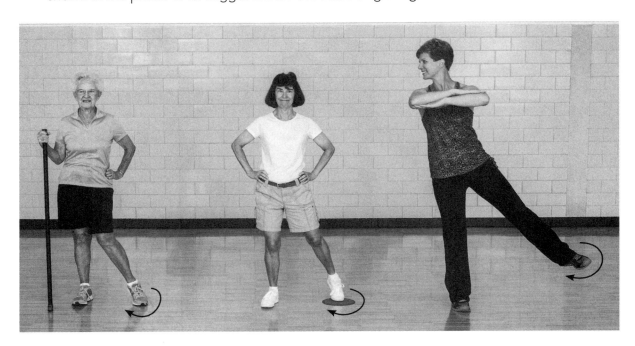

SINGLE- OR DOUBLE-LEG BALANCE WITH PERTURBATION

Have participants work in teams of two and wrap an elastic band around the waist of one participant. The other partner holds the ends of the band and exerts a random tug or pull on the band from different directions. The goal is to maintain core stability and balance no matter what.

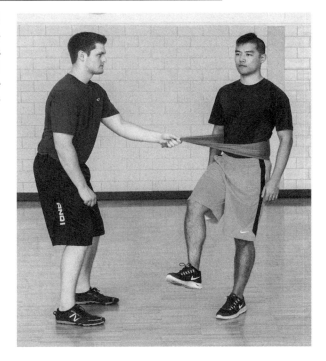

SINGLE-LEG DEAD LIFT

Stand on one leg with good alignment and hip hinge; maintain a perfectly neutral neck and spine and allow the nonsupporting leg to lift behind, ideally in a straight line with the torso. Variations include holding a dumbbell, foam roller, or stability ball.

Regress
Hold onto the back of a chair; hip hinge only slightly.

Progress
Stand on an unstable surface (foam cushion, BOSU, etc.); add rotation, reaching across the body to one side and returning.

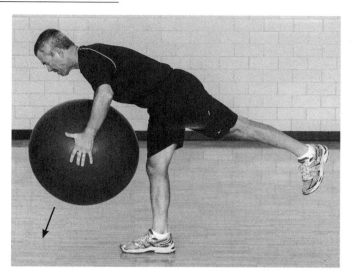

Standing and Traveling

These are dynamic balance exercises—they require participants to maintain balance while moving the body through space.

TIGHTROPE

Have participants walk along a "tightrope" on the floor. Make a line on the floor with masking tape, or if you're on a wood floor, have participants follow a line made by the wood flooring. Encourage participants to place the feet so the heel is touching, and directly in front of, the toes of the opposite foot

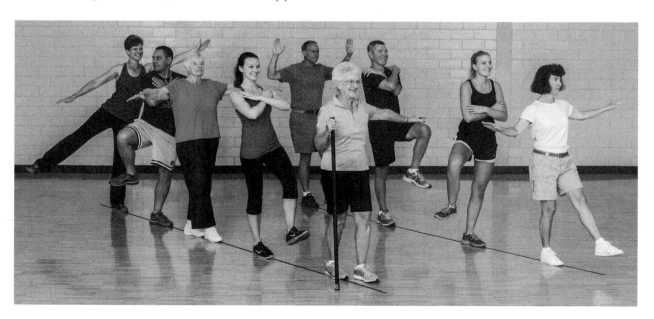

Regress
Place the tightrope 1 or 2 feet (.3 or .6 m) away from a wall so participants can use the wall with one hand if necessary; for unstable individuals, place a row of chairs on the opposite side for the other hand. Another way to regress is to make two parallel lines (like train tracks) on the floor hip-width apart; encourage participants to walk smoothly along the two lines with toes pointing straight ahead.

Progress
Have participants walk on the heels or toes along the tightrope or have them walk backward along the tightrope. Yet another progression is to have participants march along the tightrope, holding each knee high in the air and balancing for a few seconds with each knee lift.

ROCK HOPPING

Create "rocks" on the floor with agility dots or small balance pads. Have participants step from one to the other, balancing on each one as they move along.

Regress
Place dots close together, near a wall, and allow participants to move at a regular walking pace so that not much balance is required.

Progress
Place dots farther apart, necessitating a hop from one to the other. Ask participants to pause and balance on one leg at each dot. If using domed, air-filled pads, turn the pads so the flat side is up for an even greater balance challenge.

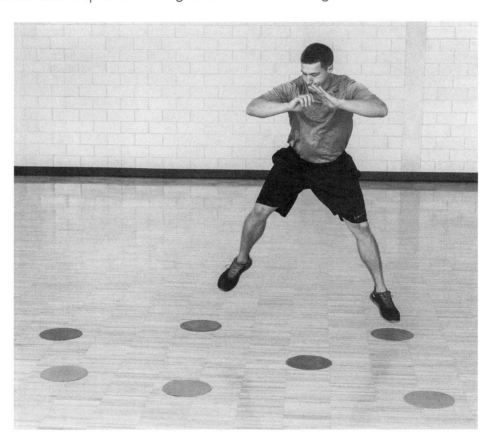

WALKING WITH ELASTIC BAND RESISTANCE

Divide participants into teams of two and wrap an elastic band around the waist of one participant. Have that person walk or march slowly while the partner pulls on the ends of the elastic band. Start with the partner standing behind, providing a straight line of pull in the sagittal plane.

Regress

Have partners stand closer; exert light force or resistance on the band; have the walking participant walk slowly with feet parallel.

Progress

Have partners stand farther apart and exert a strong force or resistance on the band. Partners can both hold the band rather than wrapping it around the waist, as shown in the photo. Have the walking participant walk on a tightrope, or line on the floor, slowly lifting one knee at a time and balancing. Additionally, the partner pulling on the band and providing the resistance may stand off to the side, exerting force in the frontal plane.

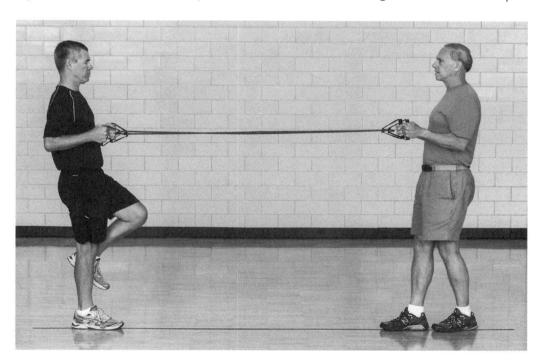

Supine Balance

The supine position is a safe and relatively more stable option, but balance can be challenged here as well.

SINGLE-LEG BRIDGE

Lie supine, knees bent, feet flat on floor, arms at sides. Evenly press up to bridge position, keeping hips level, pelvis and spine in neutral, and abdominals engaged. Lift one leg up toward the ceiling and hold (*a*).

Regress
Keep both feet on the floor for increased stability; keep both feet down on a BOSU or core board while bridging.

Progress
Perform this bridge on a stability ball, BOSU, or core board. The exercise can also be made harder by changing the arm position—from arms at the sides to arms at 90°, and eventually to arms overhead—or by dorsiflexing the ankles. Lying supine with a foam roller placed lengthwise under the spine and performing a single-leg bridge with the arms folded is a challenging balance exercise (*b*). An even harder version involves placing the foam roller under the feet.

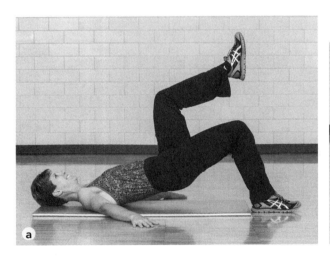

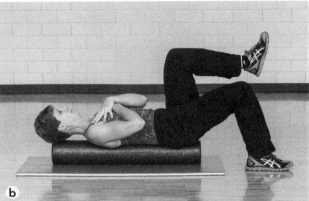

Prone or All-Fours Balance

These exercises provide a strong core stability challenge as well as a balance challenge.

QUADRUPED

Kneel on all fours with hands directly under shoulders and knees directly under hips. Maintaining neck, spine, and pelvis in neutral, lift and tighten abdominals. Smoothly raise one arm and extend the opposite hip (both in sagittal plane) without moving the torso. Hold for 10 seconds.

Regress
Lift only the arm or only the leg, not both together.

Progress
Instead of raising the arm and leg in the sagittal plane, move into shoulder and hip abduction in the frontal plane; alternatively, maintain balance and a stable torso while crossing opposite elbow to knee. The balance challenge can be greatly increased by using equipment or props; for example, kneel with one knee balanced on a BOSU and the opposite hand balanced on top of a medicine ball.

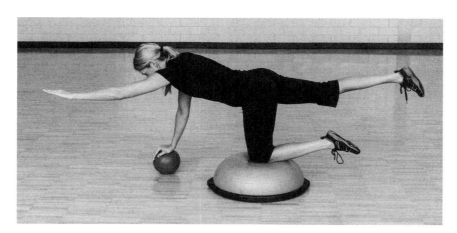

PLANK VARIATIONS

Lift up into basic full plank with abdominals engaged and neck, spine, and pelvis in neutral. Lift one leg (hip extension) and hold for 10 seconds.

Regress or modify
Modify by performing a forearm plank. Regress by performing a plank on the knees or even against a wall. Try lifting one arm or one leg.

Progress

As described for the quadruped exercise, difficulty can be increased by lifting a leg or an arm in the frontal plane or by using equipment such as the stability ball, BOSU, core board, or foam roller (a). A difficult exercise might involve placing hands on a foam roller and feet on a stability ball. Additionally, balance is significantly challenged in a side plank, especially if a prop is used (b).

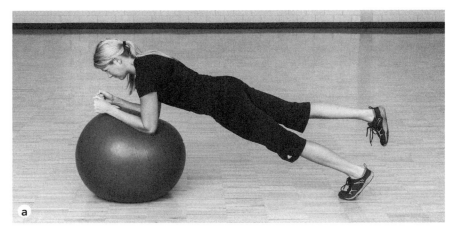

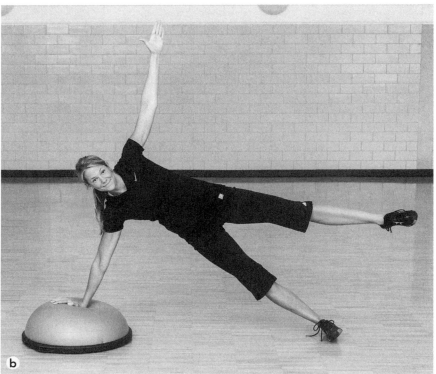

Teaching a Functional Training Class

The definition of a functional training exercise can change depending on the source. However, as discussed earlier, most experts agree that a functional exercise is multijoint, multimuscle, and multiplanar; incorporates balance; requires core stability; and is in a functional position needed for activities of daily living. The term *activation exercise* is sometimes used interchangeably, although an activation exercise can also be one used in a warm-up—something that activates the energy systems and stimulates the neuromuscular system into action. Some experts recommend training myofascial lines, arguing that movement along these lines is the most functional (Myers 2009); this thinking supports the axiom "train movements, not muscles." Anterior, posterior, lateral, spiral, and functional lines (to name a few) are identified.

Additionally, there is overlap with sport conditioning and boot camp exercise, which we discuss much more thoroughly in chapter 13. Since the functional training class format consists of specific exercise drills, you'll be using a coaching-based style of teaching for these classes. We propose that a functional training class consist of exercises that meet the criteria listed earlier (multijoint, multimuscle, etc.), that the entire class can do simultaneously (no stations), and that require a minimum of equipment. However, you can also incorporate equipment; new types of exercise equipment are constantly being developed, and many of these can be used in group exercise. Kettlebells, TRX and other suspension devices, Rip Trainers, Ballast balls, sandbags, and ViPRs (large rigid rubber tubes with handles) are a few of the newest and most popular pieces of equipment (more about these in chapter 13).

 See online video 9.2 for a sample sequence of exercises for a functional training class.

Functional Training Exercises

Here are some suggestions for exercises to incorporate into a functional training class. Appropriate exercises include standing rows (high and low) with tubing, bent-over rows (high and low) with dumbbells, planks, bridges, and quadrupeds. These exercises were either presented earlier in this chapter or are described in chapter 8. Additionally, you can create more of a sport or boot camp emphasis by incorporating exercises from chapter 13.

SQUAT

The traditional squat is a classic functional exercise. Consider how often you squat in a typical day: every time you sit down and stand up, when using the bathroom, and whenever you lift something from the floor—all frequently performed motions that require muscle coordination, strength, endurance, and balance.

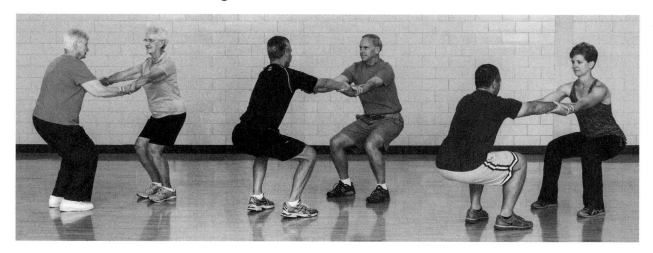

Regress

Have participants perform wall squats using stability balls behind their backs. Or, have participants try sit-back squats with partners, as shown in the photo. For knee pain, modify by reducing the range of motion—avoid flexing the knees all the way to 90°. Always keep the knees behind the toes.

Progress

There are dozens of squat variations. Have participants try big jump squats that travel across the room.

LUNGE

Lunges are also surprisingly functional. Consider how you move when quickly bending over to pick up a small object from the floor. Many people step out and bend the front knee, pick up the object, and then return back to standing with feet together—a version of a lunge! When teaching a lunge, focus on the front knee (avoid hyperflexing past 90° and keep the shin vertical) and tailbone (keep it pointing down); keep the spine vertical and neutral and lift the back heel.

Regress

Perform stationary lunges (feet do not move from their spots on the floor); stand near the wall for balance.

Progress

Step front and step back lunges are harder than stationary lunges; even harder are walking, or traveling, front lunges. For a real challenge, perform traveling Russian lunges as shown in the photos; hold weights at the shoulders and step forward into the lunge (a), then press the weight overhead in the down position of the lunge (b). Another popular lunge progression is the wheel or clock sequence (also called a lunge matrix): R leg front lunge (12:00 position), R leg front lunge to 2:00 position, R leg side lunge to 3:00 position, pivot to 5:00 position for R leg front lunge—return, R leg back lunge to 6:00 position, L leg back lunge to 6:00 position, pivot to 7:00 position for L leg front lunge, L leg side lunge to 9:00 position, L leg front lunge to 10:00 position, L leg front lunge to 12:00 position.

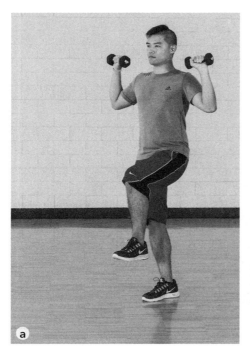
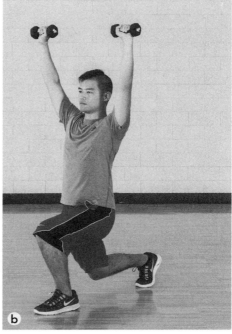

For a functional lunge variation, consider the penny pick-up; lunge forward and reach across the front foot as if picking up a penny.

STEP-UP

Step-ups are functional because they directly relate to the action of climbing stairs. Using a 4- to 8-inch (10-20 cm) step, have participants step up 8 to 20 times on one leg, then switch.

TRAVELING HOP

Traveling hops on one leg help promote balance, power, agility, and coordination. At least one source recommends no more than 8 hops in a row on one leg due to increased joint stress (Aerobics and Fitness Association of America 2010). You could ask participants to do 8 hops on the right leg, then 8 hops on the left, back and forth across the room.

WOOD CHOP AND SIMILAR MOVES

Wood chops, hay balers, and ball throws replicate potential activities of daily living and sport-specific moves. In the group exercise setting, these work well when you divide your class into duos. Partners stand approximately 4 or 5 feet (1.2 or 1.5 m) from each other; for wood chop moves, partners take turns energetically throwing a ball down and bouncing it off the floor a bit off to one side (in the direction of the partner). As the ball bounces up and away, the partner catches it up high and repeats the same diagonal wood chop move.

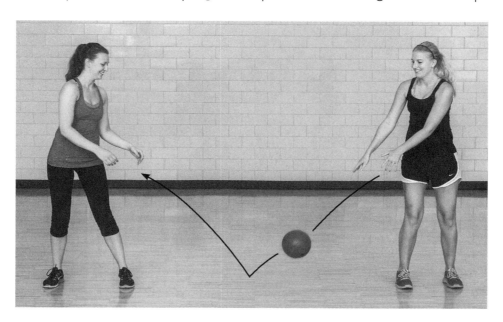

Functional Training Exercises

PARTNER STANDING CRUNCH WITH TUBING

This exercise challenges the abdominals in a functional position. Partners stand facing away from each other, each holding the handle of the tubing against the head; the distance between the partners should be sufficient so there's no slack in the tubing. Simultaneously, each partner performs resisted standing spinal flexion, along with a posterior pelvic tilt. Participants generally need a visual demonstration and several cues in order to do the exercise correctly. Watch to see that they don't perform hip flexion instead of spinal flexion.

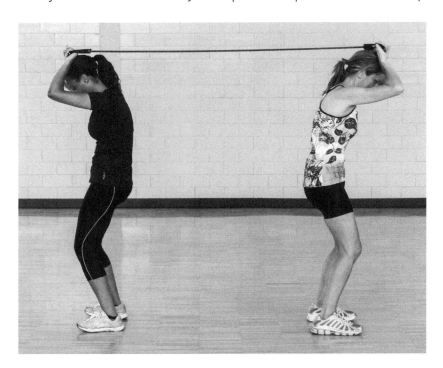

Chapter Wrap-Up

In this chapter we've covered neuromotor and functional training principles, research, and recommendations. We opted to focus primarily on balance training since a large amount of evidence-based research supports the importance of balance exercise. The chapter presented many exercises suitable for a balance or functional training class complete with regressions, progressions, and variations. We hope you'll add teaching this type of class to your repertoire of skills! Doing so connects the exercise experience with life. This concept may help participants see the value of organized exercise as they associate movements in life with movements in your class.

ASSIGNMENTS

1. Research functional training and myofascial lines and write a 1,500- to 2,000-word paper discussing your findings. Use this research to develop your own theory of what functional training is. In your analysis, cite a minimum of three articles that refer to functional training.

2. Design a balance training class. Include a warm-up and cool-down and list the exercises you'd include in the conditioning segment. Be prepared to teach a 5-minute sample of your class to your classmates.

Part III

Group Exercise Modalities

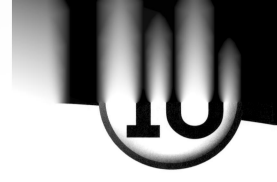

Kickboxing

Chapter Objectives

By the end of this chapter, you will be able to

- create a warm-up for a kickboxing class;
- understand alignment, technique, and safety concerns in kickboxing;
- create and instruct basic kickboxing moves;
- build kickboxing combinations and use choreographic techniques; and
- create and instruct a 2-minute kickboxing routine with appropriate content, alignment, technique, cueing, and music.

Background Check

Before working your way through this chapter, do the following:

Read

- ☐ chapter 6, "Warm-Up and Cool-Down," and
- ☐ chapter 4, the section "Applying Music Skills in Group Exercise."

Practice

- ☐ the music drills in chapter 4, in the "Applying Music Skills in Group Exercise" section, and
- ☐ chapter 4, the section "Cueing Methods in Group Exercise."

Group Exercise Class Evaluation Form Essentials

Key Points for Warm-Up Segment

- Includes appropriate amount of dynamic movement
- Provides rehearsal moves
- Stretches major muscle groups in a biomechanically sound manner with appropriate instructions

- Provides intensity guidelines for warm-up
- Includes clear cues and verbal directions
- Uses an appropriate music tempo (125-135 beats per minute) or music that inspires movement

Key Points for Conditioning Segment

- Gradually increases intensity
- Uses a variety of muscle groups
- Minimizes repetitive movements
- Observes participants' form and provides constructive, nonintimidating feedback
- Continually offers modifications, regressions, progressions, or alternatives
- Provides alignment and technique cues
- Gives motivational cues
- Educates participants about intensity; provides HR and/or RPE check 1 or 2 times during the workout stimulus

- Promotes participant interaction and encourages fun
- Provides regular demonstrations and participation with good body mechanics
- Gradually decreases impact and intensity during cool-down after the cardiorespiratory session
- Uses appropriate volume and music tempo that encourage proper movement patterns and progressions (125-135 beats per minute)

Kickboxing has grown in popularity as a group exercise modality through the late 1990s and into the 21st century. The term *kickboxing* can encompass a variety of martial arts workouts, including aeroboxing, cardio karate, box step, jump and jab, and Tae Bo. New trends include kickboxing fusion classes and the incorporation of other martial arts disciplines into the fitness setting, including tai chi, Krav Maga, Forza, jiu jitsu, and capoeira. The goal for most students in a kickboxing class is to improve health and fitness; most aren't taking the class with the intention of actually fighting. Therefore, the basic moves in a group kickboxing class are slightly modified from classical martial arts styles to enhance safety and reduce the risk of injury. We recommend that you go beyond basic group exercise training and certification and pursue additional training specific to kickboxing if you plan to teach this format. A well-taught kickboxing class can be a great workout and can also be fun and highly stimulating for you and your students (see "Kickboxing Research Find-

ings" in this chapter). The main points on the group exercise class evaluation form that relate to kickboxing are listed in the Group Exercise Class Evaluation Form Essentials.

Creating a Warm-Up

Kickboxing warm-ups follow the warm-up recommendations outlined in chapter 6 and thus include dynamic movement, rehearsal moves, and appropriate stretching. Alignment cues and a safe music speed are also very important in a kickboxing warm-up.

Dynamic Movements and Rehearsal Moves

The biggest difference between a kickboxing warm-up and other kinds of group exercise warm-ups is the inclusion of dynamic rehearsal moves specific to kickboxing. Remember that a rehearsal move is a low-intensity version of a movement that will be used later in the high-intensity cardiorespiratory portion of class. These moves prepare the body for the kickboxing workout to follow and include punches, jabs, hooks, and kicks, all performed at a slower speed than that used during the actual workout. Focus on teaching proper form and technique while your class practices these basic movements. When teaching beginners, you may even consider teaching the basic punches and kicks without music to help your students learn proper form and alignment.

Following is a simple warm-up combination that incorporates rehearsal moves:

1. Using the ready position, punch 4 times with the right arm—punch once every 4 counts (16 counts).
2. Repeat with the left arm (16 counts).
3. Perform 4 step touches (16 counts).
4. Do 4 hamstring curls (16 counts).
5. Repeat.

Practice Drill

Create your own kickboxing warm-up. Pair a basic upper-body move, such as a punch, jab, hook, or uppercut, with a basic lower-body move, such as a march, step touch, or grapevine.

Stretching Major Muscle Groups

Another important aspect of a kickboxing warm-up is the increased focus on limbering and stretching the muscles that will be heavily used in the routine that follows; these include the calf muscles, hip flexors, inner-thigh muscles, hamstrings, low-back muscles, and muscles of the anterior chest and shoulder complex. (For specific stretches, see chapter 8.) It is particularly important to include dynamic movements and full range of motion (ROM) movements. Shoulder rolls that move backward can help counterbalance all the anterior punches and jabs in the workout. Stretches held briefly (3-5 seconds) are necessary for the punching and kicking muscles because of the high number of repetitive drills found in a typical fitness-based kickboxing class. Be sure to have students stretch

the pectoralis major, anterior deltoids, triceps, hip flexors, quadriceps, hamstrings, calves, and erector spinae. As always, the warm-up is an ideal time to stress proper alignment— emphasize alignment in the punches and kicks as well as in the static stretches. Because the incidence of injury in kickboxing classes is relatively high (Davis et al. 2002), a proper warm-up and careful teaching of the basic moves are essential.

Verbal Cues and Tempo

Focus on delivering precise anatomical and educational cues when detailing alignment. Briefly review several joints or areas of the body. For example, when class members are holding a calf stretch, you can say, "Hold the head high, with ears away from the shoulders, neck in line with the spine, shoulders down and back, and abdominals in. Your body should form one long line from head to heel; stretch the heel down with the toes facing straight ahead and the hips square." Keep your cues positive, telling your class what to do rather than what not to do. Remember that pointing to or touching parts of your body can be an effective way to cue alignment visually.

A music tempo of 125 to 135 beats per minute is appropriate for most warm-ups. Movement at this tempo is fast enough to elevate heart rate, core temperature, and breathing rate but not so fast that participants will become winded or fail to complete the moves.

Technique and Safety Check

Following are recommendations for the kickboxing warm-up:

- Use at least one combination that incorporates kickboxing rehearsal moves.
- Gradually increase the speed and intensity of the kickboxing moves.
- Thoroughly prepare the hamstrings, calves, hip flexors, inner thighs, low-back, anterior chest, and shoulder muscles with both dynamic movements and light static stretches.

Kickboxing Research Findings

A number of studies have examined the effectiveness of kickboxing for cardiorespiratory training (Adams et al. 1997; Albano and Terbizan 2001; Anning et al. 1999; Bellinger et al. 1997; Bissonnette et al. 1994; Franzese et al. 2000; Greene et al. 1999; Kravitz, Greene, and Wongsathikun 2000; O'Driscoll et al. 1999; Perez et al. 1999; Scharff-Olson et al. 2000). These studies have found that kickboxing can provide a workout that is sufficient for developing cardiorespiratory fitness. Significant findings from these studies include the following: (1) increasing the music speed from 60 to 120 beats per minute during punching increased the cardiorespiratory response; (2) combining punches with vigorous lower-body moves such as shuffles, jacks, and squats resulted in a better cardiorespiratory stimulus; and (3) there was no significant difference in terms of energy cost between shadowboxing and boxing with a heavy bag. One study found that the average caloric expenditure was 7 calories per minute if the routine was predominantly leg moves combined with upper-body moves; routines using only the upper body are discouraged if the goal is weight management or cardiorespiratory fitness (Ergun, Plato, and Cisar 2006). Another study noted that kickboxing elicited a lower $\dot{V}O_2$max than treadmill running elicited at similar heart rates (Wingfield et al. 2006).

More recently, researchers have examined the effect of kickboxing on specific populations. In one study, kickboxing helped people with multiple sclerosis function better in their daily lives (Jackson 2011). Cardio–kickboxing moves can be modified so that they're viable even for people with limited mobility. Kickboxing (neuroboxing) programs have also been developed for people with Parkinson's disease.

Other researchers have examined injuries in kickboxing classes (Buschbacher and Shay 1999; Davis et al. 2002; McKinney-Vialpando 1999). A relatively high rate of injury (29.3% of participants and 31.3% of instructors) was found in the study that included 572 participants by Davis and colleagues (2002). This study also found that the risk of injury increased dramatically when the frequency of kickboxing was increased: 43% of participants who took four or more classes per week reported injuries versus 25% of participants who took only one or two classes per week. McKinney-Vialpando (1999) found that the faster the music speed, the greater the postexercise pain, and the higher the kicks, the greater the incidence of pain. Axe and crescent kicks were also found to cause pain in 22% of the study participants.

Technique and Safety Issues

Safety is always a primary concern for instructors, especially in kickboxing, where the incidence of injury has been shown to be approximately 30% (Davis et al. 2002). Another study showed that 31% of instructors and 15.5% of participants reported injuries (Romaine et al. 2003). The back, knees, hips, and shoulders were reported as the most common injury sites by instructors, whereas the back, knee, and ankle were the most common points of injury for participants. It's important to understand the common mechanisms of injury at these sites and take steps to avoid increasing your participants' risk of injury.

In the United States, 80% of people report experiencing low-back pain at some point in their lives (Frymoyer and Cats-Baril 1991. A stable spine during kicks and punches is key to preventing back problems in a kickboxing class. The abdominal and back muscles must be dynamically and statically trained to develop spinal stability, and participants must understand the concept of a neutral spine. Excessive hip flexor involvement from too many kicks can contribute to low-back pain because the iliopsoas muscles attach on the lumbar spine; constant action of those muscles may cause low-back pain. To prevent this problem, have class members stretch the hip flexors in both the warm-up and the cool-down portions of your class.

You can reduce the incidence of knee pain in kickboxing by teaching good kicking technique. Emphasize performing active retraction, or knee flexion, immediately after the knee extends in a kick. Snapping or ballistically extending the knee with excessive momentum can overstretch the knee ligaments and create knee instability. Torque, or sudden twisting moves in which the foot is anchored but the knee turns, overstretches the collateral knee ligaments and thus is another mechanism of knee injury. Remind participants to always keep the toes aligned in the direction of the knees.

Hip pain can result from a lack of muscle balance around the hip joint. Encourage students to use the hip flexors and extensors, as well as the hip adductors and abductors and the hip internal and external rotators, as evenly as possible. Provide plenty of appropriate stretches for these muscles, avoid excessive repetitions of kicks, and always teach a thorough warm-up.

Reduce the incidence of shoulder pain by teaching good punching technique (retracting the arm immediately after each punch) and by training the external rotator cuff and posterior deltoid muscles with specific exercises to counterbalance all the forward motion involved in punching. Shoulder pain is more likely to occur when the shoulder girdle isn't properly stabilized. Instruct participants to punch with the scapulae down and provide isolation exercises for the middle trapezius and rhomboids (scapular retractors) as well as plenty of stretches for the anterior chest muscles. Participating in too many kickboxing classes without proper stretching, muscular conditioning, and body awareness can result in a hunched back and rounded shoulders (excessive kyphosis). By providing proper instruction, however, you can help your students avoid this type of poor posture and thus avoid injuries.

Additionally, instructors who reported using music speeds greater than 140 beats per minute had a higher incidence of injury than instructors who used music between 125 and 139 beats per minute (Romaine et al. 2003).

Basic Moves

Although the standard kickboxing moves can be performed in a variety of martial arts styles (listed in "Martial Arts Styles"), we recommend modifying some of these traditional moves to allow for proper joint alignment and decrease the risk of injury.

Technique and Safety Check

To keep your kickboxing classes safe, observe the following recommendations.

Remember to

- provide a thorough and appropriate warm-up;
- teach proper execution of punches and kicks;
- ensure that beginners master the basic moves before progressing;
- ensure participants angle the fist in a three-quarter turn away from full pronation during punching, which places the wrist in a safer position;
- ensure students maintain muscle balance;
- remind students to maintain proper alignment, especially during kicks;
- include opportunities to cross-train;
- provide plenty of stretches for the hip flexor, hamstring, calf, low-back, upper trapezius, and chest muscles;
- provide strengthening exercises for the middle trapezius, rhomboid, posterior deltoid, abdominal, and low-back muscles;
- use exercises that have equal numbers of punches and kicks on both sides and kicks in both front and back;
- start with only one kickboxing class per week and gradually increase the number, if desired, up to three classes per week; and
- keep music tempo speed under 140 beats per minute.

Avoid

- a snapping motion when kicking and punching,
- advanced and high kicks for all but the most skilled participants, and
- music speeds greater than 140 beats per minute.

Martial Arts Styles

- American boxing
- Thai kickboxing
- Karate
- Judo
- Taekwondo
- Aikido
- Kung fu
- Jiu jitsu
- Krav Maga
- Capoeira
- Mixed martial arts (MMA)

Initial Positioning

All kickboxing moves start from one of two basic positions: the ready position (body faces forward with feet parallel) or the staggered position (body is slightly angled to the side with one foot back). In both positions, the elbows are flexed and the fists are close together to protect the face and neck (the forearms should make a

V). The core muscles (abdominals and low back) are engaged at all times, and the shoulder blades are slightly protracted (causing a slight rounding of the upper back and shoulders). The knees are slightly flexed (see figure 10.1).

Basic Punches

The four basic punches in kickboxing are the jab, cross-jab or cross-punch, hook, and uppercut. In fitness settings, these punches are performed with a concentric contraction in both directions in order to protect the upper-body joints. In other words, there are two phases to a punch:

1. The punch itself, during which the elbow extends (the triceps contracts) and the fist moves away from the body

2. The retraction phase, during which the elbow flexes (the biceps contracts) and the fist is pulled quickly back into the body

Concentric contraction in both directions prevents the elbow from hyperextending during shadowboxing (punching air) and helps protect the elbow and shoulder joints. Additionally, when punching it is safer to modify the full palm-down, pronated position of a classic martial

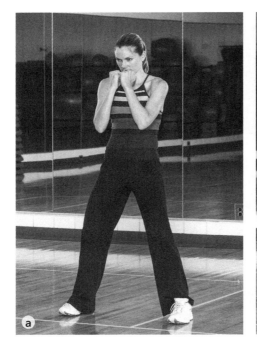 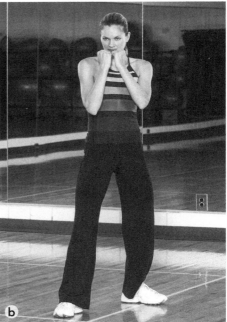

FIGURE 10.1 (*a*) Ready position and (*b*) staggered position

arts punch into a slightly angled three-quarter turn of the wrist, with the thumb slightly higher than the littlest finger (Buschbacher and Shay 1999). Be especially careful when incorporating equipment such as weighted gloves, focus mitts, or punching bags into your classes. Weighted punches and contact punches greatly increase the risk of muscle strains, ligament sprains, surface abrasions, and jamming and dislocation of the wrist and finger joints. Reserve weighted and contact punching for your advanced classes.

Jab

The jab is a straight punch to the front. When in the ready position, the torso rotates; when in the staggered position, the torso doesn't need to rotate (see figure 10.2).

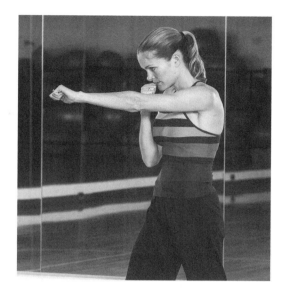

FIGURE 10.3 Cross-jab.

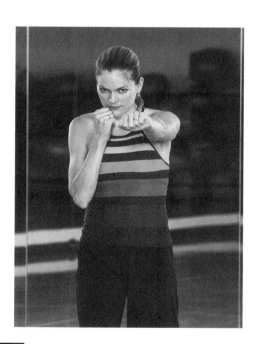

FIGURE 10.2 Jab.

Cross-Jab

The cross-jab, or cross-punch, is typically performed from the staggered position, with the heel of the back foot up so that the whole body can pivot as the punch is thrown. As the spine and hip rotate forward, the cross-jab crosses the midline of the body, and the shoulder follows through (see figure 10.3).

Hook

In the hook, the elbow is lifted and the shoulder joint is abducted at approximately 90°. The fist and arm curve around, following a horizontal line in front of the shoulders or face. The fist is kept pronated (palm facing down) or in the recommended midpronated (palm facing the body) position and the elbow flexed. The torso and hip should rotate in the direction of the punch (see figure 10.4).

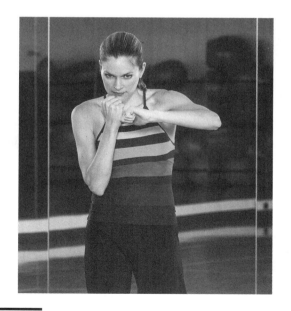

FIGURE 10.4 Hook.

Uppercut

In the uppercut, the elbow stays flexed but is kept down near the rib cage. The fist is supinated with the palm facing the body. The shoulder extends and the arm moves behind the torso (elbow remains flexed) before throwing the actual punch. Tilting the pelvis, lifting the heel, and slightly rotating the torso will increase power (see figure 10.5).

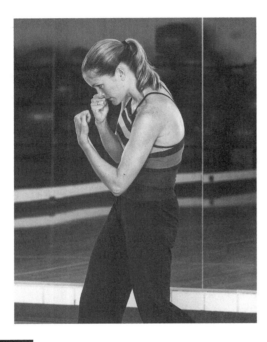

FIGURE 10.5　Uppercut.

Practice Drill

Practice the four basic punches slowly in sequence. Perform 1 punch every four counts: jab right, cross-jab left, hook right, uppercut right. Repeat with jab left, cross-jab right, hook left, and uppercut left. Choose a favorite song that is approximately 130 beats per minute to play while practicing.

Basic Kicks

The four kicks used in a typical kickboxing class are the front kick, back kick, side kick, and roundhouse kick. To decrease the risk of injury to the knee joint, the knee extension phase of the kicks should be followed immediately with a quick retraction of the leg. In other words, performing an almost reflexive and conscious knee flexion can help prevent ballistic knee hyperextension when kicking air. Proper kicks require a strong supporting leg and core (torso) as well as adequate flexibility and balance. Most martial artists take years to perfect their kicking technique, and they begin performing advanced kicks such as the crescent, axe, hitch, and spin hook only after extended study. Discourage beginners and participants who are less fit from attempting repetitive and advanced kicks too soon. Also, reserve head-high kicks for advanced participants; these kicks require great flexibility, strength, balance, and coordination, and they increase the risk of hamstring pulls and back pain. You will probably need to demonstrate kicks at waist height or lower to reduce the risk of competitive students exceeding their ROM while kicking. It's also a good idea to break down the kick movement for your students. Lead them slowly through the move as follows:

1. Flex the hip.
2. Extend the knee (avoiding hyperextension).
3. Quickly flex the knee.
4. Extend the hip and return the leg to a neutral standing position (see figure 10.6).

Front Kick

In the front kick, the kicking leg moves directly to the front while the body remains squared, with the hips and shoulders facing forward. The kicking hip flexes, but the spine remains neutral (no rounding). For advanced participants who have the flexibility and strength to kick head high, a backward lean is permitted; however, participants must maintain neutral spinal alignment throughout the movement. The ankle should be dorsiflexed so that the point of contact for the kick is at the ball of the foot, and the leg should be retracted quickly (see figure 10.6).

Back Kick

The back kick involves externally rotating the hip of the kicking leg while flexing forward on the standing hip. Again, the leg retracts immediately after kicking. A neutral spinal alignment (the spine is not flexed) is maintained while leaning forward. The point of contact is the heel of the back foot; the ankle should be dorsiflexed (see figure 10.7).

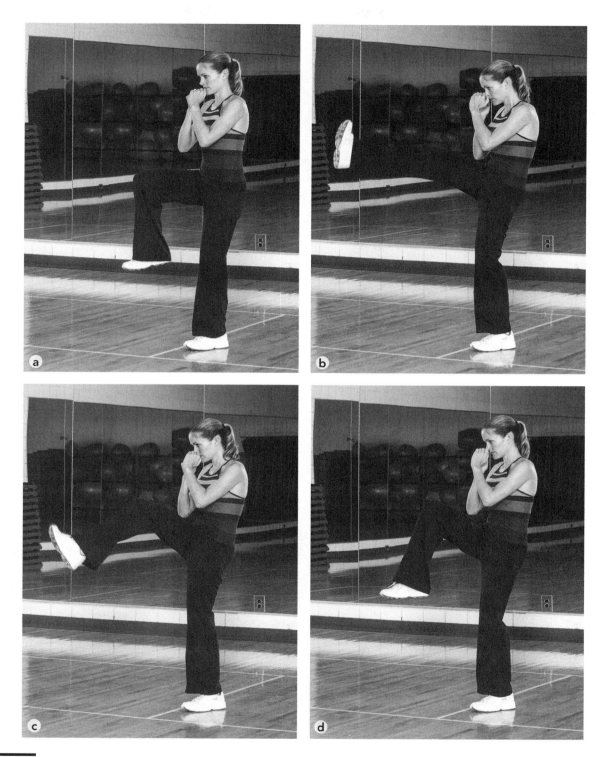

FIGURE 10.6 Phases of the front kick: (*a*) flex hip, (*b*) extend knee, (*c*) flex knee, (*d*) extend hip and return leg to neutral standing position.

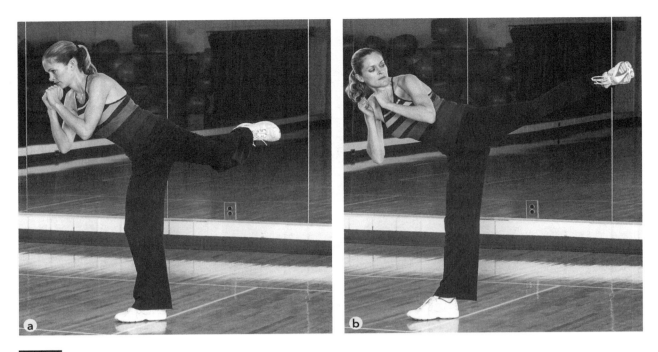

FIGURE 10.7 Phases of the back kick: (*a*) standing in hip extension and knee flexion and (*b*) knee extension at waist height.

Side Kick

In a side kick, the point of contact is the ball of the foot (again, the ankle is dorsiflexed). Depending on the height of the kick, a side (lateral) lean is acceptable; however, the spine must remain neutral without rounding. The kicking hip internally rotates so that the knee faces forward; the knee extends after the hip is abducted to the desired height (see figure 10.8).

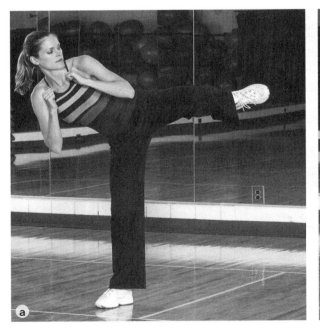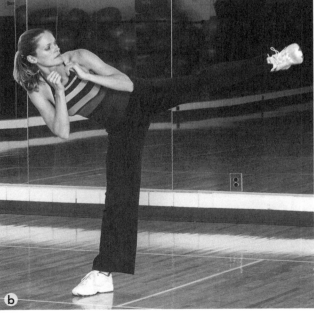

FIGURE 10.8 Phases of the side kick: (*a*) standing in hip and knee flexion and (*b*) knee extension at waist height.

Roundhouse Kick

The roundhouse kick involves working from a turned-out (externally rotated) position of both hips. The knees and toes are aligned in the same direction to avoid unnecessary torque or twisting of the knee and ankle joints. The hip of the kicking leg is externally rotated and flexed while performing lateral spinal flexion—participants should imagine making contact with the top of the foot (the forefoot)—while keeping the ankle plantar flexed. The leg retracts quickly to finish the kick (see figure 10.9).

Other Basic Moves

Other moves common to kickboxing include the boxer's shuffle, jumping rope, bob and weave, and lateral slip.

- The boxer's shuffle is a foot pattern that maintains an increased heart rate and develops speed and agility; you can use it when developing kickboxing combinations. With your feet hip-width apart and parallel, quickly move sideways without crossing the feet.
- Jumping rope is a common activity for increasing heart rate, power, stamina, and agility.

Practice Drill

Choose a favorite song (with a tempo of approximately 130 beats per minute) and practice the four basic kicks on every fourth beat as follows:

- 4 right kicks front (16 counts), 4 left kicks front (16 counts), step touch (16 counts), march (16 counts)
- 4 right kicks back (16 counts), 4 left kicks back (16 counts), step touch (16 counts), march (16 counts)
- 4 right kicks side (16 counts), 4 left kicks side (16 counts), step touch (16 counts), march (16 counts)
- 4 right roundhouse kicks (16 counts), 4 left roundhouse kicks (16 counts), step touch (16 counts), march (16 counts)

In most kickboxing classes, the jump-rope segments are in timed intervals (e.g., 3-5 minutes). During this interval, you can show different moves, including jogging, hopping twice on one foot and then the other, hop-kicking with alternating feet, bilateral jumping, bilateral jumping while twisting, and jumping jacks, all while

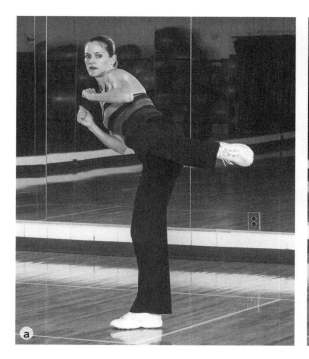
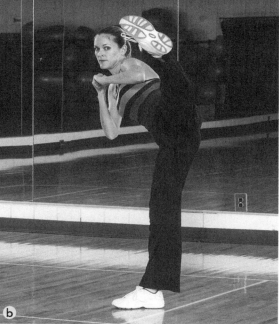

FIGURE 10.9 Phases of the roundhouse kick: (a) standing hip and knee flexion and (b) standing with knee extended.

jumping over the rope! You can have participants perform traveling moves, such as grapevines, and power moves, such as jumping high while circling the rope twice around the body (called *salt and pepper*). Participants who haven't yet coordinated the rope movement with jumping (it takes practice!) can simulate jumping rope by twirling the wrists while holding the arms close to the rib cage. Remind students to land softly and properly, rolling through the toe, ball, and heel and bringing the heels all the way down. Beginners and participants who don't want to perform the high-impact jumping can jog or simply march in place. Jump-rope intervals can be intense, so ease your participants into jumping rope with shorter intervals and be sure to spread the intervals throughout the class.

- In the bob and weave, the upper body and torso move while the feet are parallel or staggered; the upper body ducks under an imaginary punch, bobbing from one side to the other.

- In the lateral slip, the spine flexes from side to side without bobbing down and up. The feet remain anchored, usually in a parallel position.

 See online video 10.1 for a demonstration of the basic punches, kicks, and movements of kickboxing, include the jab, cross-jab, hook, uppercut, front kick, back kick, side kick, roundhouse kick, boxer's shuffle, bob and weave, lateral slip, and jump-rope moves.

Combinations and Choreography Techniques

Building combinations in kickboxing is simply a matter of combining the basic moves. Many instructors also enjoy interspersing standard high-low moves such as grapevines, hustles, step touches, hamstring curls, V-steps, and jumping jacks (see chapter 4 for a description of these moves) into the punching and kicking segments. When designing your choreography, use a variety of moves and avoid high numbers of repetitions. Because most kickboxing classes are intended to provide a cardiorespiratory stimulus, gradually increase the intensity before you include peak moves, and gradually decrease the intensity at the end of class or before participants perform floor work. Peak moves include kicks, jumping jacks, and jump-rope moves. A basic kickboxing combination is shown in table 10.1.

 See online video 10.2 for demonstrations of two kickboxing combinations.

Practice Drill

Using music with a tempo of approximately 125 to 138 beats per minute, put together your own combination of kickboxing moves. Include punches, kicks, and other basic moves.

Other Kickboxing Formats

Some instructors prefer not to teach preplanned choreography on a 32-count block (such as the routine shown in table 10.1). Instead, they may teach a more military or combat style that includes repetitive drills that may or may not use music or follow the musical beat. For example, the class might include 10 minutes of punching (with or without a bag), 3 minutes of jumping rope, 10 minutes of kicking, 3 minutes of jumping rope, 10 minutes of punching, 3 minutes of jumping rope, and 10 minutes of kicking. When using this style, have participants move in a variety of directions and limit the number of repetitions to avoid overuse injuries.

Other formats include step kickboxing classes (intervals of step alternated with intervals of kickboxing); equipment-based classes (intervals of punching with bags or focus mitts and intervals of kicking shields or bags); and classes with partner drills, circles, and other group formations. Many kickboxing classes move on to push-ups, abdominal work, or other muscular conditioning after the kickboxing portion of class.

Whatever format you choose, continuously give a variety of options in movement and intensity. For example, if you show a jumping jack followed by a jab on the right, immediately follow the introduction of this move by saying,

TABLE 10.1 Sample Kickboxing Combination

Move	Foot pattern	Upper body	Number of counts
Shuffle right	R, L, R, L, R, L, R, pause	Cross-jab L on 7	8
Shuffle left	L, R, L, R, L, R, L, pause	Cross-jab R on 7	8
Repeat			16
Front kick	R, L kick, L, R, L, R kick, R, L	Ready position	8
Repeat			8
Repeat			8
Repeat			8
Repeat			8
Bob and weave	Staggered position	Ready position	8
Lateral slip	Staggered position	Ready position	8
Repeat bob and weave			8
Repeat lateral slip			8
Jab	Ready position	Jab R, L, R, L (every 4 counts)	16
Hook	Ready position	Hook R, L, R, L (every 4 counts)	16
Repeat entire combination			

R = right; L = left.

"If this move is uncomfortable, try it without the jump—like this!" and show a lower-intensity and lower-impact option.

 See online video 10.3 for intensity and complexity options in kickboxing.

Chapter Wrap-Up

A kickboxing class can be a fun, energizing, and challenging way to exercise in a group. However, you must make safety a priority to ensure an enjoyable experience for all participants. As an instructor, learn how to throw proper punches and kicks and teach them carefully to your classes, emphasizing correct alignment and technique at all times.

Group Exercise Class Evaluation Form: Key Points

- Gradually increase intensity. In kickboxing, this means avoiding high-intensity drills, high kicks, and jump-rope intervals for the first several minutes of the cardio stimulus. Review the first practice drill in this chapter to see if you can gradually increase the intensity of this combo by increasing the ROM, traveling distance, or impact of the floor pattern.

- Use a variety of muscle groups and minimize repetitive movements. Review your combination from the last practice drill in this chapter to be sure you considered muscle balance, variety, and safety.

- Demonstrate good form, alignment, and technique for kickboxing. Keep practicing so that these become second nature to you.
- Use music appropriately. Keep the music speed under 138 beats per minute for the cardio segment. Music that is too fast makes it difficult for participants to move safely with good alignment. If you choose to teach to the music, move on the downbeat and use 32-count phrases to enhance participant success.
- Give clear cues and verbal directions. Anticipatory cues, discussed in chapter 4, are particularly important when teaching combinations. For example, cue "4, 3, 2, right hook" (the word *hook* is spoken on the last beat).
- Promote participant interaction and encourage fun. Try different arrangements such as having two groups of participants face each other while practicing punches or having the class stand in one large circle for kicking drills.
- Gradually decrease intensity during the cool-down after the cardio conditioning segment; use lower-intensity moves similar to those used in the warm-up. Decrease music speed, ROM, traveling, impact, and overhead arm motions as you return to resting conditions. Walking in place, step touches, and heel digs all can be performed at a low intensity with low arm movements.

ASSIGNMENT

Write out and create a 2-minute kickboxing routine that consists of at least two 32-count blocks (see table 10.1 or the section "Writing Out a Combination" in chapter 4 for an example of how to write out a combination). Teach your routine using the technique of repetition reduction and include upper-body and lower-body movements.

Step Training

Chapter Objectives

By the end of this chapter, you will be able to

- design a warm-up for step training;
- understand technique and safety issues in step;
- teach basic moves and patterns for step;
- create basic combinations and choreography for a step class; and
- teach a 4-minute step routine with appropriate content, alignment, technique, cueing, and music.

Background Check

Before working your way through this chapter, do the following:

Read

- ☐ chapter 6, "Warm-Up and Cool-Down";
- ☐ chapter 4, "Applying Music Skills in Group Exercise"; and
- ☐ the choreographic technique sections in chapter 4, including "Traditional Choreography", "Elements of Variation", and "Building Basic Combinations".

Practice

- ☐ the music drills in chapter 4, "Music for Group Exercise", and
- ☐ the cueing drills in chapter 4, "Cueing Methods in Group Exercise".

Group Exercise Class Evaluation Form Essentials

Key Points for Warm-Up Segment

- Includes appropriate amount of dynamic movement
- Provides rehearsal moves
- Provides dynamic or static stretches for at least two major muscle groups

Key Points for Conditioning Segment

- Gradually increases intensity
- Uses a variety of muscle groups
- Minimizes repetitive movements
- Observes participants' form and provides constructive, nonintimidating feedback
- Continually offers modifications, regressions, progressions, and/or alternatives
- Provides alignment and technique cues
- Gives motivational cues
- Educates participants about intensity; provides HR (heart rate) and/or RPE (rate of

- Provides intensity guidelines for warm-up
- Includes clear cues and verbal directions
- Uses an appropriate music tempo (118-128 beats per minute) or music that inspires movement

perceived exertion) check at least 1 or 2 times during workout stimulus

- Promotes participant interaction and encourages fun
- Provides regular demonstrations and participation with good body mechanics
- Gradually decreases impact and intensity during cool-down after the cardiorespiratory session
- Uses appropriate volume and music tempo that encourage proper movement patterns and progressions (118-128 beats per minute)

Cardio step classes have been popular since their inception in 1990; currently, approximately 58% of fitness facilities offer cardio step programs (IDEA 2011). Step classes promote cardiorespiratory fitness, muscle endurance, coordination, and balance and come with several health benefits (see "Step Training Research Findings"). Many participants enjoy the rhythmic sound, exact patterning, and high energy of a step class. Expand your options as a group exercise leader by learning how to teach a motivating, beat-driven, step class. The main points on the group exercise class evaluation form that relate to step training are listed in the "Group Exercise Class Evaluation Form Essentials."

Creating a Warm-Up

Warm-ups for step training should follow the recommendations outlined in chapter 6 and use a combination of dynamic movements and stretches to prepare the heart, lungs, and major muscles for vigorous activity. However, an optimal step warm-up also incorporates the bench, thus specifically readying the body for the workout to follow.

This is achieved by using a *floor mix*—that is, a mixture of step and low-impact moves. A simple floor mix pattern is shown in table 11.1.

Dynamic Movement and Rehearsal Moves

Table 11.1 combines low-impact and step moves: A grapevine is performed on the floor, whereas the tap-up, tap-down is a rehearsal move that uses the step. Combining the two specifically and gradually prepares the mind and body for more intense step moves. Because the warm-up is to be performed at a lower intensity than the cardio-conditioning portion of the class, the number of step moves used and the sequencing of the floor mix are important factors. Avoid continuous stepping in the warm-up because it stresses unprepared joints and can increase the heart rate too quickly. Instead, intersperse low-impact moves with step moves.

Stretching in the Warm-Up

Ideally, some of your warm-up stretches should use the step; common stretches on the bench

TABLE 11.1 Floor Mix for a Step Warm-Up

Move	Foot pattern	Number of counts
Grapevine R (on floor)	R, L, R, tap	4
Tap-up, tap-down (on step)	Up, tap, down, tap	4
Grapevine L (on floor)	L, R, L, tap	4
Tap-up, tap-down (on step)	Up, tap, down, tap	4

R = right; L = left.

Practice Drill

Design and practice a simple 32-count floor mix combination suitable for a step warm-up using no more than four moves. For example, you might combine one floor move, one step move, a second floor move, and a second step move.

include those for the hamstring, hip flexor, and calf muscles (see figure 11.1). The ideal time to increase flexibility is during the final cool-down. Therefore, stretching during the warm-up is performed to take all the joints and muscles through their full range of motion (ROM) before beginning vigorous exercise. A warm-up stretch is more about extensibility than flexibility and as such doesn't need to be held as long (8 counts are usually sufficient). Stretch the areas that are commonly tight and are used heavily in a step class: the calf (both gastrocnemius and soleus), shin, hamstring, quadriceps, hip flexor, low-back, and anterior chest muscles.

Verbal Cues and Tempo

Cueing during the warm-up is critical. You will be setting the tone for the workout, motivating class members, and educating them about safety and proper alignment. Your voice should be audible, upbeat, encouraging, and energetic. See chapter 4 for a thorough discussion of the various types of cues. Music tempo in a step warm-up is approximately the same as that in the step–cardio segment: 118 to 128 beats per minute.

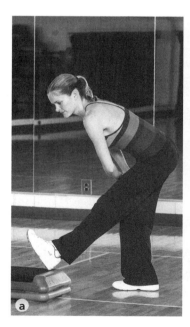 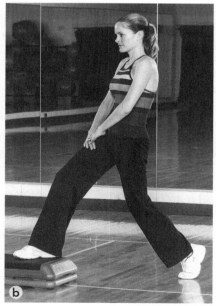 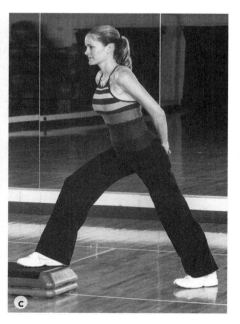

FIGURE 11.1 (a) Hamstring stretch, (b) hip flexor (iliopsoas) stretch, and (c) calf (gastrocnemius) stretch.

Step Training Research Findings

Many research studies have shown that step training can provide an excellent and predictable cardiorespiratory stimulus that results in important health benefits (Kin Isler, Kosar, and Korkusez 2001; Kraemer et al. 2001). A number of these studies have measured energy expenditure at various step heights and have found that step training meets the American College of Sports Medicine (ACSM) criteria for the achievement of cardiorespiratory fitness (Olson et al. 1991; Stanforth, Velasquez, and Stanforth 1991; Woodby-Brown, Berg, and Latin 1993). A recent study examined the effect of 12 weeks of step training on older women (average age: 62) and found a significant improvement in maximal aerobic capacity for that population (Hallage et al. 2009). In another study, researchers found improvements in functional fitness as a result of step (Hallage et al. 2010). Among women ages 50-75, step aerobics was also shown to improve static balance (Clary et al. 2006).

Research shows that intensity and caloric expenditure increase with step height (Wilson et al. 2010; Stanforth, Stanforth, and Velasquez 1993; Wang, Scharff-Olson, and Williford 1993; Woodby-Brown, Berg, and Latin 1993). Specific moves and patterns as well as the inclusion of arm movements influence the energy cost (Calarco et al. 1991; Francis et al. 1994; Olson et al. 1991), as does adding propulsion to common step moves (Greenlaw et al. 1995). Some researchers have found that a faster music tempo results in increased energy consumption (Wilson et al. 2010; Scharff-Olson, Williford, Duey, et al. 1997; Stanforth, Velasquez, and Stanforth 1991), whereas others have found that holding 2-pound (1 kg) hand weights while stepping does not significantly influence the energy cost (Kravitz et al. 1995; Olson et al. 1991; Workman, Kern, and Earnest 1993). The continual use of vigorous arm movements, however, has been shown to result in a disproportionately high heart rate relative to $\dot{V}O_2$max (Lloyd 2011); this is known as the pressor effect. Researchers, therefore, do not recommend using heart rate to assess intensity during step training. Alternating step training with high-low impact (for 45 minutes of cardio) has been shown in one training study to significantly increase high-density lipoprotein (HDL) cholesterol (Mosher, Ferguson, and Arnold 2005). Yet another study found significant body composition changes (weight, percent body fat, waist-to-hip ratio, waist circumference, and BMI [body mass index]) after 8 weeks of step aerobic exercise (Arslan 2011).

Other studies have measured the impact forces experienced by the feet during step training. Francis and colleagues (1994) found that the feet undergo approximately the same peak vertical forces when stepping on a 10-inch (25 cm) step as when walking at 3 miles per hour (5 kph), which is roughly 1.25 times body weight. However, the lead foot (first foot down off the step) absorbs a greater impact force—1.75 times body weight. This is one reason why it's so important to change the lead foot frequently during step. Other researchers have found that vertical ground reaction forces increase with increasing step height and with the addition of propulsion (Wilson et al. 2010; Johnson, Johnston, and Winnier 1993; Moses 1993; Scharff-Olson, Williford, Blessing, et al. 1997). The forces on the knees during stepping also have been examined (Francis et al. 1994), and researchers have found that greater forces are incurred with an increasing angle of knee flexion. A 24-week study looking at the health benefits of step training found that step training had significant positive effects on bone density in postmenopausal women (Wen et al. 2007), and a study on women aged 50 to 75 years found that balance improved as a result of a step program (Clary et al. 2006).

Data have been collected on step instructors (Kravitz 1995); it was found that instructors have a relatively low percentage of body fat and favorable upper-body and lower-body strength. Other researchers have examined the effect of step intensity on mood; they found less fatigue and anger in participants who exercised at higher intensities and reduced state anxiety in participants who had just finished step training (Hale and Raglin 2002).

Technique and Safety Check

Following are warm-up recommendations for step training:

- Use the step for at least one low- to moderate-intensity floor mix.
- Avoid continuous stepping until the body is thoroughly warm.
- Use the step for some short-term static stretches.
- Briefly stretch the areas that are commonly tight or are heavily used in step: calves, hip flexors, hamstrings, low back, and chest.

Practice Drill

Design a warm-up segment that incorporates the step to provide short-term stretches for the calf and hip flexor muscles. Before students do the calf stretch, have them limber the ankle by lifting and lowering the heel; before they do the hip flexor stretch, have them limber the pelvis and hip.

 See online video 6.2 for a sample step warm-up. This warm-up is also outlined in appendix F.

Technique and Safety Issues

Good alignment and technique for step training include maintaining a neutral spine and neck, with the head and eyes up, and keeping the abdominals lifted and contracted. As always, remind students to avoid hyperextending, hyperflexing, or twisting the knees (see figure 11.2). All joints face the same direction, and the shoulders are down, even, and relaxed. Have students use a full-body lean when stepping up—visualizing one long line from heel to head and avoiding leaning from the hips or waist (see figure 11.3).

You can greatly enhance the safety of your class by not stepping forward off the step; research has shown that stepping forward off the bench rather than stepping backward while facing the bench generates much greater impact forces (Francis et al. 1992). Always step lightly on the platform and avoid pounding the feet. In addition, step to the center of the bench and make sure the heel doesn't hang off the back; this helps protect the Achilles tendon. When stepping up, extend the knees fully without hyperextending them. To minimize the risk of patellar tendinitis, always keep the angle of knee flexion greater than 90°. Stay close enough to the step that you can bring the heels comfortably all the way to the

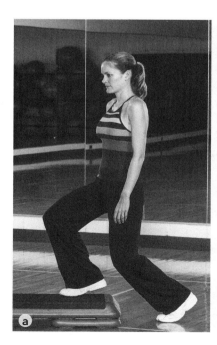
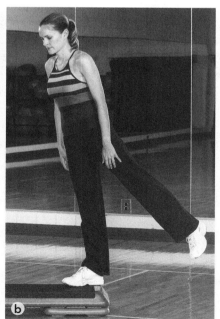
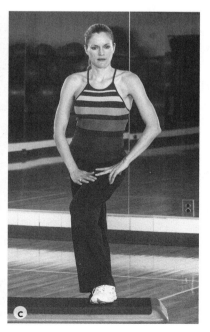

FIGURE 11.2 Avoid (a) hyperflexion, (b) hyperextension, and (c) twisting of the knees.

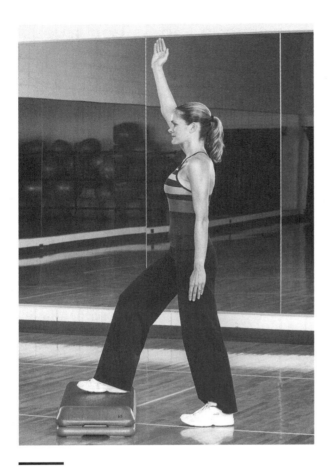

FIGURE 11.3   Good alignment on a step.

floor when stepping down (landing and rolling through the toe, ball, and heel). Your feet should land approximately one shoe length away from the step. Step down without bouncing. Bouncing when you land on the floor increases the eccentric muscle loading and forceful stretching of the Achilles tendon and may lead to Achilles tendinitis. Encourage participants to jump up on the step instead! Have students avoid forcing heels down to the floor during lunges and repeaters.

In this case, encourage students to use the ball of the foot to make contact with the floor and keep the heel lifted. Forcing the heel down may increase the risk of Achilles tendinitis due to the forceful stretching and eccentric loading of the tendon. When performing pivot turns on the step, show students how to unload the lower leg by simultaneously hopping so that the foot is not in contact with the step during the actual turn.

Help participants choose the proper step height. Step heights greater than 8 inches (20 cm) should be reserved for exercisers with long legs or who are at an advanced fitness level (see table 11.2). It's also a good idea to change the lead leg frequently to minimize repetitive stress to the leg stepping down off the bench. Finally, keep the tempo of your music slow enough that all participants are able to step safely with good technique and alignment. Several organizations recommend step speeds no greater than 128 beats per minute. Music tempo can be a challenging issue in clubs where participants are used to stepping at much faster speeds. However, research clearly shows that effective workouts are possible at speeds under 128 beats per minute, and these slower speeds have the added benefit of decreasing impact forces and enhancing safety for participants. Model looking where you are stepping by glancing down occasionally with your eyes while keeping your head up. In your classes, avoid high numbers of moves that stress the musculoskeletal system, such as repeaters with more than five repetitions. Limit lunges and other propulsive moves to 1 minute or less, depending on your participants. Avoid using hand weights while stepping; while caloric expenditure increases are minimal, the risk of injury is significantly greater (Olson et al. 1991; Step Reebok 1997; Workman, Kern, and Earnerst 1993).

TABLE 11.2   Guidelines for Step Height and Step Speed

Participant level	Step height	Step speed
Novice (new to exercise)	4 in (10 cm)	118-122 bpm
Beginner (regular exerciser who has never done step)	<6 in (15 cm)	<124 bpm
Intermediate (regular stepper)	<8 in (20 cm)	<126 bpm
Advanced (regular, skilled stepper)	<10 in (25 cm)	<128 bpm

Adapted from the revised *Guidelines for step Reebok* 1997.

Technique and Safety Check

To keep your classes safe, observe the following recommendations.

Remember to

- maintain a neutral spine and neck, with the head and eyes up;
- keep the abdominals lifted and contracted;
- keep all joints facing the same direction;
- keep the shoulders down, even, and relaxed;
- use a full-body lean when stepping up;
- step to the center of the platform;
- keep the angle of knee flexion greater than 90°;
- help participants choose the proper step height; and
- change the lead leg frequently.

Avoid

- hyperextending, hyperflexing, or twisting the knees;
- stepping forward off the step;
- pounding the feet; and
- using step speeds greater than 128 beats per minute.

Basic Moves and Step Patterns

There are six basic locations around the bench from which to perform step moves. The six basic approaches to the step are front, side, end, corner, top, and astride (see figure 11.4).

Lower-Body Moves

Using a step in group exercise classes presents many options for basic lower-body movements. The online video accompanying this text presents the basic lower-body moves in step training; table 11.3 also lists these moves. Those moves

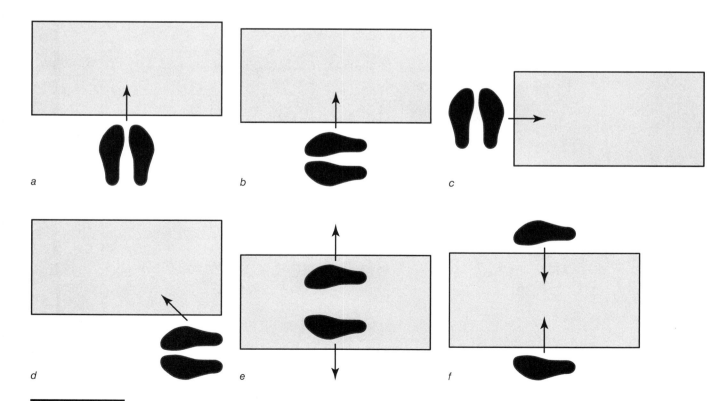

a   b   c   d   e   f

FIGURE 11.4 Step approaches: (*a*) front, (*b*) side, (*c*) end, (*d*) corner, (*e*) top, and (*f*) astride.

Practice Drill

Take a step class and write down the instructor's approaches to the bench. How many of the six approaches were used? Did they flow well? Put together two lower-body moves that share the same approach. Practice alternating these two moves so that you create a simple combination on the step.

near the bottom of the list may be more difficult to teach, may be more complex, or may require other approaches and are better suited for a more experienced instructor. Lower-body moves on the step are all 4-count moves unless otherwise noted.

 See online video 11.1 for basic lower-body step moves and variations.

Most of the moves and patterns in table 11.3 can be performed with either a single lead or an alternating lead. A single lead means that the move is executed in such a way that the same foot continues to lead. An example is a V-step with no tap-down: up with the right foot, up with the left, down with the right, down with the left, up again with the right foot, and so on. In a V-step performed with an alternating lead, however, a tap-down is performed on the fourth count, which changes the lead foot: up with the right foot, up with the left, down with the right, down tap left, up with the left foot, up with the right, down with the left, down tap right, and so on.

Additionally, propulsion, or power, can be added to many moves to increase the intensity if desired. Adding propulsion simply means jumping up on the step, which requires significantly more energy (never jump off the step because doing so increases joint stress—see "Technique and Safety Check" earlier in this chapter). Good moves for adding propulsion include the basic step, lift step, over-the-top, across-the-top, L-step, tap-up, lunge, and pivot turn.

Upper-Body Moves

As in high-low impact cardio workouts, there are endless variations of upper-body moves in step. Review chapter 4 for a discussion of unilateral and bilateral, complementary and opposition,

TABLE 11.3 Basic Step Moves

Move	Typical approaches
Basic step	Front, end, corner
V-step	Front
Tap-up, tap-down	Side, end, corner, front
Lift step (a knee lift to the front, side, or back; a kick to the front, side, or back)	Front, side, end, corner, astride, top
Turn step	Side
Over-the-top	Side
Repeater	Front, side, corner, end, astride (8 counts)
Lunge	Top (2 counts); can face front or side
Straddle-down	Top
Straddle-up	Astride
Across-the-top	End
Corner-to-corner	Corner
L-step	Front, end, side
A-step	Corner, side
Charleston	Front, corner, side
Over-the-top pivot	Side

and low-, mid-, and high-range arm movements. Common arm moves and step patterns include the following:

- Bilateral biceps curls with the basic step
- Externally and internally rotated shoulders (out, out, in, in) with the V-step
- Overhead press (clap on count 4) with the turn step
- Bilateral shoulder circumduction with over-the-top
- Chest presses with lunges facing front

It's generally easiest for participants if you teach the lower-body movements first. Add the arms only when everyone is comfortable with the lower-body patterns.

Practice Drill

Practice the short combination you designed after observing a class in the previous drill; this time, add simple upper-body moves.

Basic Combinations and Choreography Techniques

The elements of variation discussed in chapter 4 provide an unlimited number of variations for step moves and patterns. You can vary your moves by changing the

- lever,
- plane,
- direction (and, in step, the approach),
- rhythm,
- intensity (add propulsion), and
- style (see "Elements of Variation" in chapter 4).

For example, let's see how a hamstring curl (knee lift to the back) performed with a front approach to the step can be varied. Begin by performing the hamstring curl and then (1) increase the lever, which results in hip extension, (2) change the plane for a side-out (long-lever leg lift to the side, hip abduction), (3) add the element of direction by angling the body diagonally

to alternating corners, (4) change the rhythm by performing a hesitation move before each alternating side-out, (5) increase the intensity by adding propulsion (jump up) on each side-out, and (6) play with the style by performing a funky shimmy movement with the shoulders on the hesitation and then dorsiflexing the foot and pressing the heels of the hands down on the side-out.

Drilling the elements of variation can result in entirely new moves and even new combinations! It's easiest to transition smoothly when one move begins where the previous move finishes (i.e., when the end point and starting point of the two moves connect). Moves that share the same approach usually connect well; for example, both over-the-top and tap-up, tap-down can be performed from the side approach, and thus they flow together.

Practice Drill

Begin by performing one basic move and then add (or subtract) an element of variation. Perform each move you create at least 4 times (16 counts) before adding or subtracting another element of variation. Make your transitions smooth and natural by finding moves with connecting end points and starting points (see the section "Creating Smooth Transitions" in chapter 4). Challenge yourself by changing first an element of variation for the upper body, then one for the lower body, and then one for the upper body, building a linear progression.

Teaching to Music

It is essential to teach with the music in a step class. Because almost all step moves are 4 or 8 counts, participants will naturally want to initiate moves on the first downbeat of 8-, 16-, and 32-count phrases. Find some step music with a strong beat and practice finding the beats until hearing the downbeat and the musical divisions into counts of 4 becomes second nature for you. Teaching on the beat and with the music keeps you and your students from becoming frustrated and discouraged; your patterns will be easier to follow and more enjoyable. Many students, although they may not be able to articulate why, instinctively feel that something is wrong when an instructor is not on the downbeat. Refer to chapter 4 for a thorough discussion of beats, downbeats, measures, and 8-, 16-, and 32-count phrases. Teaching with the music and on the beat means mastering anticipatory cueing: the ability to smoothly and easily move your entire class at the same time on a particular musical beat (see chapter 4). You let them know at just the right moment what to do next. Good anticipatory cueing eliminates participant anxiety, helps them relax and get a better workout, and helps keep your class safe (there's less chance they'll stumble or run into each other).

32-Count Blocks

As in high-low impact choreography step choreography usually consists of blocks of 32-count combinations. These blocks can be repeated over and over, expanded or reduced, or linked together to create long, complex combinations. Movements within the blocks can be layered for increasing complexity or changed using the elements of variation (see chapter 4 to learn about different choreographic techniques). Here's an example of a 32-count block in step training:

1. Facing front, perform 3 basic steps, leading right (12 counts; to increase complexity, add a different arm movement with each basic step).
2. Perform 1 half-time squat with the right foot on the bench (face the left side for the squat, then face the front on the return; 4 counts).
3. Repeat to the other side, leading left (for a total of 16 counts).

This first block could be linked to another 32-count block:

1. Facing front, perform 2 alternating knee lifts (8 counts).
2. Complete 1 three-knee repeater (8 counts).
3. Perform 2 alternating knee lifts (8 counts).
4. Complete 1 three-knee repeater to the other side (8 counts).

You could alternate these two blocks with each other, or you could link them to more blocks to create a longer combination.

 See online video 11.2 for a demonstration of 32-count step combinations.

Practice Drill

Using a favorite premixed step CD with a strong beat (see chapter 4 for a list of companies that produce step music), put together two 32-count blocks of simple choreography for step. Be sure to start your routine at the top of the phrase, which is the first downbeat of the 32-count phrase.

Repetition Reduction

Repetition reduction is another important technique in skillful step teaching. As discussed in chapter 4, to use repetition reduction, repeat each move several times until participants are comfortable, and then gradually reduce the number of repetitions. This technique can result in a complex combination that requires everyone to concentrate! Here's a relatively simple example:

1. Start with 4 alternating V-steps and 4 alternating knee lifts.
2. Reduce to 2 alternating V-steps and 2 alternating knee lifts.
3. Reduce to 1 V-step and 1 knee lift.

Holding Patterns

A holding pattern is a move (e.g., basic step, or an over-the-top) that is repeated over and over for a brief time to allow the instructor and the participants to collect their thoughts and return to the desired intensity level. Performing a holding pattern provides an ideal time for you to communicate with your students, giving alignment, technique, educational, or motivational cues as necessary.

Step Intensity

Compared with traditional cardio floor choreography, step training has workloads that are easier to measure because of the known variable

Writing Out a Step Combination

	Lead	Movement	Counts
A	Lead R	3 basic steps, 1 4-count squat facing side (R foot on bench)	1-16
	Lead L	3 basic steps, 1 4-count squat facing other side (L foot on bench)	17-32
B	Lead R	2 alternating knee lifts to the corners, 1 three-knee repeater	1-16
	Lead L	2 alternating knee lifts to the corners, 1 three-knee repeater	17-32

Note that A and B signify different moves: Each designates the lead leg, indicates the numbers of each move and the moves themselves, and gives the number of counts. Such a chart helps make the combination clear and easy to understand. Technically, we've shown two 32-count blocks of choreography, which can then be linked to other blocks, as you will see.

When writing out cues, the following model may be helpful:

Move: 4 basic steps R; (the next move will be 4 basic steps L)

Cue: "4, 3, 2, tap switch L"

Counts: 1, 2, 3, 4; 1, 2, 3, 4; 1, 2, 3, 4; 1, 2, 3, 4 (= 16 counts)

Remember that almost all step moves take 4 counts. In the previous example, where four basic steps are planned, the anticipatory cue comes on the last basic step, alerting participants that a change is coming. Additionally, it's very helpful to play traffic cop with visual cues and count down with your fingers held up in an exaggerated gesture. Writing out your combinations and cues will help you to be more prepared and confident. Providing clear anticipatory cues will help keep your class safe and help participants feel more confident and successful.

of the step height. As you might suspect, the higher the step, the greater the intensity and the higher the vertical ground-reaction forces (Wilson et al. 2010; Johnson, Johnston, and Winnier 1993). Have students use a step that provides a sufficient cardiorespiratory challenge but also allows them to move with good form and alignment and minimize the risk of injury. Higher platform heights have been associated with knee discomfort that is attributable to the increased angle of knee flexion (Francis et al. 1994). It is recommended that beginner steppers start with a 4-inch (10 cm) platform and gradually progress to a higher step as they become more conditioned and familiar with proper step biomechanics (Aerobics and Fitness Association of America 2010).

Intensity is also affected by the specific step moves and sequences being used and by increased lever length, elevated arm movements, increased traveling, and a greater number of propulsion moves. Moves that involve more traveling over and around the step or more vertical displacement, such as lunges, have been found to have a greater energy cost than moves that involve less knee flexion and extension, such as basic steps. The energy costs of common step moves are listed in table 11.4. Interestingly,

TABLE 11.4 Energy Costs of Step Moves

	Basic step	Traveling with alternating lead	Over-the-top	Knee lift	Lunges	Repeaters
$\dot{V}O_2$max (ml · kg^{-1} · min^{-1})	26.2	35.5	26.6	28.7	32.7	32.0
METS	7.5	10.1	7.6	8.2	9.3	9.1

METS = metabolic equivalents; HR = heart rate; RPE = rating of perceived exertion

Adapted from Calarco et al. 1991.

there's often a negative correlation between complexity and intensity: The more complicated the choreography, the lower the intensity for all but the most skilled participants.

The music speed can affect the intensity, although most experts do not recommend using a music tempo above 128 beats per minute because of the increased risk of injury. At faster tempos, participants have a more difficult time completing their movements with full ROM and may end up compromising their alignment and stepping technique. Compromised technique increases the likelihood of injuries such as Achilles tendinitis (see "Technique and Safety Check" earlier in this chapter).

 See online videos 11.3 and 11.4 for additional step training combinations.

Websites for Choreography Ideas

- www.turnstep.com
- www.fitnesstrainingdownloads.com
- www.stepcenter.com
- www.dailymotion.com
- www.fitmoves.com

Training Systems

Step classes can be formatted in several ways, including step supercircuits, step intervals, step alternated with high-low impact intervals, double step (participants use more than one step), and various step fusion options (e.g., step combined with slide or glide, step combined with Pilates, or step combined with stability ball training). Following are descriptions of step circuit and step interval formats.

Step Circuit

In a step circuit or supercircuit class, several minutes of step may be alternated with several minutes of muscular conditioning to create a complete workout (Kraemer et al. 2001). Here's a sample step circuit: Warm up for 10 minutes; step for 4 minutes; perform weighted squats, pliés, and lunges on the floor for 4 minutes; step for 4 minutes; perform weighted latissimus dorsi and deltoid exercises for 4 minutes; step for 4 minutes; perform standing chest exercises such as wall push-ups plus upper-back exercises with tubing for 4 minutes; step for 4 minutes; perform biceps and triceps exercises with weights or tubing for 4 minutes; step for 4 minutes; perform a cool-down after the cardio segment for 4 minutes; work abdominals and lower back on the floor for 5 minutes; and stretch on the floor for 5 minutes. Total circuit time is 60 minutes. This type of class efficiently addresses all the components of fitness and is also quite fun!

Step Intervals

In this type of class, power intervals are randomly or regularly interspersed throughout the step session. The power interval typically lasts 30-60 seconds and consists of a simple move or pattern repeated over and over. Participants are given intensity options that allow them to work at higher levels during the interval if desired. A good example of a power interval is as follows: Facing front, perform 2 lift steps (knee lift with a tap-down) with the right foot leading for 8 counts and follow with 4 jumping jacks on the floor for 8 counts. Repeat the 2 lift steps with the left foot leading for 8 counts, and then do 4 more jumping jacks for 8 counts. Then demonstrate this simple combination with at least three intensity options: (1) without jumping—the jacks become low-impact toe touches to the side, (2) with a jump-up on the step (arms low) during the lift steps and regular jacks on the floor, and (3) with a jump-up on the step (arms high) and fly or cheerleader jacks on the floor with the arms circumducting. Allow your students to select the intensity option that requires more work than during the regular step portion of class but is still appropriate for them. For more information on Tabata and high-intensity interval training (HIIT) see chapters 7 and 13. When adding high-intensity intervals to step (or any other format), always provide lower-intensity options in order to accommodate all your participants' needs.

Chapter Wrap-Up

The basic teaching strategies for step include providing a warm-up that incorporates rehearsal moves (generally in the form of a floor mix) and teaching a combination in small parts, usually in 8- or 16-count blocks. Drill these parts, using the principle of repetition, until participants have learned the movements. Teach the lower body first and then add the upper body. Then teach the 32-count block, using repetition reduction until participants have learned the movements. Layer your combination with the elements of variation, changing the lever, plane, direction or approach, rhythm, style, or intensity. Repeat this process with the next 32-count block and add more blocks onto your first block as desired (A + B + C + D). Use holding patterns between blocks to enhance your communication with your class and to avoid brain strain. Practice these teaching techniques, as well as proper anticipatory cueing, so that you become a creative and effective step instructor.

Group Exercise Class Evaluation Form: Key Points

- Gradually increase intensity. After the warm-up, when you are beginning the cardio segment, gradually increase intensity until you reach the peak part of the cardio stimulus. Do not have the class perform plyometric intervals, lunges, and other high-intensity moves near the beginning of the cardio segment.

- Use a variety of muscle groups and minimize repetitive movements. Avoid performing high numbers of any move in a row since doing so can lead to overuse injuries and muscle imbalances. Follow 4 knee lifts on the step with 4 hip extensions on the step, for example.

- Demonstrate proper form, alignment, and technique on the step. Be a good role model for your students because they will unconsciously copy your form and alignment. Stand tall, move with precision, and avoid bouncing down off the step.

- Use step music appropriately. Use a recommended tempo (118-128 beats per minute) that allows all participants to complete full ROM safely and with control. Keep practicing to get better at moving on the beat, initiating new moves at the beginning of phrases, and using the 32-count phrase.

- Give clear cues and verbal directions, including anticipatory cues, safety and alignment information, directional cues, and motivational cues. Remember that for big anticipatory cues, you usually count backward starting with "4," as in, "4, 3, 2, knee lift." That way, class members will perform the knee lift together on the downbeat of the next phrase.

- Promote participant interaction and encourage fun. Have participants call out their names, greet their neighbors, and occasionally count down with you. Ask questions such as, "Everybody feeling fine?"

- Gradually decrease intensity during the cool-down after the cardio segment by avoiding high-intensity moves and eventually moving off the step. A simple example is to march for 4 counts on the step and then march for 4 counts on the floor, repeat several times, and finish by marching only on the floor. Incorporate some static stretches while standing, especially stretches for the calves, hip flexors, hamstrings, and low back.

ASSIGNMENT

Prepare a 4-minute step routine that consists of four 32-count blocks. Teach your routine using the techniques of repetition reduction and changing the lead leg. Prepare an outline of the routine on paper to use when you lead the class (this can be on a notecard).

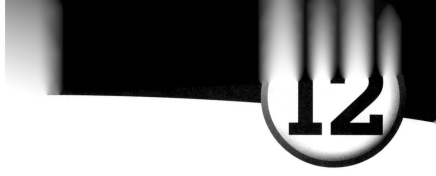

Stationary Indoor Cycling

Chapter Objectives

By the end of this chapter, you will be able to

- understand proper positioning on a bike, including alignment and safety issues;
- create a warm-up for stationary indoor cycling;
- apply basic indoor cycling class techniques and music;
- format different indoor cycling classes;
- use cueing and coaching techniques on and off the bike; and
- teach a 4-minute indoor cycling segment with appropriate content, technique, cueing, and music.

Background Check

Before working your way through this chapter, we suggest you do the following:

Read

☐ chapter 5, "Coaching-Based Concepts,"

☐ chapter 6, "Warm-Up and Cool-Down," and

☐ chapter 7, "Cardiorespiratory Training."

Group Exercise Class Evaluation Form Essentials

Key Points for Warm-Up Segment

- Includes appropriate amount of dynamic movement
- Provides rehearsal moves
- Provides dynamic or static stretches for at least two major muscle groups

- Provides intensity guidelines for warm-up
- Includes clear cues and verbal directions
- Uses appropriate music and movement

Key Points for Conditioning Segment

- Gradually increases intensity
- Uses a variety of muscle groups
- Minimizes repetitive movements
- Observes participants' form and provides constructive, nonintimidating feedback
- Continually offers modifications, regressions, progressions, or alternatives
- Provides alignment and technique cues
- Gives motivational cues

- Educates participants about intensity; provides HR (heart rate) or RPE (rating of perceived exertion) check at least 1 or 2 times during the workout stimulus
- Promotes participant interaction and encourages fun
- Provides regular demonstrations and participation with good body mechanics
- Uses appropriate movement and music

Stationary indoor cycling (known by such trademarked names as *Spinning, SchwinnFitness, RealRyder, Kranking,* and *Power Pacing)* is another popular modality for group exercise. Although Thompson's (2012) worldwide fitness trends list eliminated indoor cycling from the top 20 programs offered by fitness programmers, the IDEA Fitness trends survey (Schroeder and Donlin, 2013) describes indoor cycling as being offered in 55-60% of facilities that offer fitness services. Many fitness programs designate a room specifically for indoor cycling, complete with specialized indoor bikes, sound systems, microphones, cycling DVDs, or even candles. Unlike group exercise classes such as kickboxing or boot camp, indoor cycling classes may be held in darkened rooms without mirrors. The focus is less on how you look or if you remember the combination of movements and more on how you experience the workout. As some instructors like to say, "It's about the ride or journey and not about the final result." Because there are no choreographed moves that all participants perform at the same time, it's much easier for indoor cyclists to personalize their workouts. Hence, indoor cycling classes easily accommodate several fitness levels, with elite cyclists working next to deconditioned novices. In fact, this type of class may be one of the most user-friendly and nonintimidating group exercise formats.

Nevertheless, researchers caution that this activity may be a high-intensity cardiovascular choice for participants, and particularly for beginning and middle-aged exercisers. This could be why the current trends in indoor cycling identify this activity as not making the top 20 programs in the ACSM (Thompson, 2012) trends report. It is well documented in the research literature that high intensity exercise can discourage participation. Lopez-Minarro and Rodriguez (2010) studied 30-year olds and found that indoor cycling can be considered a high-intensity exercise mode for novice subjects. Caria and colleagues (2007) found that indoor cycling represents a significant challenge for the cardiovascular system. These authors suggest that indoor cycling is not suitable for unfit or sedentary individuals, especially if they're middle aged or elderly. Finally, Battista and colleagues (2008) wrote that indoor cycling should be considered a high-intensity exercise mode of cardiorespiratory training since it provides an excellent cardiorespiratory workout, burning

400 to 550 kilocalories per 45-minute ride, not counting the warm-up and cool-down. What is important is that instructors identify any deconditioned individuals and provide special instructions on intensity monitoring.

Two new types of cycling workouts, Kranking and RealRyder, use equipment that is different from a typical indoor cycling bike. Kranking resembles a conventional upper-body ergometer (UBE) in which you sit and pedal with your hands. Boyer, Porcari, and Foster (2010) contend that Kranking is an intense, effective workout that may build upper-body muscular fitness and boost aerobic capacity. RealRyder bikes (figure 12.1) have a unique articulating frame that allows the bike to steer, lean, and feel like an actual road bike. The RealRyder simulates the experience and the benefits of riding a bike in the real world. Little research has been conducted on either the Krankcycle or the RealRyder, but both are gaining in popularity as modalities in the group exercise cycling arena. For information on Kranking and RealRyder, see the following websites:

www.krankcycle.com

www.realryder.com

Many fitness programs require specific training and equipment in order to teach a cycling class (see "Indoor Cycling Product Vendors and Training Programs" in this chapter). Before addressing specific class content, we'll review preclass bike set up in the "Positioning, Alignment, and Safety" section later in this chapter. Setting up the bike properly helps enhance the enjoyment of a cycling class.

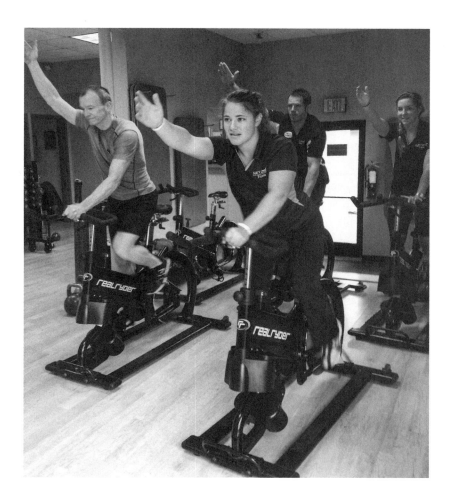

FIGURE 12.1   A RealRyder class.

Indoor Cycling Research Findings

Many studies have examined the cardiorespiratory and metabolic responses to group indoor cycling. Virtually all researchers have found that a stationary indoor cycling workout can provide a stimulus sufficient to meet American College of Sports Medicine (ACSM) guidelines for the development and maintenance of aerobic fitness, and most have reported high levels of caloric expenditure, up to 550 kilocalories per 45-minute ride. One study by Hotting and colleagues (2012) noted that improvement in memory correlated positively with the increase in cardiovascular fitness related to cycling training. Several investigators have measured responses to the various positions and activities found in a typical cycling class. Standing, climbing, high-resistance settings, and jumping maneuvers elicited the maximal heart rate (MHR), RPE, oxygen consumption, and caloric expenditure (Chinsky et al. 1998; Flanagan et al. 1998; Francis, Witucki, and Buono 1999; Williford et al. 1999). Williford and colleagues (1999) found that speed play and vigorous jumps or lifts may produce transient maximal effects.

Several studies have examined the effects of cadence on performance at specific workloads. Mora-Rodriguez and Aguado-Jimenez (2004) concluded that a high pedaling cadence (>120 rpm) reduces performance in well-trained cyclists. In studies of elite cyclists, Foss and Hallen (2004) and Lucia and coworkers (2004) found that when cadence increases along with workload, work efficiency (defined as a low level of oxygen consumption at any given workload) also increases. And in one study (Francis, Witucki, and Buono 1999), energy cost was found to be unrelated to cadence: Higher pedaling speeds did not appear to increase caloric expenditure as long as the workload was maintained.

John and Schuler (1999) reported that the 6- to 20-point Borg RPE scale may be inaccurate when used by novices during group cycling; thus, these participants may require either heart rate monitors or more detailed instruction regarding the RPE scale. Novice cyclists were also found to have movements and muscle recruitment patterns that were less refined than those of trained cyclists; researchers surmised that the neuromuscular system was not yet sufficiently adapted in new cyclists (Chapman et al. 2004). Finally, Olson and colleagues (2012) surprisingly found that in a spin class, class duration had more of an influence on joint angles and proper form than did the instructor's cues.

Indoor Cycling Product Vendors and Training Programs

Mad Dogg Athletics, Inc.
2111 Narcissus Ct.
Venice, CA 90291
800-847-SPIN
www.spinning.com

Keiser
800-888-7009
www.keiser.com

Schwinn
800-605-3369
www.Schwinnfitness.com

Livestrong & Kranking
Matrix Fitness
1600 Landmark Drive
Cottage Grove, WI 53527
866-693-4863
www.matrixfitness.com
www.krankcycle.com

RealRyder
RealRyder International
3200 Airport Ave., Suite 21
Santa Monica, CA 90405
800-976-6280
www.realryder.com

Positioning, Alignment, and Safety

Before beginning a cycling class, make certain that each participant is properly aligned and adjusted on the bike. Show up 15 minutes before class to assist participants with bike setup, answer any questions, get to know new participants, and set up your own equipment (including the music and microphone). The three main bike adjustments are the seat height, the fore and aft seat position, and the handlebar height. The correct seat height depends on the cyclist's leg length: the longer the leg, the higher the seat. In general, when the rider is seated on the bike with the balls of the feet on the center of the pedals, there should be a slight bend in the knee of the extended leg when pedaling. Experts suggest this knee flexion should be anywhere from 5° to 30°. If the seat height is too low, inadequate leg extension may cause knee problems, especially in the front of the knee. If the seat is too high, the rider's hips will rock back and forth; in addition, the risk of knee hyperextension is increased, which may cause pain at the back of the knee. Most beginning participants err on the side of setting the seat too low in an effort to minimize saddle soreness. Proper seat height is the key to healthy knees.

For proper fore and aft positioning, adjust the saddle so that the cyclist's front kneecap is aligned directly above the center of the pedal when the pedal is forward and the crank is horizontal (the nine o'clock position). Cycling with the saddle too far forward can cause anterior knee problems. The correct fore and aft positioning also should allow the arms to comfortably reach the handlebars with the elbows slightly flexed. In addition, a proper position of the fore and aft seat setting will reduce the sitting-bone pain beginners often feel when first starting an indoor cycling class, particularly if they do not have cycling shorts.

Handlebar height is mostly a matter of personal preference. Some experts have shown that a higher handlebar height puts riders in a better posture position to help minimize low back pain while riding. Beginners are encouraged to put the handlebars higher so the torso is more upright. The upright, neutral spine position is recommended for participants with back or neck problems. The lower the handlebars, the more the cyclist simulates a racing position, which creates favorable aerodynamics when cycling outdoors but is unnecessary when riding indoors. Teach participants to ride with a relaxed grip and neutral wrists and to vary their hand positions.

Additionally, encourage participants to wear stiff-soled shoes that remain rigid over the pedals; students should position the feet so that the balls of the feet, not the arches, contact the pedals. Clipping the shoes onto the pedals or securely strapping the shoes into the foot cages can enhance pedaling efficiency. Because most bikes are fixed gear and have pedals that continue to rotate after the feet are taken off, remind your class members to keep their feet on the pedals until the pedals stop moving, or to hold their feet away from the bike if they must detach from the pedals before the pedals come to a complete stop (alternatively, many indoor cycling bikes have an emergency brake that can be pressed to instantly stop the flywheel and pedal rotation).

Remind participants to maintain neutral spinal alignment on the bike. The rider is in a neutral spine position (also known as *ideal alignment)* when the four natural curves of the back are in their proper relationship to each other. Maintaining this position is easiest when the rider is sitting upright with the torso perpendicular to the floor. When the rider is seated and riding with a forward lean, the spine is in a neutral position, albeit inclined at a 45° angle, depending on the activity. Tucking the hips under (creating a posterior pelvic tilt) causes the back to round (or flex) and places much more strain on the structures of the back and should be avoided. When using proper form, the shoulder blades are kept down and slightly retracted in a position known as *neutral scapular alignment.* Rounding or hunching the shoulders or allowing the shoulder blades to come up by the ears should be avoided (see figure 12.2).

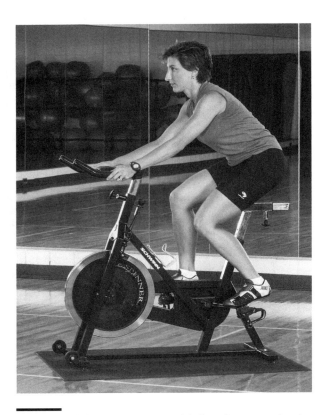

FIGURE 12.2 Proper seated bike alignment in the inclined position.

 See online video 12.1 for a cycle setup demonstration.

Remind participants to ride with a full water bottle and a towel. As with any new activity, recommend that participants gradually increase the frequency of their classes, starting with one or two per week and slowly increasing to three or four classes per week if desired.

Creating a Warm-Up

A stationary indoor cycling warm-up generally follows the warm-up recommendations in chapter 6. It consists primarily of dynamic movements, rehearsal moves, and some light upper-body preparatory stretching, all taught with skillful cues at the appropriate intensity for a warm-up. The key points for a warm-up follow the same principles we've reviewed in previous chapters. The main points of the "Group Exercise Class Evaluation Form" that relate to stationary cycling are outlined at the beginning of this chapter.

Dynamic Rehearsal Moves

The focus of a group cycling warm-up is on gradually increasing the intensity to elevate heart rate, ventilation, and oxygen consumption—all preparations for the cardiorespiratory workout to follow. Have participants sit upright on their bikes and keep their spines in neutral alignment while cycling and loosening up their legs. Bikes should be adjusted so there is light resistance and just enough tension on the flywheel for participants to stay in control. A typical indoor cycling warm-up lasts approximately 4 to 8 minutes; intensity may be gradually increased toward the end of the warm-up by changing either the resistance or the pedaling speed. Rehearsal movements in an indoor cycling class warm-up may include

- teaching participants how to ride out of the saddle for 1 or 2 minutes, thus simulating a hill cardio segment;

Technique and Safety Check

To help keep your classes safe, observe the following recommendations.

Remember to
- undertake a thorough, appropriate warm-up;
- maintain a neutral spine whether sitting upright, inclined forward, or standing;
- keep the neck in line with the spine;
- adjust the bike properly;
- keep the wrists in neutral and maintain a relaxed grip;

- wear proper footwear and contact the pedals with the balls of feet; and
- stay hydrated.

Avoid
- tucking the hips under or
- hyperextending the neck.

- introducing a short jump series where participants ride out of the saddle for 10 seconds and then back down in the saddle for 10 seconds, particularly if a series of ups and downs will be used later in the cardio segment;
- practicing increasing and decreasing intensity while using the resistance knob so participants become familiar with bike tension (each bike has a slightly different tension setting); or
- teaching cadence drills so participants can later identify a slow, moderate, and fast cadence during the workout.

Stretching Major Muscle Groups

We recommend performing some light preparatory stretching and dynamic movements for the upper body while cycling during the warm-up. Ideas for moves and stretches include rolling the shoulders backward, stretching the pectoralis major (chest), and stretching the upper trapezius

(neck) to counteract the rounded, hunched posture so often seen in cycling classes (see figure 12.3). Most instructors reserve lower-body stretching for the end of a cycling class when everyone is warm and psychologically ready to relax and hold the static stretches. Also, participants enjoy getting off the bicycle at the end of the workout. Stopping the rhythmic rehearsal movements of cycling to perform lower-body static stretches would have the negative effect of decreasing heart rate and oxygen consumption, exactly the opposite of the warm-up's purpose. Therefore, we suggest waiting to stretch the lower-body muscles until the end of class.

Verbal Cues and Tempo

The warm-up is an ideal time to teach proper alignment and riding technique as well as review intensity guidelines. Teach your class about neutral spine and scapulae, and proper neck, elbow, and wrist alignment. Give pedaling pointers such as, "Visualize your feet spinning in separate

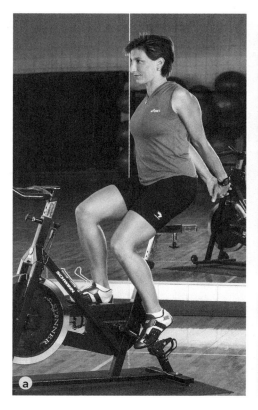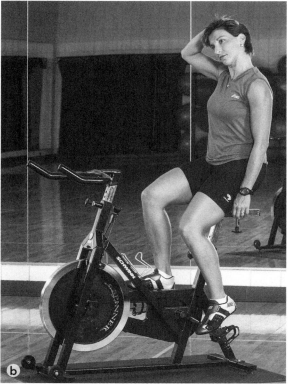

FIGURE 12.3 Upper-body stretches for indoor cycling: (*a*) pectoralis major stretch and (*b*) upper trapezius stretch with neck laterally flexed.

perfect circles" or "Feel each foot moving front to back with each revolution" or "Create a perfect balance between your right foot and left foot." Additionally, many participants need instruction regarding proper intensity. Address heart rate issues, perceived exertion, cadence and resistance, and the concept of listening to your body and working at the level that is right for you. Some instructors suggest that participants silently create an intention, or a personal focus, for the workout ahead to help them self-regulate through the course of the workout. For example, Gollwitzer and Sheeran (2006) suggest that using "if . . . then" planning will help support a participant's intention when problems arise during the workout. An example of "if . . . then" planning specific to indoor cycling might be this: "If my gluteus maximus starts to hurt, then I will get out of the saddle for a minute to reduce the pain and enjoy the experience of the class more fully." Finally, make certain that all participants can hear you; be sure music volume and microphone volume are well balanced.

Music and movement that allows participants to work comfortably at a low to medium intensity and enjoy the music during the warm-up is important. There are no set guidelines for music tempo, and participants can pedal either on or off the beat. There are three ways to pedal on the beat: (1) One leg completes a downstroke on every other beat (slow), (2) one leg completes a downstroke on each beat (faster), or (3) both legs complete a downstroke on each beat (very fast, or double time). Because of the variability in how music is used, rigid tempo guidelines are somewhat meaningless. Instead, select warm-up music that is motivating, is fun to listen to, and that encourages a comfortable pace at a low to moderate intensity.

Basic Moves

The typical indoor cycling class is divided into several segments, or drills, that are usually designed to simulate aspects of an outdoor ride. These segments may be linked to specific songs or cuts of music and are often attached to specific goals for intensity (heart rate or cadence). Segments may include

- seated flats;
- seated climbs (hills);
- standing flat runs or jogs;
- standing climbs (hills);
- seated downhills or flushes;
- rebounds, jumps, or lifts; and
- seated and standing sprints (also known as *spin-outs, fast hammers,* or *power drills*).

Participants are often asked to visualize themselves performing these segments outdoors on various types of terrain. Many instructors create imaginary journeys and scenarios for cyclists to visualize. Images of tropical islands, mountain roads, green forests, sandy beaches, open fields, and grassy meadows can all be conducive to improving the workout and creating an enjoyable class experience. Visualization can also be used to improve breathing, alignment, muscle focus, mental awareness, and even self-empowerment! Have participants picture the goal they wish to accomplish and see themselves being successful. This can be a very powerful aspect of a group cycling class.

 See online video 12.2 for a demonstration of basic seated flats and seated climbs.

Seated Flats

The seated flat is the most basic cycling technique. Participants can work at a variety of speeds, and the flat road can be used in the warm-up, cardio stimulus, and cool-down phases of class. The seated flat is perfect for cadence drills, alignment and pedaling work, endurance work, and rhythm presses (a pulsating, wavelike movement of the upper body). Recommended cadences for a seated flat ride run from 80 to 110 revolutions per minute. During the cardio stimulus especially, the seated flat is usually performed in the basic riding position, in which the body is inclined at approximately 45°.

Climbs

Seated and standing hill climbs are simulated by increasing the resistance on the bike. When performing seated climbs, the rider shifts the hips to the back of the saddle to avoid putting excessive pressure on the knees (figure 12. 4a). When climbing and standing, the rider moves the hands forward on the handlebars and keep the hips in line over the seat, maintaining hip flexion (figure 12.4b). These segments are usually performed with a slow cadence of 60 to 80 revolutions per minute and can be quite strenuous, with the primary focus on strength. Avoid having participants perform cadences under 60 revolutions per minute with heavy resistance as this may contribute to back and knee injuries.

Flat Runs

In the standing flat run or jog, the focus is on endurance; the resistance is light to medium, and the cadence is typically 80 to 95 revolutions per minute. The cyclist's weight is balanced over the lower body while the hands rest lightly on the handlebars (figure 12.4c). Instructors may require that participants remain vertical or are slightly flexed at the hips, keeping the spine in neutral.

Downhills

The downhill, or flushing, segment is usually short, lasting 1 to 3 minutes, and is used for recovery after a strenuous uphill climb. The flywheel tension is low, the cyclist is seated, and the breathing rate and heart rate return to more moderate levels.

Rebounds, Jumps, and Lifts

Rebounds, jumps, or lifts are advanced moves occasionally used to increase intensity. Participants need to be completely familiar with seated and standing positions before attempting jumps. Jumps or lifts are most often taught on the beat at regular intervals: Participants stand up for 8 counts, then sit down for 8 counts. The intervals can be short or long. An entire song or just part of a song may be used for jumping. Participants need to keep the lifting and lowering fluid and even, working for smooth knee transitions between sitting and standing. Jumps are usually accomplished without changing the pedal cadence. Jumping can be hard on the knees. Most cycling organizations recommend limiting or avoiding jumps due to the increased intensity of these types of movements, particularly for the beginning exerciser.

 See online video 12.3 for a demonstration of a standing climb and rebounds, with cues for cadence and resistance.

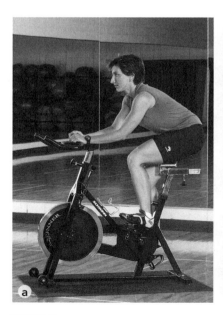 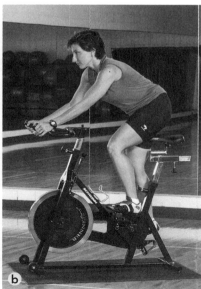 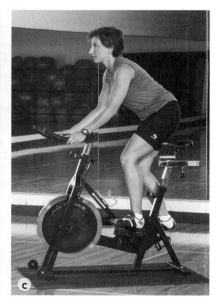

FIGURE 12.4 (a) Seated climb, (b) standing climb, and (c) standing flat run on the bike.

Sprints

Sprints, also known as *spin-outs, fast hammers,* and *power drills,* may be performed while seated or standing. They may be used in intervals or randomly dispersed throughout a segment. During a sprint, the cadence changes to a fast pace of 100 to 120 revolutions per minute and the resistance is set from light to moderate—just enough to keep the hips from bouncing. Experienced participants may cross the anaerobic threshold and cycle with a near-maximal effort, focusing on speed and power. Participants need to be careful when pedaling over 110 revolutions per minute; little resistance is possible at such high speeds, and the flywheel develops such a high momentum that it is doing almost all the work of turning the pedal arms. Interval training is highly effective as a method of improving cardiorespiratory training and can be used effectively in indoor cycling classes through a combination of seated climbs or standing climbs.

Practice Drill

Using your favorite music, practice seated flats, seated and standing climbs, combo hills, standing runs, and sprints. Work on positioning your body in ideal alignment as you experiment with these positions and riding techniques.

Formatting Indoor Cycling Classes

Formatting an indoor cycling class is a matter of combining the basic moves or drills. These combinations become the ride profile, which is the structure, or organization, of the cycling workout. The ride profile, with the accompanying music selections, needs to be prepared in advance. However, be ready to modify your plan depending on the fitness and skill levels of the individuals in class; the profile is only a guideline and will be subject to change. Each class will be different, and participants will have different needs. If you teach indoor cycling classes regularly, you will eventually accumulate many class profiles and a large selection of music from which to choose. You can be spontaneous and creative! Just remember to gradually increase the intensity at the beginning of class and gradually decrease the intensity at the end of class. A sample 45-minute profile is shown in table 12.1.

The music you choose for your cycling class is key to making your class a success. Unlike group exercise formats that require music to be metered into even 32-count phrases for choreography purposes, group cycling can be paired with virtually any style of music. Songs may have an even number of beats or not. You can choose from pop, disco, rock and roll, rhythm

TABLE 12.1 Sample Ride Profile

Segment	Body position	Resistance	Cadence (rpm)	Intensity (%MHR)	Music tempo	Music selection	Duration (min)
1. Warm-up	Seated	Light	80-90	65	Moderate	New age	5
2. Climb	Standing	Moderate	70	80	Slow	Rock and roll	4
3. Climb	Standing	Heavy	60	85	Slow	Rhythm and blues	4
4. Flat road	Seated	Moderate	90	75	Moderate	Rock and roll	6
5. Flat road	Standing	Moderate	90	75	Fast	Latin	4
6. Jumps	Seated or standing	Moderate	90	75	Moderate	Pop	4
7. Climb	Seated	Heavy	60	85	Slow	Funk	6
8. Downhill	Seated	Light	100	70	Slow	Classical	2
9. Sprints	Seated or standing	Moderate	110	85	Moderate	Rock and roll	5
10. Cool-down	Seated	Light	80	60	Moderate	Pop	3
11. Stretch	Off bike				Slow	New age	>2

and blues, jazz, reggae, rap, Latin, country, folk, gospel, classical, new age, world, and movie sound tracks. Find music that makes everyone smile and want to work. It's usually best to include several kinds of music in your workout so you can fit varying participant preferences and match the various class segments and moods you'll be creating. Connecting the music with the segments, mood, intensity, and journey can be the most fun yet challenging aspect of teaching an indoor cycling class.

Some instructors prefer to cross-train with their cycling classes. One way is by varying the focus of the classes held throughout the week. For example, the class might focus on strength (hills) on Monday, endurance on Wednesday, and speed on Friday. Another approach is to combine indoor cycling with a different exercise modality such as muscular conditioning, Pilates, or yoga. In this type of fusion format you might lead cycling for 30 minutes followed by yoga for another 30 minutes. The Keiser Power Pace cycling program has recommended using free weights, rubber tubing, and bands to incorporate muscular-conditioning exercises into the bike workout itself.

Intensity Monitoring

Another important training issue is intensity. As mentioned earlier in the chapter, research has shown that this type of group exercise is high intensity; therefore, intensity needs to be monitored on a regular basis. One of the benefits of group indoor cycling is that participants can work at their own levels, and the pressure to conform to the group is much less than it is in a traditional cardio class with mirrors. Even so, give your students target heart rate zones, RPE guidelines, and cadence goals and help them learn to pay attention to their intensity levels.

Many indoor cycling instructors strongly recommend the use of a heart rate monitor. Using heart rate monitors has a number of advantages as well as some disadvantages. Heart rate monitors can be useful if students know their actual training zones, as they might if they have had a graded exercise stress test (see the section "Intensity Monitoring" in chapter 7). The monitors make it easy to keep track of heart rate at any time during the class and do not require participants to stop moving in order to

check the rate. They can also provide an incentive to work harder when motivation falters. Unfortunately, most exercisers who use heart rate monitors do not know their actual training zones and assume that the standard suggested training zones are accurate; in fact, standard heart rate formulas are suitable for only 75% of the population (McArdle, Katch, and Katch 2009). In the other 25% of the population, the target heart rate zones are either overestimated or underestimated, sometimes significantly. Another limitation of the heart rate method involves the effects of medications (many either decrease or increase heart rate). No one heart rate formula will fit every participant, so it's wise to use other methods as well. Help your students establish a workout intensity zone—a heart rate training zone, a perceived exertion zone, or both.

During the workout, you can suggest that participants work at a low level (at the low end of the target heart rate zone or at 8 through 12 on the 6 to 20 Borg RPE scale) during the warm-up, cool-down, and downhill segments; a moderate level (at the middle of the zone or 12-14 RPE) during seated flats and standing runs; and a high level (at the top of the zone or 15-18 RPE) during climbs, jumps, and power intervals. Some participants may choose to push past the anaerobic threshold during power surges; this should be reserved for advanced students only.

The Schwinn Cycling program uses four zones for intensity cueing and assessment:

Zone 1	Easy and comfortable	50%-65% MHR	5-6 RPE (10-point scale)
Zone 2	Challenging but comfortable	65%-75% MHR	6-7 RPE
Zone 3	Challenging and uncomfortable	75%-85% MHR	7-8 RPE
Zone 4	Breathless (not max) but winded	85%-90% MHR	8-9 RPE

Remind your students that they can modify their cycling intensity by changing

1. the position (e.g., sitting instead of standing),

2. the resistance, or

3. the pedaling cadence.

Cadence is a widely used method for establishing intensity. Many bikes now come equipped with cadence computers and usually heart rate, distance in miles or kilometers, and estimated caloric expenditure information. Without such a device, cadence can be counted manually by tapping the thigh on each revolution. A slow cadence is 60 to 80 revolutions per minute (rpm), a moderate tempo is 80 to 100 revolutions per minute, and a fast cadence is 100 or more revolutions per minute. Being able to suggest cadence goals for each segment enhances your ability to guide and coach participants through a class. Let students know that even though you'll be giving intensity suggestions and goals, they still must exercise at their own pace. In addition to knowing the suggested cadence, many participants appreciate knowing how long each segment will last, so consider making announcements such as, "We'll be working hard on the next hill for 5 minutes" before leading into the more difficult sections. Or better yet, post an outline of your plan for all participants to see so they will know what to expect in the class.

Include a thorough cool-down at the end of class. Gradually decrease the intensity to little to no resistance while continuing to ride so that your participants' heart rates, breathing rates, oxygen consumption, and caloric expenditure can return toward normal values. We recommend statically stretching all major muscle groups at this time as well. Many instructors prefer to stretch the upper body while slowly cycling on the bike and then dismount to stretch the lower body. In addition to the upper-body stretches, be sure to include stretches for the hamstrings, quadriceps, hip flexors, calves, buttocks, and low back (see figure 12.5).

 See online video 12.4 for a demonstration of a cycling cool-down.

Cueing and Coaching Techniques

Leadership skills are all-important in an indoor cycling class. In many other group modalities (e.g., step, kickboxing, sport conditioning) instructors need to be concerned with getting all participants to move together at the same time. This is not necessary for group cycling. Instead, focus on motivating, coaxing, encouraging, and setting the mood with your voice and cues. Use plenty of motivational cues such as, "You can do it!" "Altogether!" "Drive it forward!" Pull your class through difficult segments with positive affirmations such as, "We are strong!" "We are committed!" "You can climb this mountain!" Suggesting that your students set goals for their workouts is another effective strategy to help them succeed. Ask them during the warm-up to create a focus or an intention for the class. For example, "If I still have energy during the last 30 seconds of any out of the saddle work, I will increase the resistance by a slight turn of the resistance knob." Then remind them of their focus during the challenging segments. For example, you can tell them, "Hang onto that goal!"

Indoor cycling classes are perfect for promoting a sense of teamwork within the class. One popular method for doing so is to divide the class into two or three pods, or small teams, and have the teams take turns sprinting or drafting as if in a race. You can use humorous techniques for dividing the group: for example, you could say everyone who prefers chocolate ice cream is on team one, and everyone who prefers strawberry ice cream is on team two. You can ask for sport team or color preferences and more. Be sure to ask your participants what *they* would like to do as well. Many in your class will want to suggest workout songs—when possible, incorporate their suggestions! The more input you get from participants about music and format the more buy in you get from them concerning coming back to class on a regular basis.

Remember to use visualizations during cycling classes. Many instructors suggest that riders picture themselves following the yellow line straight down the highway while feeling the wind in their faces or smelling the clean ocean air. Some instructors create an entire trip within the class, taking participants to Hawaii, down the beach, or through rolling hills.

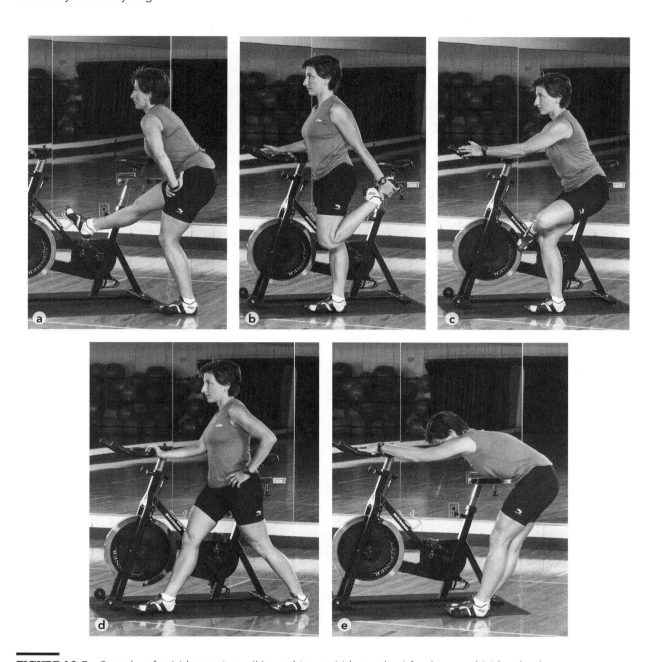

FIGURE 12.5 Stretches for (*a*) hamstrings, (*b*) quadriceps, (*c*) buttocks, (*d*) calves, and (*e*) low back.

Take advantage of the opportunity to get off the bike and teach. Walk through your class to check form and alignment and to support and encourage participants when the going gets tough. A simple "Hang in there!" to a fatigued class member can make all the difference.

Participants usually enjoy making noise while riding; you might try getting them to count the number of jumps they're performing or asking them to call out refrains to familiar songs you are playing. Theme classes are a great way to build camaraderie and fun; try picking your music around a special event, theme, or holiday. You can play scary music on Halloween, seasonal music for Christmas, love songs on Valentine's Day, or patriotic music on Memorial Day or the Fourth of July. For times when there aren't any holidays coming up, you can create a Motown music day, disco day, or beach music day. Encourage your students to relax and party!

Chapter Wrap-Up

In this chapter we covered indoor cycling, including proper positioning on the bike and cycling safety issues. We also covered warm-up, basic moves, programming, intensity recommendations, and cueing for stationary indoor cycling classes. Mastering this information is fun and rewarding and can definitely expand your teaching horizons!

Group Exercise Class Evaluation Form: Key Points

- Gradually increase intensity. Include rehearsal movements such as getting out of the saddle or low-level interval work for 30 seconds during the warm-up to begin to gradually increase intensity.
- Use a variety of cycling techniques. Avoid 10-minute segments; instead use a combination of movements such as seated flats for 3 minutes, standing jogs or runs for 3 minutes, and seated and standing climbs intermixed for 30-second intervals If you are out of the saddle for more than 50% of the class, you are using one technique for too long.
- Promote participant interaction and encourage fun. Have one side of the room rest while the other side engages in sprints. Encourage the rest group to cheer on the group performing sprints.
- Demonstrate good form and alignment for indoor cycling. Be sure to come early to class to help participants get properly set up on their bikes. If you see people struggling with their bike, get off your bike and help them so they are comfortable.
- Give clear cues and verbal directions, including intensity instructions, affirmations, visualizations, goal-setting reminders, and team-building statements. Use a microphone and tell participants often that they're doing a good job or have them set personal goals for class. Suggest they share goals with each other at the end of class.
- Help students monitor their intensity during the cardio segment, either with heart rate checks or perceived exertion checks or both. Bring heart rate monitors to class one day and allow participants to experiment with their HR and RPE estimates so they can get an idea of where their target heart rate (THR) range is during indoor cycling class.
- Gradually decrease intensity during the cool-down after the cardio segment and include some static stretches at the end of class. Have the last song of the cardio series be less intense, with a relaxing tempo. Encourage participants to get off their bikes for stretching at the end of class to enhance the effectiveness of stretches.
- Use music appropriately. At times, encourage participants to stay with the music tempo; other times have them pedal slower than the music, and at other times pedal faster than the music.

ASSIGNMENTS

1. List 15 motivational cues and affirmations appropriate for coaching a cycling class.
2. Prepare a 45-minute indoor cycling profile with music suggestions similar to those in table 12.1. Include music artists in the music selection section as well as the beats per minute. Write out all the details of class content, including the warm-up and cool-down.

Sport Conditioning and Boot Camp

Chapter Objectives

By the end of this chapter, you will be able to

- create a warm-up for a sport conditioning or boot camp class;
- understand what equipment to use for a sport conditioning or boot camp class;
- plan safe and effective movements for a sport conditioning or boot camp class;
- investigate current research in sport conditioning and interval training;
- apply leadership and team-building skills; and
- analyze and create a sport conditioning or boot camp group exercise class.

Background Check

Before working your way through this chapter, do the following:

Read

- ☐ Chapter 3, "Foundational Components";
- ☐ Chapter 5, "Coaching-Based Concepts";
- ☐ Chapter 6, "Warm-up and Cool-Down";
- ☐ Chapter 7, the section "Intensity Monitoring"; and
- ☐ Chapter 9, the section "Functional Training Principles."

Practice

- ☐ monitoring intensity using rating of perceived exertion (RPE),
- ☐ movement options and exercises on equipment used in sport conditioning and boot camp classes, and
- ☐ participant interaction as discussed in chapter 5.

Group Exercise Class Evaluation Form Essentials

Key Points for Warm-Up Segment

- Includes appropriate amount of dynamic movement or rehearsal moves
- Provides dynamic or static stretches for at least two major muscle groups

- Provides intensity guidelines for warm-up
- Includes clear cues and verbal directions
- Uses movements that are at an appropriate tempo, intensity, and impact level

Key Points for Conditioning Segment

- Gradually increases intensity
- Uses a variety of muscle groups
- Uses a variety of sport conditioning and functional training techniques
- Minimizes prolonged emphasis on any one technique and repetitive movements
- Observes participants' form and provides constructive, nonintimidating feedback
- Continually offers modifications, regressions, progressions, or alternatives
- Provides alignment and technique cues as well as provides written cues and pictures of exercises at each station

- Gives motivational cues
- Educates participants about intensity; provides HR (heart rate) or RPE check 1 or 2 times during the workout stimulus
- Promotes participant interaction and encourages fun
- Provides regular demonstrations and participation with good body mechanics
- Provides clear cues and verbal directions
- Uses appropriate movement and music tempo
- Gradually decreases impact and intensity during cool-down at end of the workout stimulus

Key Points for Cool-Down, Stretch, and Relaxation Segment

- Includes static stretching for the major muscles worked
- Demonstrates using proper alignment and technique
- Observes participants' form and offers

modifications, regressions, progressions, or alternatives
- Provides alignment cues
- Ends class on a positive note and thanks class

Fitness professionals often begin their careers working one on one with clients, only to find that their clients' routines would benefit from workout options. Sport conditioning or boot camp–style classes can provide that variety and add a dimension of competition and social interaction with others that assists with motivation. Fitness programming schedules refer to such classes as boot camp, sport conditioning, cross-conditioning, HIIT (high-intensity interval training), Tabata training, or metabolic conditioning. Many of these were developed by fitness professionals who sought a less choreographed approach to the group exercise experience, or by personal trainers who discovered that training several clients at one time can be more lucrative, breed less dependence on the trainer, and create

fun movement experiences in a group setting.

Instructors can take boot camp classes outdoors or use the track in their facility—either way, they move out of the four walls of the traditional group exercise setting and into an environment that is more natural for human movements. Cook (2010) believes that stabilizer muscles used in natural human movement are multitaskers and need to be used within movement experiences that mimic how we live, move, and work. Thus, working out in more natural environments may help train the body to move in more natural environments. Also, the class format of boot camp or sport conditioning classes often appeals to participants who have been involved in a structured sport workout with an athletic team or who seek variety and purposeful movement experiences.

The setting of these classes often eliminates the need for a microphone and even music. Unlike step and kickboxing, this type of class is not driven by the 32-count phrase. Rather, sport conditioning and boot camp–style classes often use interval training and mix the components of cardio, strength, and endurance training while incorporating movements and drills that are easy to follow and more athletic in nature (figure 13.1). Additionally, class participants can work as a team, which creates a sense of group cohesion.

According to Zuhl and Kravitz (2012), traditional low-intensity exercise can produce significant gains, but improvements from interval training can happen in a shorter time with fewer sessions. With time being the number one reason people give for not getting involved in an exercise program, sport conditioning and boot camp classes that emphasize interval training are on the rise. Bartels, Bourne, and Dwyer (2010) report that interval training crosses the spectrum of fitness conditioning: cardiac rehabilitation programs have included low-level interval-style group exercise experiences in their clients' workout plans for decades. New on the scene are drill-based interval classes using suspension training (e.g., TRX), ropes, ViPR, or the Gravity Training System. According to the 2013 IDEA Fitness Programs and Equipment Trends Report (Schroeder and Donlin 2013), 47% of respondents offer classes using one or more of these types; 73% offer indoor boot camp classes while 40% offer outdoor boot camps. Group exercise instructors are becoming increasingly versatile as more equipment suitable for the class setting is developed. Fitness facility owners will attest to the value of sport conditioning and boot camp classes as being important for member retention (Tharrett 2012). These formats also appeal to men and thus attract more men into the predominantly female world of group exercise.

When people first hear the term sport conditioning, they often ask, "What sport are you conditioning for?" It would be nice to include conditioning classes specific to tennis, basketball, golf, skiing, and more in fitness facility programming. Unfortunately, doing so is usually not practical and may fail to appeal to enough participants to fill such classes. Therefore, the term sport conditioning, or cross-conditioning, was created to refer to general training for sport movements rather than participation in a group exercise format such as water exercise or stationary indoor cycling. Also popular with the baby boomer generation are programs that train participants for week-long bike rides, or a hike up a 12,000-foot (3,658 m) mountain peak. This type of conditioning may be called sport conditioning, but it could also be called adventure conditioning. Many active-minded participants remember conditioning for a particular sport when they were younger. Whether conditioning for a sport or an adventure trip, this type of program adds more purpose and outcome to traditional workouts that in the past were more aesthetically based.

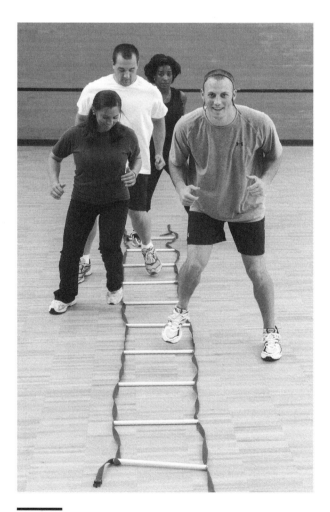

FIGURE 13.1 An exercise typical of a sport conditioning–type class: using ladders to enhance footwork.

Sport Conditioning and Boot Camp Research Findings

The following research studies include findings that can be applied to sport conditioning and boot camp classes. For example, golfers improved their swing and their daily living activities after participating in three 90-minute functional training sessions for 8 weeks (Thompson, Cobb, and Blackwell 2007). Sport conditioning instability resistance training, (which uses lower forces and more bodyweight exercises) was found to increase strength and balance in previously untrained young individuals, similar to training with more stable machines employing heavier loads (Sparks and Behm 2010). However, there was no overall difference between unstable and stable resistance training, and the training effects were independent of gender. Instability resistance training should be incorporated in conjunction with traditional stable training in order to provide a greater variety of training experiences without sacrificing training benefits (Kibele and Behm 2009). Additionally, high muscle activation with the use of lower loads associated with instability resistance training suggests that this type of program can play an important role within a periodized training schedule, in rehabilitation programs, and for nonathletic individuals who prefer not to use ground-based free weights to achieve musculoskeletal health benefits (Behm et al. 2010). Another study found that circuit weight training that does not include aerobic stations can elicit a cardiorespiratory response that meets the minimal American College of Sports Medicine (ACSM) guidelines for cardiorespiratory fitness (Gotshalk, Berger, and Kraemer 2004). A few studies have been performed on the efficacy of TRX (suspension) training. One study (Cayot et al. 2011) evaluated muscle activation in a TRX biceps curl versus a standard free weight curl; the results showed that the anterior deltoid exhibited greater activation during the TRX suspended curl. Another study (Fernando et al. 2012) found that push-ups performed with TRX invoked more lumbopelvic muscular activation than standard floor push-ups or push-ups performed on wobble boards or other unstable devices. Scheett and colleagues (2010) examined heart rate and lactate responses during a TRX workout using 30-second work intervals; the results indicated a moderate level of intensity was elicited.

Creating a Warm-Up

Warming up for sport conditioning and boot camp is somewhat similar to warming up for other formats (see Chapter 6). However, moves are obviously more sports based, are more like drills, and are not taught on the beat. Music is optional, although most participants find music with a strong rhythm and upbeat lyrics to be motivating. We recommend using music whenever possible. Crews (2008) suggests basic movements be included that increase mobility and release the low back as well as simple athletic movements that elevate core temperature and prepare the joints for work as well as prepare the brain for fun! We suggest that warm-ups include dynamic and/or rehearsal moves performed at a lower intensity and dynamic or static stretches for at least two major muscle groups. A related and important concept for this type of class is providing mobility (limbering) exercises for key joints. Since the hips, ankles, thoracic spine, and shoulders tend to be tight, appropriate mobility exercises are recommended. See the following exercises for examples of limbering exercises.

 See online video 6.3 for a sample warm-up for a sport conditioning–style class.

Hip Circle Warm-Up

When leading a good hip circle warm-up, start by walking slowly and rotating the hip through multiple planes while explaining to participants that the hip is a ball-and-socket joint that will work better throughout the boot camp class if it is moved through its full range of motion. For safety, remind participants to choose which level of stability and balance they need and encourage them to work toward not holding onto the wall while warming up in order to improve their neuromotor ability.

In a front leg swing (see figure 13.2) the knee is extended and the hip flexes and extends in the sagittal plane. To add the upper body, the hand from the same or opposite side may be stretched forward to touch the calf or toes of the swinging leg, increasing the difficulty of this total body warm-up movement. Participants can walk, stand, or use a wall or partner for support as long as they move both the lower body and upper body through full range of motion.

Lunge Warm-Up

Partial lunges in several planes provide limbering for the hip and knee joints and help to warm up the large leg muscles prior to a sport conditioning class. Make certain the knee faces the same direction as the toes and does not overshoot the toes.

This sequence constitutes a matrix, utilizing partial lunges in the sagittal, frontal, and horizontal planes: partial lunge in the sagittal plane; partial side lunge in the frontal plane, toes facing forward; and rotational lunge in the horizontal plane, feet positioned perpendicular to each other.

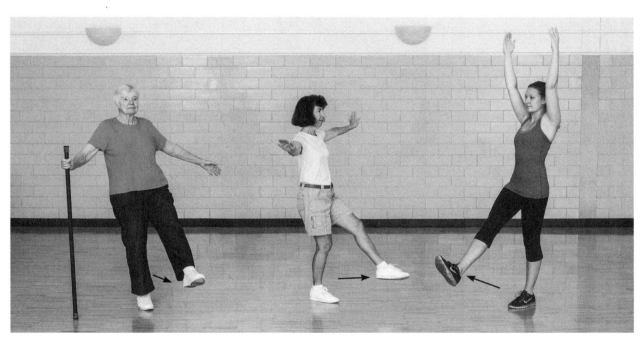

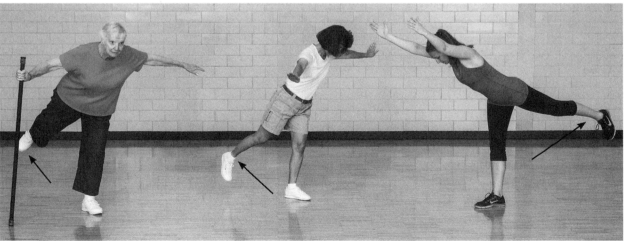

FIGURE 13.2 Leg swing variations from easiest to hardest.

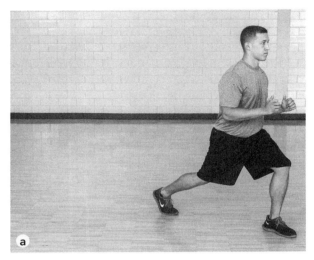

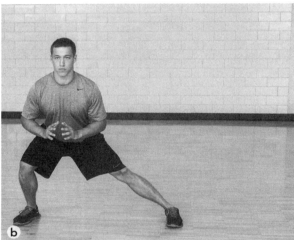

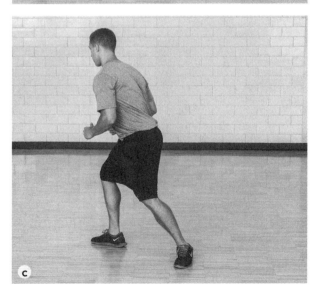

FIGURE 13.3 Integrating sagittal (*a*), frontal (*b*), and horizontal (*c*) plane movements collectively enhance the neuromotor system warm-up.

Ankle Warm-Up

Walking in a circle on the toes, and then the heels, increases blood flow to the lower extremities. Balance can also be challenged by standing on one leg while performing circles and figure eights with the other ankle. A dynamic standing calf stretch is performed by bending and straightening the front knee while keeping the back heel down (see figure 13.4 a-b). Rising up on the toes and then rocking back on the heels helps warm up both the anterior (shins) and posterior (calves) parts of the lower leg.

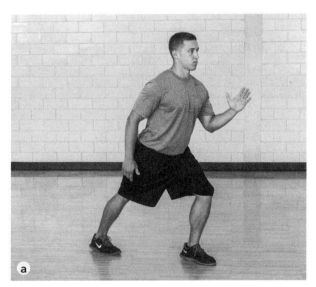

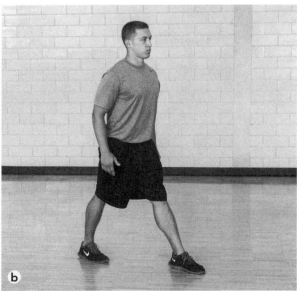

FIGURE 13.4 Dynamic calf stretch.

Thoracic Spine Warm-Up

Walking forward several paces while holding hands behind ears and turning the upper body first to one side, then the other helps warm up the thoracic spine (see figure 13.5). These combined movements help improve the transverse plane action of the spine, a motion that can be lost when participants sit for much of the day.

Shoulder Warm-Up

Upper body wall slides provide an effective warm-up movement for the shoulders. In this exercise, the back is flat against the wall with knees slightly bent, feet a few inches away from the wall, and abdominals engaged. A 90/90 (goalpost) position is created with both shoulders and elbows; arms are pressed back against the wall. In this move, the arms slide slowly and smoothly up and down while maintaining contact with the wall (see figure 13.6).

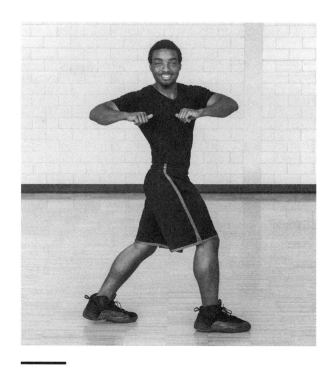

FIGURE 13.5 Walking while warming up the thoracic spine.

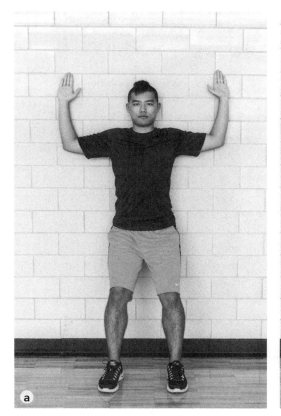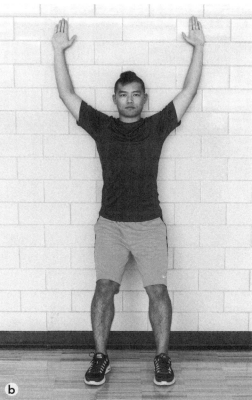

FIGURE 13.6 Upper body wall slides to warm up the shoulder complex.

Equipment and Setup

Choosing how to teach your sport conditioning or boot camp class ultimately depends on your personality, teaching philosophy, and clients' response to various formats. Your background as a group exercise leader and perhaps as a personal trainer will also influence how you teach your class (Vogel 2006). It is rare to find any two classes that are formatted the same way. Typically, sport conditioning classes use the equipment available within the group exercise facility. For example, McMillan (2005) decided to turn her step class into a sport step class. She noticed that many participants had drifted away from traditional step classes because such classes contain complex choreographed movements that require a lot of skill. To appeal to a different audience, McMillan called her classes *Power Step* and *Sport Step*. She made her movements feel like sport moves by incorporating variations such as adding a reach toward the ceiling during a basic step, imitating a jump shot in basketball. She also changed some traditional step names, for example across the step became man-to-man defense. Changing a few simple moves and using creative and purposeful cues made all the difference in her class. Baldwin (2007) suggested an H_2O Boot Camp style class combining athletic training formats in the water in order to bring the boot camp format into the aqua environment.

McLain (2005) used a different approach and created an outdoor boot camp class. He held the class in neighborhoods and parks rather than fitness facilities. His goal was to create a club without walls by taking programs out of the facility. This concept is what many health educators are suggesting in order to reach the general public more effectively. Francis (2012) envisions fitness professionals reaching out through community organizations, faith-based community programs, and other local neighborhood groups to reach more people who might not venture into a fitness facility. Many of these participants begin their movement experiences through participating in a boot camp or sport conditioning neighborhood class. Rather than expecting participants to drive to a facility, many contemporary professionals consider going to the people and using public resources and facilities, such as local parks and open green spaces, for sport conditioning and boot camp classes. There are issues with this concept, such as addressing liability concerns and obtaining appropriate informed consents, but ultimately the outdoor boot camp concept has been a proven success for McLain and others.

Some professionals purchase equipment or provide outdoor facilities to enhance the sport conditioning or boot camp experience. Crews (2009) took her baby boomer class outside and ran a Zoomer Boot Camp class. She focused on balance and rotation exercises using the BOSU ball for balance exercises and a medicine ball for rotation exercises. The equipment you use will depend on what is available to you and what population you are serving. Many fitness professionals prefer to use little or no gym equipment, relying instead on body-weight and plyometric moves; some of these ideas are discussed in chapter 9, "Functional Training Principles." In this chapter, "Sport Conditioning and Boot Camp Equipment" provides equipment ideas for sport conditioning or boot camp classes; various types of equipment are shown in figure 13.7.

 See online video 13.1 to get an idea of what sport conditioning equipment you can use in your classes. Notice how the instructor in this demonstration teaches the class differently from the way traditional high-low impact step, or kickboxing classes are taught.

Another important organizational element for group sport conditioning and boot camp classes is to have placards that help inform the interval or workout stations (figure 13.8). Often instructors will move around the room, explaining the various movements at each station, and then start the workout. This can make it difficult for participants to remember which movement is to be performed at which station. A detailed explanation of the exercise, placed at each station, will assist participants in understanding how to perform the movement correctly. For a brain activity while moving, you could eventually turn over every other placard after moving through the first round, but we recommend for safety to

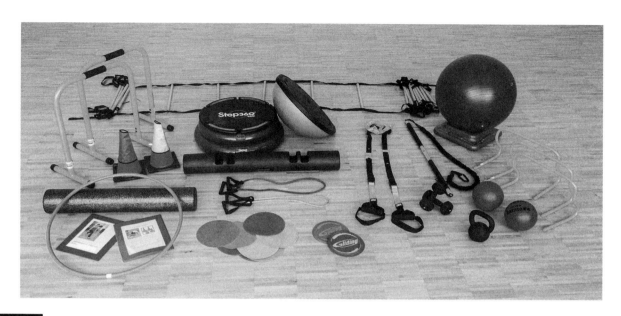

FIGURE 13.7 Sport equipment for indoor workouts.

Sport Conditioning and Boot Camp Equipment

Indoors

- Agility ladders
- Low hurdles
- Equalizers (Lebert Equalizers)
- Steps, step 360, and plyo boxes
- Slideboards and gliders
- Cones
- Jump ropes
- Medicine balls
- Reaction balls
- Kettlebells
- Dumbbells and weighted bars
- Exercise tubes and resistance bands
- Stability balls
- BOSU balance trainers
- Hula hoops
- TRX
- RIP Trainers
- Ropes
- Tires
- ViPR tubes
- Sleds
- Sandbags
- Agility dots and pads

Outdoors

- Running trails or tracks
- Stairs
- Benches
- Hills
- Playground equipment
- Cement walls
- Fitness trail stations
- Logs
- Sand

have cues and pictures available for participants during the first round of movement options. Products, designed by physical education vendors, are available to help make station labeling easier.

Two products we find useful are cones that have insert sleeves for instructional pieces of paper and rubber bases that contain sleeves for inserting placard instructions (shown in figure 13.9).

Station # _____

Place a photo or illustration of the exercise or movement here

Name of the exercise _____

Description of move _____

Alignment Cues _____

Safety Cues _____

Modifications, Regressions, Progressions _____

_____

FIGURE 13.8   Sample placard template for a sport conditioning station.

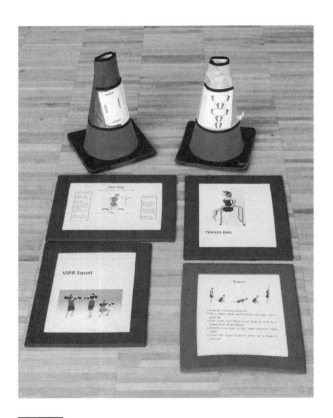

FIGURE 13.9   Products like these placard holders make station labeling easier.

Having a plan, with your exercise options clearly written out, is key to offering a professional sport conditioning or boot camp class.

Planning Safe, Effective Movements

One of the great advantages of a sport conditioning or boot camp class is the flexibility it provides you as the instructor. You are free to include whatever sport-specific exercises you like. Workouts can include functional training moves (discussed in chapter 9), balance exercises, boxing moves, traditional muscle-conditioning exercises, foam rollers, and more. Entire classes can be designed around certain pieces of equipment. For example, if your facility has invested in an S-frame with multiple TRX stations, you can structure a boot camp class around the large variety of TRX exercises. As you choose your format and your exercises, however, make sure each class includes a warm-up and cool-down and addresses the skill-related and health-related components of fitness (American College of Sports Medicine 2014).

Skill-related components of fitness

- Agility (including acceleration, deceleration, and change of direction)
- Balance (including static and dynamic)
- Coordination
- Power
- Speed
- Reaction time

Health-related components of fitness

- Cardiorespiratory training (including aerobic and anaerobic)
- Muscular strength and endurance (including core stability)
- Neuromotor fitness (including balance, stability, and mobility)
- Flexibility (including dynamic flexibility)

When teaching a sport conditioning or boot camp class, show exercise modifications for varying levels of fitness as discussed throughout this book. We can't assume that all participants will have the same fitness level or sport skill level. Cueing options for different movements are the key to leading a successful class. Instructors who demonstrate the intermediate option while suggesting advanced and beginner options will create a sense of comfort that allows all participants to have a good experience. The video clip showing sample drills also shows how to cue modifications for various participant levels. Notice how the instructor chooses to demonstrate the intermediate option in the video segment.

Let's discuss how some basic locomotor patterns can be modified for various fitness levels. Most of the locomotor patterns taught in our physical education classes were high impact and high intensity, such as broad jumps, burpees, and mountain climbers. These movements are fine when we're young but may become too stressful on the body as we age. Table 13.1 takes these basic locomotor patterns and presents high-impact, moderate-impact, and low-impact options for them. Lead the class through the intermediate modifications but demonstrate the other options so participants can choose the level of impact and intensity right for them.

The functional exercise continuum (see figure 13.10) continues to be important here. A skilled instructor is prepared to move left or right along the continuum, depending on the needs of participants. As you move to the left, you're making the exercise easier (a regression) or safer and more appropriate for a person's needs (this could also be a modification). If you move to the right, you're making the exercise harder, more sport-specific, and potentially higher risk. When planning your class, keep in mind how you'd regress (i.e., modify) or progress all your moves and drills. In this way you will provide appropriate exercise at the right time for each participant, thus helping each one enjoy the exercise experience and potentially prevent an injury from occurring.

TABLE 13.1 Modifications of Basic Locomotor Patterns for Sport Conditioning and Functional Training Classes

Low impact and intensity	Moderate impact and intensity	High impact and intensity
Walking using large arm movements	Walking with alternating slight hop	Skipping
Tapping side to side	Tapping side to side with a jump in the middle	Jumping in place
Walking using large arm movements	Walking 10 steps followed by running 10 steps	Running
Carioca without jumping	Sliding without the jumping or carioca	Sliding by hopping laterally
Knee lift without hopping	Knee lift with alternate hopping	Knee lift with a hop
Galloping with both feet performing a low-impact gallop	Galloping with only back leg hopping	Galloping with both legs hopping

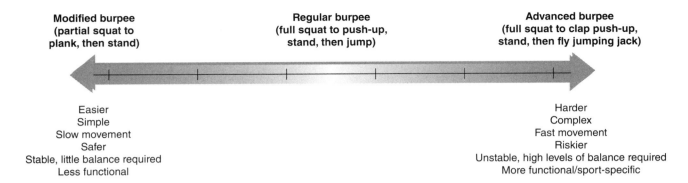

| Modified burpee (partial squat to plank, then stand) | Regular burpee (full squat to push-up, stand, then jump) | Advanced burpee (full squat to clap push-up, stand, then fly jumping jack) |

Easier
Simple
Slow movement
Safer
Stable, little balance required
Less functional

Harder
Complex
Fast movement
Riskier
Unstable, high levels of balance required
More functional/sport-specific

FIGURE 13.10   The progressive functional training continuum.

Basic Moves

Burpees (squat thrusts), bear crawls (mountain climbers), plyo lunges, pyramid planks (alternate downward dog with plank), alternating front kick with squat, and push-ups are all typical movements used in sport conditioning and boot camp classes. We encourage you to think beyond these traditional movements and consider organized drills and activities that incorporate a sport along with conditioning exercises; be sure to include modifications for each movement so participants are successful and will want to return. For example, in a cardio tennis class, rather than having participants perform line drills, organize the participants to have continuous tennis play rotating from court to court, with a ladder sequence in between the courts to keep cardio conditioning as a part of the playing experience. You can even have them play a game and keep score with the winners running to the next court to play the next round and the losers staying on the initial court. Whatever moves you choose, make sure you are visible for demonstration and motivation purposes.

There are a number of options for positioning yourself and your participants. In sport conditioning classes, standing in front of the participants is not the norm. Here are some alternative positioning ideas:

- Circle: You stand in the middle of a circle created by your participants.
- Circle: The participants form a circle and you stand still (off to the side) as they pass by you in small groups.

- Groups: The participants form two or three groups when they perform various drills. For example, two groups of participants could line up and face each other on opposite sides of a gym.
- Open or traditional: The participants spread out across the room or outdoor space but do not form lines.
- Relay: One participant at a time performs the exercise.

Sport conditioning and boot camp classes can be formatted so that the entire group performs the various drills together, or so that participants rotate though a variety of stations in small groups or teams. If your group is performing all the moves together, then you'll need to have enough equipment for everyone to use at the same time. For example, if using TRX exercises, then you'll need one TRX for each person in the class. If your group is rotating through stations in small groups, however, then you may only need 3 or 4 pieces of each type of equipment. See figure 13.11 for an example of a sport conditioning circuit or station class setup. If you had 30 participants, you could divide them into groups of three and have each group start the workout at a different station, using 10 stations. After 1 minute, each group would rotate to the next station, and so on.

Let's review some specific exercise ideas that address the basic components of a sport conditioning or boot camp class. Note that these exercises also include suggestions for participant positioning.

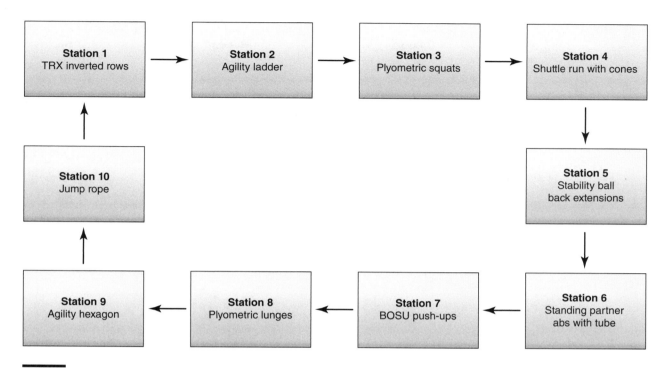

FIGURE 13.11 Sample setup for a sport conditioning class.

 See online video 13.2 for an example of a class that uses a station setup.

Agility, Coordination, and Reaction Time Drills

Cone drill. Using an open format or a relay format with participants standing next to each other in one line, have participants run forward 10 feet (3 m), touch a cone, turn around and run back, then run forward 20 feet (6.1 m), touch a cone, turn around and run back, run forward 30 feet (9.1 m), touch a cone, and turn around and sprint back. This activity is like the shuttle run you may have experienced in physical education classes, in which you picked up an eraser rather than touched a cone. If you have two to three people in the relay line, they will get a rest as other participants run, and so this would be an interval exercise for them. The relay format also can build team camaraderie since it encourages participants to cheer on their team members as they perform the drill. Repeat the drill 3 or 4 times; team members will improve as they learn the activity.

Ladder and jump rope drill. Drills using ladders or jump ropes are good ways to develop coordination and reaction time. Ask participants to line up in groups of three and then walk through a ladder series, alternating right and left legs with one foot in each ladder square. You will need enough ladders to accommodate groups of three. Place a couple of jump ropes at the ends of the ladders and ask participants to jump rope with both feet while they wait their turn to go through the ladder again. You can instruct participants going through the ladders to hop on one leg per square, hop on both legs per square, or use any other combination of movements. These neuromuscular movements require the mind and body to work together; they build both mental and physical outcomes from physical activity training.

Balance and Neuromotor Exercises

Ask participants to form a circle. Encourage them to jog or walk forward and then ask them to stop and stand on their right legs for 30 seconds; you can suggest that they close their eyes if they need more of a challenge and stand that way until they hear a whistle blow. Have them begin another movement such as the grapevine and then stand on the left foot for 30 seconds the next time they hear the whistle. Have participants change directions and perform this drill again. Incorporating balance movements into cardio segments is a good way to cross-train because you're combining skill-related components with health-related components of fitness. You can find many more balance exercise ideas in chapter 9.

Cardiorespiratory Training

Our lives are a blend of aerobic and anaerobic movements. We walk from our cars to the front doors of our office buildings and then take the stairs up to work. Sports also involve a blend of the aerobic and anaerobic. We serve a tennis ball, run to get it, and then rest when the point is over. Short bursts of exercise combined with longer aerobic movements make up many sport conditioning and boot camp drills. Place a bench at the end of your exercise area and have your participants stand at the opposite end. Ask the participants to walk or jog to the bench, walk up 10 flights of stairs (step up, up, down, down on the bench for 10 counts), and then walk or jog back. You can change this format and have them walk or jog for 10 to 40 seconds; you can also increase or decrease the number of times they step up on the bench. If you are performing this drill outdoors, you can have participants walk or jog on a track and then go up and down a nearby set of stairs. These types of movements fit well in both functional and sport-specific training.

Recently, high-intensity interval training (HIIT), sometimes known as metabolic training, has become very popular. The purpose of metabolic training (as well as HIIT) is to dramatically and radically kick-start the metabolism, ideally helping to quickly improve fitness and burn large numbers of calories. Slordahl and colleagues (2004) and Burgomaster and others (2008) demonstrated that HIIT training can increase fat-burning mechanisms and can be more effective than traditional continuous training. While some of the claims appear to be true, the high-intensity and high-impact nature of these workouts may be too much for many beginning participants. Remember, too much, too soon is

the major cause of injury and drop out. Consider reserving HIIT and metabolic training programs for fit and motivated participants. Some sample HIIT drills include these:

1. Have participants sprint down one long side of the gym (or football field), then jog across the short end, sprint down the other long side, and jog across the short end.

2. Place a cone in each of the four corners of the room. Have participants sprint between the cones; at each cone, have them stop and perform an exercise for 30 to 60 seconds. For example, Cone a: burpees, Cone b: plyo squats, Cone c: jumping jacks, Cone d: mountain climbers.

3. Use the form of high-intensity training known as the Tabata method, which uses Tabata drills. In this method, participants are asked to perform 20 seconds of all-out, very high-intensity work, then rest for 10 seconds. This sequence is usually repeated 6 to 8 times: 20 seconds of work, 10 seconds of rest, 20 seconds of work, 10 seconds of rest, and so on. Then a new move is introduced and the same 6 or 8 Tabata interval sequence is performed, and so on. Examples of moves that are used include burpees; one big plyo squat forward, two jumps back; butt kickers; one squat followed by a kickboxing-style side or roundhouse kick; push-ups; forearm planks pressing up to full plank (up, up, down, down rhythm), and so on. Obviously, it's critical to provide a proper warm-up and cool-down and to constantly suggest regressions and progressions. You can read more about HIIT and Tabata training in chapter 7.

 See online video 13.3 for sample high intensity interval training using Tabata drills.

Core Strengthening

Building core strength and stability is essential for any group exercise class. The core (i.e., the scapular, abdominal, and low-back musculature) supports most standing activities; since humans spend much of their lives standing on two feet, strengthening the core muscles will improve posture and athletic performance. It is important to strengthen the core while in a standing position for both functional and sport conditioning exercises (see figure 13.12.) However, finishing with plank exercises to recruit the transverse abdominis (see figure 13.13) and train the spine in neutral, or moving into a prone position and performing back extension exercise variations, are other effective strategies for core strengthening.

Muscular Strength and Endurance

In chapter 8 we reviewed muscle strength and conditioning exercises using body weight or external resistance. Many of these exercises are used in sport conditioning and boot camp classes. Here are a few suggested guidelines to follow when selecting exercises.

- To emphasize maintaining muscle balance, whenever you pick a pushing exercise, also select a pulling exercise. For example, if you incorporate an exercise that works the pectorals

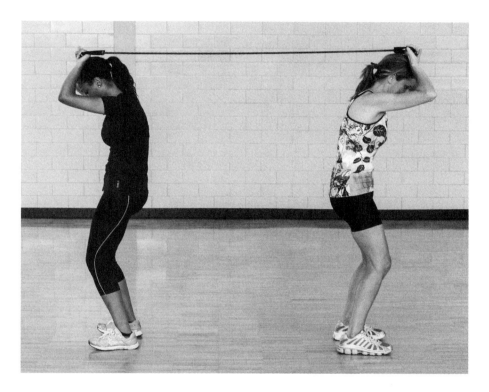

FIGURE 13.12 Cue this exercise as "Feel how this move helps counteract the tendency to stand with your low back arched."

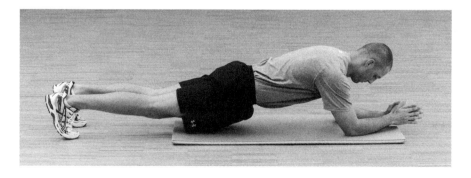

FIGURE 13.13 The plank position is a core-strengthening exercise often used in sport conditioning classes.

(pushing muscles), also include an exercise that works the rhomboids, middle trapezius, and posterior deltoids (pulling muscles).

• For comfort, plan to work larger muscle groups (such as the quadriceps) before working smaller muscle groups (such as the tibialis anterior) so that the larger muscle groups can recover while you work on smaller muscle groups.

• If your focus is on functional training, concentrate on working the muscle groups that do not get used as much throughout the day. For example, when performing daily activities, people often lift items with their biceps. Therefore, focus your class on the triceps muscle, which is assisted by gravity all day and rarely gets used with daily activity.

You can also cue exercises in ways that draw participants' attention to their functional value. Try calling a sit-to-stand exercise a *get-out-of-your-chair exercise* rather than a *squat* so participants see the connection between their workout and their daily movements (see figure 13.14). An overhead press with hip abduction (see figure 13.17) can strengthen the gluteal muscles in an upright position in order to improve walking gait.

Figures 13.15 and 13.16 give additional functional muscular strength and endurance examples.

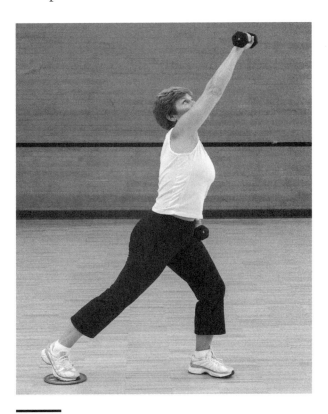

FIGURE 13.15 Cue this exercise as "Reach into your cupboards!" rather than "Do an overhead press."

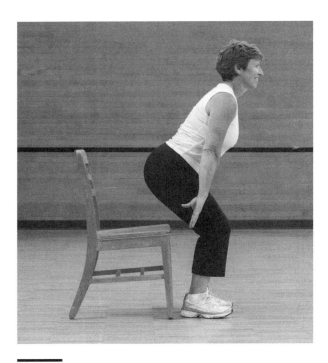

FIGURE 13.14 Cue this exercise as "Get out of your chair" versus "Do a squat."

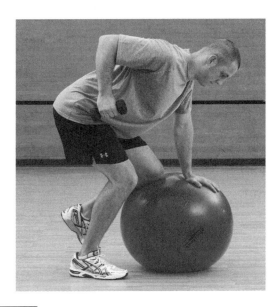

FIGURE 13.16 Cue this exercise as "Start the lawn mower!" rather than "Perform a bent-over row."

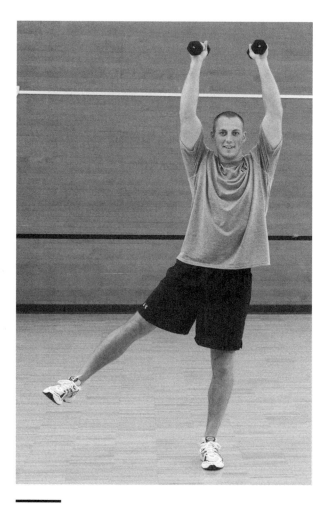

FIGURE 13.17 For this exercise, cue your participants, "Alternating hip abduction in a standing position helps you strengthen your gluteal muscles for standing. Because your gluteal muscles keep your hips in line when you walk and run, it's important to strengthen them in an upright standing position."

Flexibility

In chapter 8 we also reviewed stretching exercises for each major muscle group. Many of these stretches are appropriate for sport conditioning or functional training classes (see figure 13.18). Refer to table 3.2 for an overview of the muscles that are recommended for stretching in a sport conditioning or boot camp exercise class. Stretching the muscles that are used throughout the day will enhance overall relaxation. Since interval training is a primary format for boot camp and

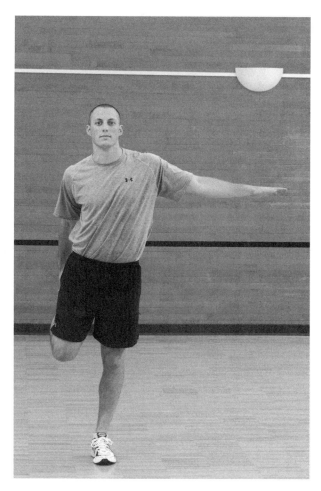

FIGURE 13.18 Stretching the quadriceps is a great functional stretch since the quadriceps is a strong muscle used in many daily and sport activities.

sport conditioning classes, flexibility exercises may even be performed in between intervals. For example, after your participants finish a high-intensity walking or jogging interval, lead them in a calf stretch against the wall while they wait for the next cardiorespiratory interval to begin. While incorporating stretching throughout the workout is effective, spending the last 5 minutes of class stretching on the ground, where the body is relaxed against gravity, improves flexibility and provides a chance for participants to recover completely from the workout before leaving. Remember to hold stretches for 15 to 60 seconds during this final segment.

Chapter Wrap-Up

A sport conditioning or boot camp class offers a unique opportunity to improve a participant's enjoyment in a sport or enhance a participant's daily living activities. Participants are seeking group exercise that is more purposeful, which is why these types of formats are gaining in popularity. Rather than focusing on improving their looks, many participants are becoming more concerned with how easily they perform their daily routines, as well as how comfortably they engage in leisure pursuits. A sport conditioning or boot camp class can be a purpose-driven experience that can make a difference in the health and wellness of participants. Plus, it can bring out the kid in us as we remember playing as a form of physical movement.

Group Exercise Class Evaluation Form: Key Points

- Include an appropriate amount of dynamic movement. For the warm-up, use dynamic movements such as walking in a circle on the toes.
- Provide rehearsal moves. Introduce rehearsal moves by showing a modification of one of the basic locomotor patterns.
- Stretch major muscle groups in a biomechanically sound manner with appropriate instructions. Stretch the major muscle groups throughout the workout and especially at the end or between intervals.
- Give clear cues and verbal directions. Modify exercises for participants by giving movement intensity options.
- If music is used, choose appropriate music that inspires movement and may have beeps for timed interval changes.
- Gradually increase intensity during the workout stimulus.
- Use a variety of sport conditioning and functional training movements; match movements to purposeful activity when possible.
- Minimize prolonged emphasis on any one locomotor pattern or sport conditioning component.
- Demonstrate good form and alignment for all exercises and participate with clients.
- Promote participant interaction and encourage fun. Use relay race formats, among others, to engage your participants in your class.
- Gradually decrease impact and intensity during the cool-down after the conditioning segment.

ASSIGNMENTS

1. Write a complete outline for a 10-minute sport conditioning or boot camp class that includes a 2-minute warm-up, a 6-minute combination cardio and strength segment, and a 2-minute cool-down that includes stretching. List the specific exercises to be performed, the purpose of each exercise, how you'll regress or modify each one, and the titles of any music pieces. Prepare yourself to present the workout.

2. Research an online sport conditioning or boot camp workout. Describe the exercises and methodology shown and evaluate the instructor using the Group Exercise Class Evaluation Form (appendix A). Do you think the workout was safe? Effective? Appropriate (for whom)?

Water Exercise

Chapter Objectives

By the end of this chapter, you will be able to

- identify the benefits of water exercise;
- understand the properties of water and Newton's laws of motion;
- analyze and apply water exercise research principles to class instruction;
- create a water exercise class using progressive resistance training principles;
- apply appropriate use of training systems and water-specific equipment to water exercise; and
- modify the group exercise class evaluation form for water exercise.

Background Check

Before working your way through this chapter, do the following:

Read

- ☐ chapter 3, "Foundational Components,"
- ☐ chapter 5, "Coaching-Based Concepts," and
- ☐ chapter 8, sections titled "Recommendations and Guidelines on Muscular Conditioning," Cueing Muscular Conditioning Exercises," and "Demonstrating Progressions, Regressions, Modifications, and Alternatives."

Practice

- ☐ monitoring intensity using rating of perceived exertion (RPE) (see chapter 7),
- ☐ showing various movement options for intensity levels, and
- ☐ encouraging participant interaction as discussed in the chapter 5, in particular the section "Motivational Strategies for Coaching-Based Group Exercise."

Group Exercise Class Evaluation Form Essentials

Key Points for Warm-Up Segment

- Includes appropriate amount of dynamic movement
- Provides rehearsal moves
- Stretches major muscle groups in a biome-

chanically sound manner with appropriate instructions

- Includes clear cues and verbal directions
- Uses music and movements at an appropriate tempo and intensity

Key Points for the Conditioning Segment

- Gradually increases intensity
- Uses a variety of water exercise techniques
- Minimizes prolonged emphasis on any one technique
- Offers modifications, regressions, progressions, or alternatives
- Promotes participant interaction and encourages fun

- Demonstrates good form and alignment and provides clear verbal cues
- Educates participants about intensity; provides RPE check at least 1 or 2 times during workout stimulus
- Gives motivational cues
- Gradually decreases intensity during cooldown after the cardiorespiratory session
- Uses music appropriately

As we strive to make the exercise experience more purposeful and fun for our participants, we need to consider water exercise. Water exercise is growing in popularity in the United States as the population ages and participants seek nonintimidating and nonimpact exercise. The World Health Organization's (WHO 2010) latest projections estimate that the world population will grow from 6 billion in 1999 to 9 billion by 2042. In about 5 years' time, the number of people aged 65 or older will outnumber children under age 5, and the over-65 segment of the population will grow from an estimated 524 million in 2010 to nearly 1.5 billion in 2050, with most increases occurring in developing countries. According to the U.S. Census Bureau (2010) between 2010 and 2050, the United States is projected to experience rapid growth in its over 65 year old population. In 2050 the number of Americans aged 65 and older is projected to be 88.5 million, more than double its projected population of 40.2 million in 2010. Water exercise will be a natural medium for the baby boomers to experience group exercise. Vogel (2006) believes that despite the emerging popularity of water exercise, many fitness consumers still view it as a specialized or overly gentle activity. However, the Aquatic Exercise Association (2010) touts

the activity as having a far-reaching impact on the population, from older adults to athletes. Sanders (2010) reports that water exercise has shown promise as an effective, yet comfortable and safe, movement option for people who are unable to exercise on land regardless of age or fitness ability. As consumers become aware of the many facets of water exercise, they will be more likely to view it as an effective way to enhance their health and wellness.

Benefits of Water Exercise

Pools are often viewed as a place for obtaining a cardiorespiratory workout by swimming. Unfortunately, pools are expensive to maintain when used only for lap swimming because each person requires a large amount of space to benefit from exercise. In a water exercise class, more than 25 participants can work out in the pool together, enjoy the benefits of the water's resistance, and not even get their hair wet. Water exercise can also be a most effective form of group personal training if the right equipment is available. We need to think of our pools as giant resistance machines. In fact, research tells us that pools can be great for muscular strength and conditioning. Tsourlou and colleagues (2006) studied the training effects of a 24-week aquatics class on muscular strength in healthy elderly women and found that the water provided an alternative to traditional resistance training as well as enhanced the social environment for this population. D'Acquisto, D'Acquisto, and Renne (2001) found that water exercise is effective for cardiorespiratory and weight-management training. Pools provide overload from the water's resistance; muscles are trained while at the same time stress on the joints is reduced through buoyancy assistance. In the strength and conditioning area, variable resistance machines overload the muscles by using weights that are designed to move against gravity. In the pool, the viscosity and other properties of water can create overload for the muscles.

Group water exercise instructors often see many newcomers who want instruction on how to move properly in the water. Many participants who try water exercise for the first time find that the pool environment allows them to set their own pace and intensity and to rest when necessary. On the other hand, people who need a more intense workout find that the resistance that water provides acts in all directions (and not just in the direction of gravity), no matter what the movement. In some ways, water exercise is safer than land-based activity—falls don't carry the same threat of injury, and joints receive less stress from impact. Furthermore, water cools participants as they work out, so sweating is not a problem (Gangaway 2010).

Water is particularly kind to people who are overweight and also to women (Brown et al. 1997), who are genetically programmed to carry more stored energy and thus more body fat. When overweight participants enter a traditional group exercise class, they are often intimidated by the mirrors and the fact that other people may be looking at their bodies. In a water exercise class, the body is covered up by water, and extra body fat actually makes the person more buoyant. Nagle and coworkers (2007) found that aquatic exercise, in combination with walking, can serve as an alternative to walking exercise alone for overweight women who are losing weight; thus, aquatic exercise can be a useful method to improve functional health status. The current obesity pandemic in the United States

will undoubtedly cause a continual increase in the popularity of water exercise.

As the focus of exercisers shifts from aesthetic fitness to functional fitness, use of the water for exercise will increase because it is one of the best environments to accomplish functional and specific resistance training (Bravo et al. 1997; Simmons and Hansen 1996; Suomi and Koceja 2000). Sport scientists know that to improve sport performance, it is best that muscles are trained with movements that are as similar as possible to the desired movements or skills required in a specific sport. A movement performed in a sport can be replicated in water for added resistance. It is important to note that as with any other mode of exercise, consistency of participation and enjoyment of the activity are key components to continued adherence. In fact, Bocalini and colleagues (2010) studied healthy older women who had not exercised previously but were willing to participate in a water exercise class. After 12 weeks the women had improved in neuromuscular patterns and quality-of-life measurements. Making sure your classes are fun is important for continued participation and for maintaining gains in health parameters.

Water exercise is also a wonderful medium for injury rehabilitation and provides a way to gradually progress to functioning on land (Sanders and Lawson 2006). From a health perspective, skills that enhance proper posture are critical to daily functioning. Many movements performed on land do not functionally train the muscles for improved posture. For example, performing supine curl-ups on land does not prepare the abdominals to be strong in a functional, upright position—rather, these curl-ups strengthen the abdominals in a forward, flexed position. This abdomen-forward flexed position can be observed in older adults in retirement homes who walk bent over at the waist. It's important to strengthen and stretch the body in an upright position to improve daily living activities for life. In the pool, simply walking against the natural resistance provided by the water works the abdominals in an upright position and thus strengthens the abdominals and low back collectively to improve daily functioning (Kennedy and Sanders 1995). It is important to note that once participants are trained, they can be

Water Exercise Research Findings

- When the chest cavity is immersed in water, heart rate decreases, and so it is not appropriate to use land-based target heart rates when monitoring exercise intensity (Craig and Dvorak 1968; D'Acquisto, D'Acquisto, and Renne 2001; Svedenhag and Seger 1992; Benelli, Ditroilo, and DeVito 2004).

- Training from water exercise can carry over to improve function and health on land (Bushman et al. 1997; Davidson and McNaughton 2000; DeMaere and Ruby 1997; Eyestone et al. 1993; Frangolias et al. 2000; Gehring, Keller, and Brehm 1997; Raffaelli, et al. 2010; Takeshima et al. 2002; Tsourlou et al. 2006; Gulick, 2010).

- When running in deep water, women experience less physiologic stress than men experience (Brown et al. 1997). Deep water running improves cardiorespiratory fitness (Loupias and Golding 2004).

- Aquatic exercise can serve as an alternative to walking exercise alone for overweight women who are losing weight (Nagel et al. 2007). Water exercise improved $\dot{V}O_2$ in older women (62-65 years old) more than a land walking program (Bocalini et al. 2008). A short-term water-based exercise intervention on overweight older women was useful in improving aerobic capacity, muscle strength, and quality of life (Rica et al. 2012).

- Walking performed in chest-deep water had a better effect on exercise-induced hypotension in untrained healthy women than walking at a similar intensity on land (Rodriguez et al. 2011).

- Pool exercises targeting activities of daily living can improve performance of these activities on land (Templeton, Booth, and O'Kelly 1996; Jentoft, Kvalvik, and Mengshoel 2001). Participating in water exercise 2 times per week for a year was necessary for maintaining adult daily living ability for frail elderly during a 1-year exercise period and for 1 additional year afterward (Sato 2009). It is also possible to plan and execute a water exercise program that has a positive effect on bone status of postmenopausal women (Rotstein, Harush, and Vaisman 2008).

- Interval training in the water is recommended for beginners to reduce local muscular fatigue, increase duration, and make the workout more enjoyable (Frangolias, Rhodes, ands Taunton 1996; Michaud, Brennan, et al. 1995; Quinn, Sedory, and Fisher 1994; Wilbur et al. 1996).

- Water exercise has a greater anaerobic demand (in untrained water exercise participants) and therefore provides muscular strength and endurance training throughout the entire session (Brown et al. 1997; Evans and Cureton 1998; Frangolias and Rhodes 1995; Michaud et al. 1995; Wilbur et al. 1996). Killgore (2009) stated that proper biomechanics must be factored into an appropriate exercise prescription when performing deep-water running.

- Reducing the speed of movements performed in water is essential. It is recommended that movements be performed approximately one-half to one-third slower than movements on land (39 % slower) for equivalent energy expenditure (Frangolias and Rhodes 1995). Allow students to adjust their speed based on their RPE (Gehring, Keller, and Brehm 1997; Hoeger, Warner, and Fahleson 1995).

challenged with increasing resistance just as is done in traditional strength and conditioning programs. Equipment overload (usually provided by surface area) and speed adjustments need to be applied progressively (Mayo 2000).

Performing basic locomotor patterns (i.e., walking and running) using the water's resistance enhances functionality as the body stabilizes itself against resistance; plus, there is little load on the body's lower-extremity joints.

Thus, water exercise provides specific resistance in an upright, functional position while at the same time unloading the musculoskeletal system (Norton et al. 1997). Finally, many land-based activities such as tai chi and Pilates can provide increased solace and relaxation when they're moved into the water (Archer 2005). Overall, water exercise is transitioning from an emphasis on its traditional clients (older adults and younger adults with injuries) to newer markets that include athletes, younger adults, and mind-body enthusiasts (Vogel 2006) due to its ability to provide a functional training outcome. See "Group Exercise Class Evaluation Form Essentials" for the main points on the evaluation form that apply to water exercise.

Properties of Water and Newton's Laws of Motion

Let's examine some general properties of water that make water exercise different from land exercise. Then we can move on to reviewing the muscular requirements of water exercise and Newton's laws of motion as they apply to water. Knowing the principles that govern movement in water is important to maximizing the success of your water exercise classes.

Viscosity, or the friction between molecules, causes resistance to motion. Water is more viscous than air, just as molasses is more viscous than water (Aquatic Exercise Association 2010). Because water is more viscous than air, it provides greater resistance to motion. When a person walks forward in the water, the viscosity (cohesion and adhesion of the water molecules) creates a block of water that must move with the person. This block of water, often called a *drag force,* adds overload that increases energy expenditure.

Buoyancy is a force experienced in water that is analogous to experiencing the force of gravity on land. Buoyancy pushes the body upward and has the opposite effect of gravity. An object's buoyancy depends on its density relative to its size; the relative density of an object determines whether it will sink or float (Bates and Hanson 1996). Thus, body composition, because it affects body density, affects a participant's buoyancy. Participants with greater amounts of body fat (or stored energy) have greater buoyancy. On the other hand, participants with less body fat have a greater relative density and thus are less buoyant. Leaner participants may need the assistance of buoyant devices when exercising in deep water. For example, a lean athlete running in deep water requires a different flotation device from the one used by a female with average body fat. Buoyancy will also affect range of motion (ROM) when exercising in water. In an exercise such as standing hip abduction (figure

14.1), buoyancy will push the leg toward the top of the water. If the leg goes beyond the 45° ROM of the hip abductors, the rectus femoris and iliopsoas and not the hip abductors will act as the primary mover of the exercise. Clasping the hands in front helps keep the body from going underwater with this movement. If a regular jumping jack move were performed, the participants would submerge and get their hair wet. Typical land movements need to be modified so they are water friendly and will keep participants comfortable. ROM and direction of resistance are important to keep in mind when cueing water movements. Practice the movement in the water before instructing participants from the deck. In the example shown in figure 14.1, cue participants to keep the hip abduction movement to 45° and press the hands together

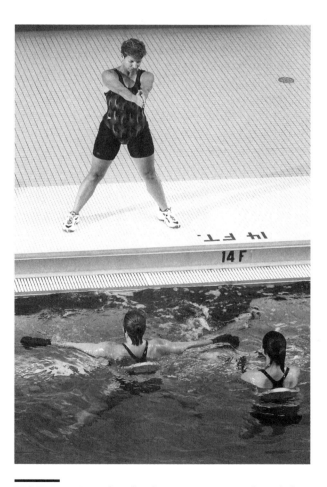

FIGURE 14.1 When leading participants in hip abduction, cue them to keep their ROM to 45° and press their hands in front so they do not become submerged and get their hair wet.

firmly in front to prevent the head from going underwater.

Differences in Muscle Action

One reason why exercising in water is comfortable and relatively pain free is because movement in water requires little eccentric muscle action (however, equipment that requires eccentric muscle actions can be added). Eccentric muscle actions are often associated with delayed onset muscle soreness (DOMS) (Byrnes 1985). DOMS can set in 1 or 2 days after an exercise experience and cause muscular discomfort that can lead to a lack of adherence. A meta- analysis of 10 randomized, controlled clinical trials that compared land to aquatic exercise for adults with arthritis found no difference in outcomes between land- and water-based exercise (Batterham, Heywood, and Keating 2011); however, most of the studies in this meta-analysis did not reflect on the "comfort" of the participants but rather on the health and musculoskeletal outcomes. Many regular water exercise participants report how "good" movement in the water makes them "feel." It's important to note that looking to the research to guide program design related to muscle action will be difficult until more qualitative measures of the impact of how participants "feel" in the water becomes available in published literature, particularly from older adults who value comfort as an important part of their movement experience. However, coupling the fact that movement in water involves predominantly concentric muscle actions with the fact that activity in water

is nonimpact in nature and can be more comfortable for those with special needs, we know the pool provides a safe and comfortable workout environment. To become an effective instructor in water exercise, it is important to understand these and other implications of movement in water. Table 14.1 shows the differences between muscle actions on land and muscle actions in water for standing shoulder abduction and adduction. Adding equipment changes which muscle is used. Understanding Table 14.1 will help you describe to participants which muscle groups are being used with each movement.

Progressing Water Exercises

Progressive resistance in water exercises is created by varying speed, surface area, travel, and work against buoyancy to gradually increase muscular overload in order to achieve training effects. Being able to vary the plane of motion during a resistance exercise, which can be more difficult to do in a traditional group exercise class, is one of the most important benefits of water exercise. For example, if a participant horizontally adducts the shoulders (thinking the pectoral muscles are being worked) by performing a basic dumbbell fly while standing on land, gravity forces the deltoid muscles to be the prime movers instead (since the deltoids must work to keep the dumbbells lifted in the air). For this movement to be effective for the pectoral muscles, the participant must lie in the supine position and perform the dumbbell fly. When the participant performs a dumbbell fly while

TABLE 14.1   Standing Shoulder Abduction and Adduction on Land Versus in Water

Environment	Equipment	Joint action	Anterior or middle deltoid muscle action	Latissimus dorsi muscle action
Land	None	Shoulder abduction	Concentric	None
Land	None	Shoulder adduction	Eccentric	None
Water	None or surface-area device	Shoulder abduction	Concentric	None
Water	None or surface-area device	Shoulder adduction	None	Concentric
Water[a]	Bouyant device	Shoulder abduction	None	Eccentric
Water[a]	Bouyant device	Shoulder adduction	None	Concentric

Participants should stand upright, with hands at sides and feet shoulder-width apart.

[a]Slow speed to resist buoyancy.

standing in water, however, the pectorals are the prime mover because the deltoids are assisted by buoyancy. Because in water gravity does not affect the direction of resistance, movements and planes can be varied while working in an upright, functional position. In other words, water exercise allows more options for upright overload.

A suggested water exercise progression for increasing and decreasing movement intensity for the pectoralis major is illustrated in figure 14.2, which depicts this movement in action with participants in a deep water exercise class.

Figure 14.2 shows a pectoral progression using a breaststroke. At first, the participant marks the move performing horizontal shoulder adduction in place; next the participant moves backward to assist the move (figure 14.2a).

Then, to overload the movement, the participant jogs forward to create resistance against the breaststroke (figure 14.2b).

Let's use this knowledge and the progression model in figure 14.2 to build a resistance intensity progression targeted toward working the pectoral muscles. As with any group exercise format, it is important to warm up before beginning any exercise progression series. First, warm up the pectoral muscles by standing or marching in place and horizontally adducting the shoulder joints in a relaxed fashion, using functional ROM. Then, increase the speed or force of the movement following the progression model, pushing the body backward. Next, increase the surface area of the movement by putting on webbed gloves and increase the speed

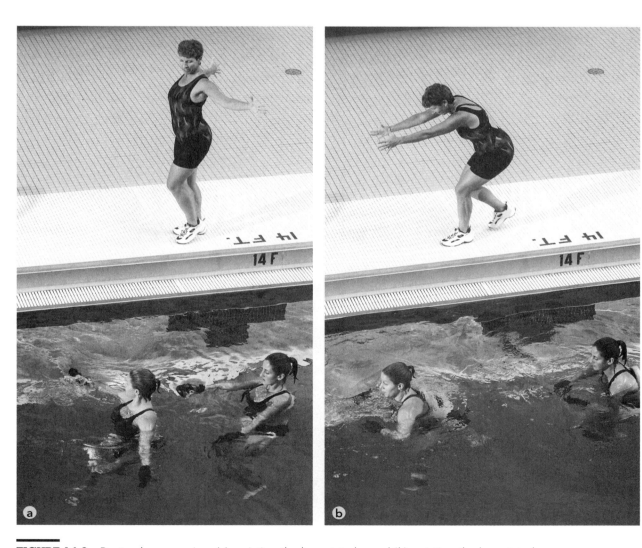

FIGURE 14.2 Pectoral progression: (a) assisting the breaststroke and (b) resisting the breaststroke.

again. Next, begin to jog forward while traveling against the current and performing horizontal adduction of the shoulder joint. Increase the speed of travel again. Finally, suspend the body by lifting the feet off the bottom of the pool to drag the surface area of the body through the water. Contract the trunk stabilizers to add more drag with the body and to stabilize against the effects of buoyancy. This is an example of using the progression model in figure 14.3 to gradually increase the movement's intensity. The movements can also be performed in reverse to decrease movement intensity. Figure 14.3, representing a model for resistance intensity progression, can be applied to exercises for all muscle groups to increase and decrease exercise intensity in a water exercise class.

Newton's Laws of Motion

A general understanding of Newton's laws of motion is essential for providing safe, effective water exercise instruction. Remember learning these in physics class? Now it's time to put them to practical use. Let's take a moment to review these laws while applying them to water exercise movements.

Inertia is the subject of Newton's first law of motion. Inertia is the tendency of a body to remain in a state of rest or of uniform motion until acted on by a force that changes that state. When the human body moves through water, it creates currents because of the water's inertial tendency to remain in motion. The movement of the water currents influences the effectiveness of an exercise. For example, running in circles in water reduces the work of moving because the person is moving with the currents, whereas turning around and running against the currents just created increases the work. If a person stands in place in the water, there is little resistance against the body. Therefore, standing in place is easier than moving. Short-travel moves, such as running 10 feet (3 m) and turning around and running back for 10 feet (3 m), use the water's

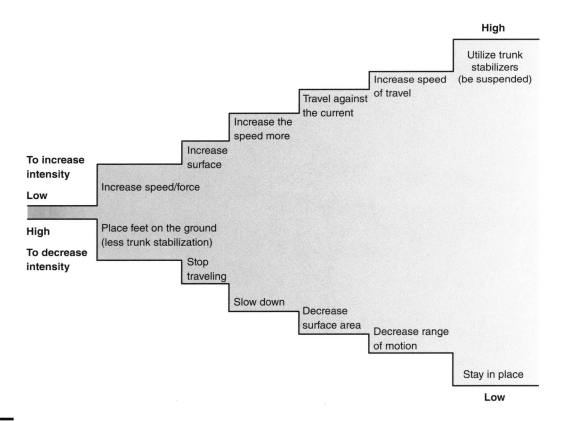

FIGURE 14.3 Water resistance intensity progression model. Increasing and decreasing water exercise intensity can be accomplished by using a progression model to guide your movement selection.

Reprinted, by permission, from C. Kennedy and M. Sanders, 1995, "Strength training gets wet," *IDEA Today* May: 25-30.

inertia to create overload. Beginners need to do most of their exercises in place in order to gain balance and skill without having to deal with inertia currents. Once they progress, traveling through the water can be introduced.

Acceleration is mentioned in Newton's second law of motion, which states that force equals mass times acceleration. Thus, this law says that speed (acceleration) can be used to create resistance overload. For example to increase intensity while walking in water, walk faster without changing the ROM. Doing so will be moving the same amount of water, but it will be harder to move because you are moving faster. When you add acceleration to the moves, you introduce the element of power because power is defined as resistance times speed. Be careful not to compromise range of motion when introducing acceleration; shortening the ROM makes the muscle movement more isometric and results in greater pain due to lack of blood flow. Using full ROM is the optimal way to train muscles.

Action and reaction are tied together in Newton's third law of motion, which states that for every action, there is an equal and opposite reaction. For example, when you reach out in front with extended arms and push the water behind you, the body moves forward. The action is the arm movement, and the reaction is the full-body movement. Use this concept to analyze what is wanted and what can be gotten out of a movement. For example, when adducting the shoulder (a latissimus dorsi frontal plane movement) in deep water, the concept of action and reaction means that the body will pull up slightly. This reaction can be used to overload the shoulder muscles instead of allowing the body to come up. By holding the body steady, you will be challenging the action and reaction law and therefore performing more work. The same can be done in shallow water by bending the knees to bring the arms beneath the water. The key is to determine the reaction direction of the action and then work against it for overload, or with it for recovery.

Creating a Warm-Up

Warming up for a water exercise class is slightly different than warming up for a land-based class. In water, dynamic ROM exercises replace static stretching movements. For example, in a land class, the hamstrings are warmed up dynamically and then can be stretched statically depending on participant preference. In a water class, hip flexion and hip extension exercises warm up and stretch both the quadriceps and hamstrings; there are no eccentric muscle actions occurring due to the lack of gravity. If participants are in cool water that is below 86°F (30°C), a vigorous warm-up may be appropriate to promote thermoregulation of the body. If the pool temperature is 86°F (30°C) or above, which is considered thermoneutral, it may not be necessary for moving vigorously to keep the body warm. Full ROM total-body exercises are appropriate and encouraged in a water exercise warm-up.

Following are samples of dynamic warm-up and rehearsal movements that target specific muscle groups. Have participants perform each of these movements through their full ROM. Keep increases in tempo to a minimum during the warm up period.

Figures 14.4 through 14.8 show total-body movements that can be used for thermoregulation purposes. These exercises will increase core temperature through increased energy expenditure. With these moves, participants can travel against, and then with, the inertia currents by practicing traveling and changing directions. Taking the muscles through their full ROM replaces static stretching in water exercise. The muscles do not have to work against gravity. When a muscle contracts, the opposing muscle is automatically stretched. Therefore, a stretching segment within the warm-up portion is not needed when teaching a water exercise class. Encourage and instruct participants that full range of motion movements are to be performed in a slow and controlled manner within the warm-up portion.

Formatting Water Exercise Classes

Teaching from the deck is important in water exercise since visual cues are as important as verbal cues for participants. We recommend demonstrating moves on the deck and allow

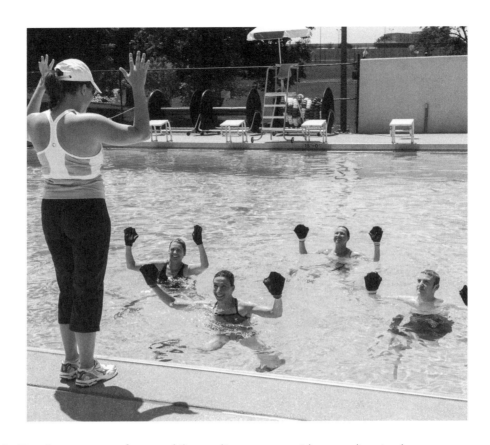

FIGURE 14.4 Keeping arms out of water while treading water provides a cardio stimulus.

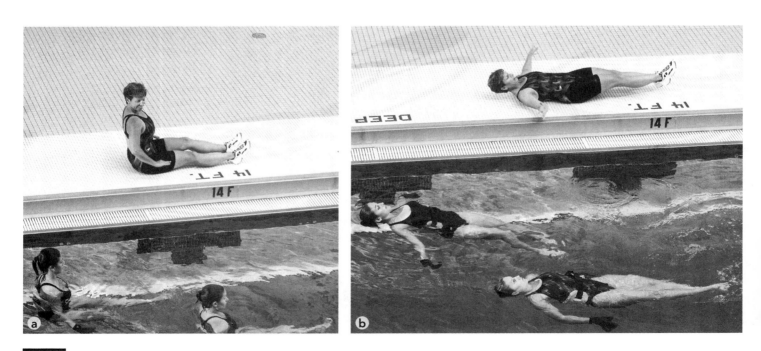

FIGURE 14.5 Seated flutter kick with (*a*) backward movement and (*b*) lying supine to change the surface area and move faster (works the quadriceps and abdominal and low-back muscles).

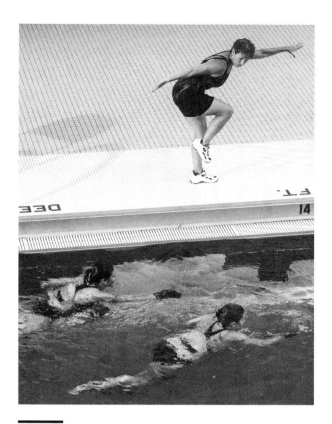

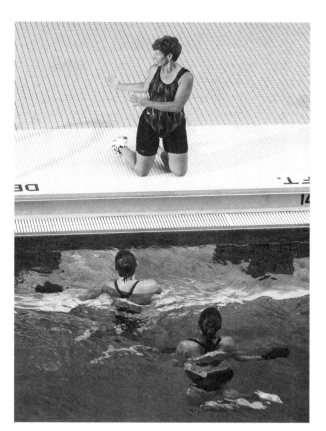

FIGURE 14.6 Total-body rock climber movement in which resistance is created by pushing the hands down in the water and traveling against the water's resistance (works the gluteal, abdominal and low back, and posterior deltoid muscles).

FIGURE 14.7 Washing machine: Arms (tucked into the sides) and legs are rotated in opposite directions, alternatively contracting the core and rotator cuff muscles.

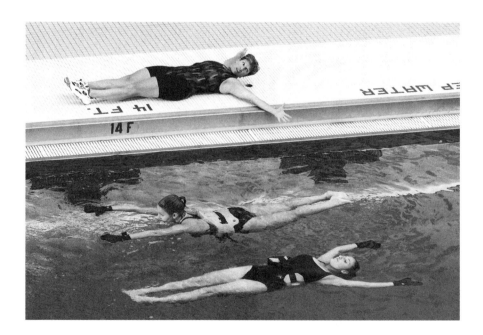

FIGURE 14.8 Lie supine, tuck the knees, and stretch out in a prone superman or superwoman position (works the abdominal and low-back muscles); reverse, tuck the knees, and lie supine (lie in the sun).

Key Points for Warm-Up Segment

- Uses appropriate speed when demonstrating movements on the deck
- Emphasizes full ROM with each movement
- Keeps participants moving and checks for water temperature comfort
- Points out individual muscle groups to the participants and uses total-body movements to keep the body warm
- Demonstrates how to use music tempo as a gauge by moving on the beat, moving faster than the beat, and moving slower than the beat

participants to practice moves within the water before getting into the water with them. Instructing a class while in the water does not assist in teaching the participants how to perform the movements in a biomechanically correct way. In terms of music, water exercise is a lot like indoor cycling or sports conditioning: Use the music to set the mood and not necessarily the tempo. If you move on the beat all the time, you will not progress participants properly. Use the tempo of the music as a gauge. For example, start with the beat and then ask participants to work faster than the beat for 15 seconds, if your goal is to increase the intensity of the class, or work slower than the beat if you want participants to recover.

Before teaching a water exercise class, make sure a lifeguard is present so you can focus on your instruction. You cannot be responsible for both safety and instruction. However, do discuss safety issues, especially for participants who are not comfortable in the water. Believe it or not, many people cannot swim. If you are teaching in deep water, make sure participants have their flotation devices adjusted properly. Review how each piece of equipment should be worn before starting the class. For example, there are different levels of buoyancy belts for deep water exercise. A participant who is lean needs a belt that provides more buoyancy, whereas a participant with more body fat needs less buoyancy. In fact, some participants who have a lot of stored energy (body fat) may not even need a buoyancy belt. Once the class has started, take a moment to remind participants of safety skills, especially when working in deep water. While exercising, some participants may fall forward

and not be able to get their faces out of the water. Others may fall backward and not be able to get their legs down. Teach recovery skills for these situations, and throughout the workout remind participants to engage their abdominal muscles to stay upright. Inform the lifeguard of any participants who are not comfortable in the water so that the lifeguard can watch them closely. Finally, if you are working in a pool that has a drop-off into deep water, be sure the lane lines separate the shallow and deep areas.

Understanding that most movements in the water entail using all the health-related components of fitness (cardio, strength, flexibility, and neuromotor) will help you create an effective water exercise routine and thus improve the quality of your participants' lives.

There are three water depths we suggest you teach in:

1. Deep water, in which flotation devices are used
2. Transitional water, in which feet are on the pool floor but lungs are submerged
3. Shallow water, in which the water depth is below the xiphoid process

When teaching in the shallow depth, there are three ways to use the water:

1. Rebound a move and jump, which creates more impact and more intensity.
2. Stay neutral with the shoulders at the water surface and use the resistance of the water with less impact.
3. Suspend the move, which is more difficult but has the least impact.

Technique and Safety Check

To help keep your water exercise classes safe, observe the following recommendations.

Remember to

- encourage full ROM movements before speeding up,
- use different movement planes,
- encourage participants to maintain a neutral spine and neck and keep the head and eyes up,
- encourage participants to keep abdominal muscles lifted and contracted,
- strive to work all major muscle groups and identify them to participants to increase body awareness,
- make sure a lifeguard is on duty and water safety practices are introduced,

- demonstrate movements visually on deck so participants understand what to do, and
- encourage individuality and proper progression throughout the workout by allowing participants to work at their own levels.

Avoid

- following the tempo of the music for the entire class,
- speeding up your deck demonstrations to land speed, and
- getting in the water with participants before performing visual deck demonstrations.

Understanding the basic total-body movements will get you started on appropriate movement combinations. Some sample total-body movements are illustrated in "Basic Moves" later in this chapter. These movements use large muscle groups to increase energy expenditure and are also functional. For example, the mall walk is a basic walking movement named after a popular leisure activity—shopping! Another total-body move, the cross-country skier, mimics the motion of cross-country skiing. Any time a functional movement can be brought into a water activity, participants will benefit and find that the same movement is easier to perform on land.

Training Systems

According to Weltman (1995), $\dot{V}O_2$max may not be the best predictor of endurance performance on either land or water. He believes that the blood lactate response to submaximal exercise may be a better indicator of endurance performance. Studies (Brown et al. 1997; DeMaere and Ruby 1997) on water exercise have verified that blood lactate responses to an exercise in the water are greater than responses to the same exercise performed on land. The resistance of the water creates an anaerobic response to

exercise that is similar to what happens physiologically during resistance training on land. A large increase in blood lactate levels, especially in deconditioned participants, can be uncomfortable and lead to exercise adherence problems. Thus, because of the resistance properties of water, interval training has been recommended for water exercise, especially for beginners. A person does not go into a weight room and continuously lift weights. Rests are incorporated between exercises for muscle groups or sets to allow the blood lactate to be recycled within the body. Resistance exercises are usually performed in sets. Frangolias and colleagues (2000) determined that when participants train in water, eventually they adapt to the environment and stop showing increases in blood lactate levels. That is, once participants gain the strength to overcome the resistance of the water, they won't see the big increases in blood lactate levels they saw when they began exercising in the water. Progressive overload is important to the success of a water exercise class because it provides a way for participants to keep improving.

Because participants who are new to water exercise experience an increase in lactate that is greater than what is experienced when moving on land, the workout plan can be modified to couple interval exercise with continuous movement (Eyestone et al. 1993). Interval training in the water helps participants adapt to the increased blood lactate levels and makes the activity more enjoyable. The premise of interval training is that an individual can produce a greater amount of work if high-intensity bouts are separated by times of rest (Kravitz 1994). Many people find the resistance of the water too challenging for continuous work and so may get more out of their water exercise class through interval training. Following are terms you should know in order to understand interval training:

work interval—The time of the high-intensity work effort

recovery interval—The time between work intervals. The recovery interval may consist of light activity (sculling only) or moderate activity (easy jogging).

work-recovery ratio—The time ratio of the work and recovery intervals. A work-recovery ratio of 1:3 means that the recovery interval is 3 times as long as the work interval. An example of a 1:3 ratio is jogging 1 minute and recovering 3 minutes.

cycle (repetition)—A work interval combined with a recovery interval. Since a recovery interval follows a work interval, some resources report the number of work intervals as repetitions.

set—The number of cycles performed for an exercise. A series of 4 work-recovery cycles makes one set of 4 cycles.

It's best not to perform interval training during the entire time of the group exercise class. Rather, insert smaller segments of interval training when you can. See chapter 7 for more information on interval training or chapter 13 for more ideas on drills. A sample series for interval training in the water is outlined in table 14.2.

Benefits of Interval Training

- Increased enjoyment due to added variety
- Potential for greater total work in a shorter amount of time
- Improved anaerobic and aerobic power and capacity
- Potential for fewer injuries and reduced participant burnout
- Increased participant adherence to exercise

Water Exercise Equipment

Once participants have been involved in a water exercise class for 6 to 8 weeks, they will adapt to the resistance of the water, and eventually they will need to use equipment to overload the muscles. There are several types of overload devices available. This section reviews surface area devices and buoyancy devices. Using buoyancy devices over long durations and for full-body support (without a belt) can be detrimental to the shoulders when working in deep water because buoyancy assists the deltoids and thus pulls the shoulder joint into a horizontal position. These devices are best used in shallow water, where they are less burdensome to the shoulder joint. Figure 14.9 shows examples of buoyancy devices. Surface area devices are fine to use in both deep and shallow water.

Surface area devices predominantly elicit concentric muscle contractions of the agonist and antagonist muscle groups. They also help provide overload since they require a greater amount of water to be moved. Many surface area devices also offer progressive resistance. For example, when using webbed gloves, participants can choose to open the fingers for more resis-

TABLE 14.2 Interval Training Series for Water Exercise

Segment	Total time	Cycles	Recovery and work
1	3 min	3 cycles	40 s recovery and 20 s work
2	3 min	3 cycles	30 s recovery and 30 s work
3	3 min	3 cycles	20 s recovery and 40 s work

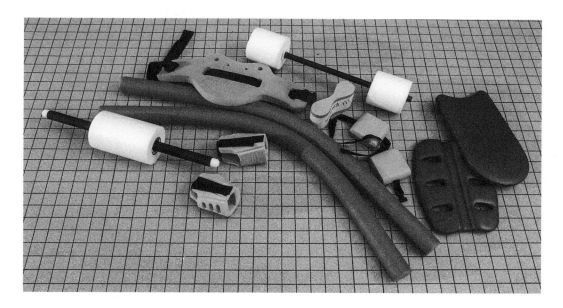

FIGURE 14.9 Buoyancy devices.

tance or make a fist for less resistance. Figure 14.10 shows examples of surface area devices.

Encourage slow speeds when participants are working with buoyancy equipment; moving too quickly will cause the equipment to bounce right out of the water, just as a dumbbell on land falls to the ground if it is lowered too rapidly. Buoyancy devices allow eccentric muscle actions to occur in the water. Stabilizing the core is crucial because the core serves as the base for many exercises. Water equipment companies are beginning to develop surface area and buoyancy devices that can be individualized to the person, just as a 5-, 10-, or 15-pound (2.3, 4.5, and 6.8 kg) handheld weight can be used to individualize resistance in a land class. Keep in mind that proper muscular strength and endurance training begins with a focus on progression of movements. Check out the "Water Exercise Resource List" for providers of water fitness products.

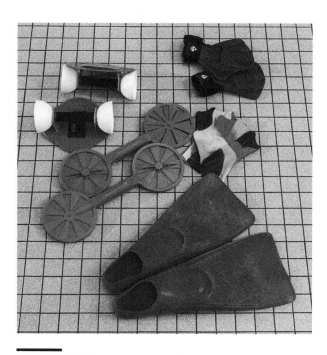

FIGURE 14.10 Surface area devices.

Water Exercise Resource List

- www.sprintaquatics.com
- www.aquajogger.com
- www.waterfit.com
- www.aquatherapeutics.com
- www.aeawave.com
- www.waterart.org
- www.poolates.com
- www.uswfa.com
- www.waterfitness.co.uk/index.html
- www.waterwellnessworkouts.com

BASIC MOVES

All the following exercises are excellent total-body conditioning moves for a water exercise class. See appendix G for a sample water exercise routine.

 See online video 14.1 for a sample class that demonstrates basic movements in water exercise.

Basic Progressions

The following exercises are total-body conditioning movements that involve the upper and lower body and the core. These movements fit well into the conditioning segment of the water workout that includes cardio, strength, flexibility, and neuromotor movements. Remember to use acceleration, inertia currents, and progressive resistance, as discussed earlier in the chapter, in order to challenge participants.

GENERAL JOGGING AND WALKING

This works the quadriceps, hip flexors, hamstrings, abdominals and low-back muscles; simulates walking or jogging functional movements that can carry over to improve movement on land.

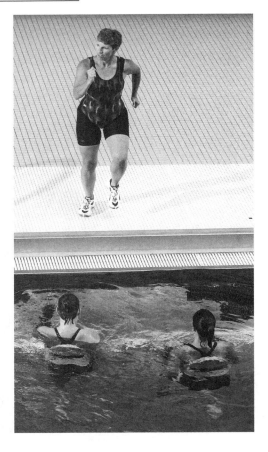

MALL WALK

This exercise progresses the jogging and walking movements by increasing lever length and is functional for shopping (and other walking activities). Flex the foot for less resistance and point the toes for added resistance.

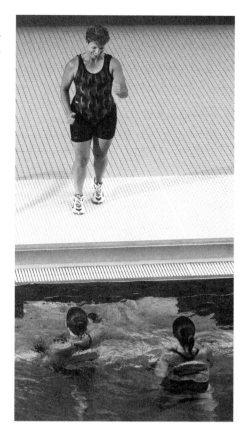

CROSS-COUNTRY SKIER

This works the hip flexors, gluteal muscles, hamstrings, deltoids, and latissimi dorsi. Start the movement by placing the right arm straight out in front and the left leg extended behind. Simultaneously alternate the movement as if cross-country skiing. Add gloves to increase upper-body resistance.

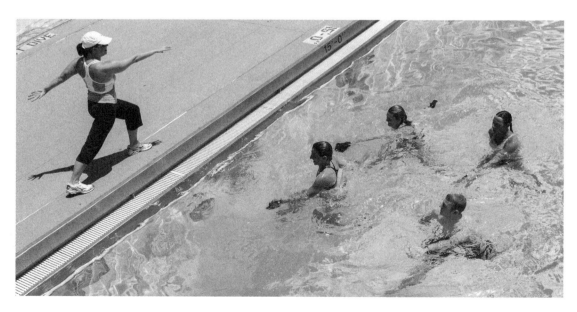

STRAIGHT-LEG RAISE WITH OPPOSITE HAND AND FOOT

This exercise works the hip flexors, hamstrings, latissimi dorsi, and posterior deltoids. Reach the right arm to the left toe. In one smooth movement switch to the left arm touching the right toe. To enhance the stretch on the hamstrings and posterior deltoid, lengthen the opposite arm and leg and lean the chin into the movement, keeping shoulders over hips for good posture.

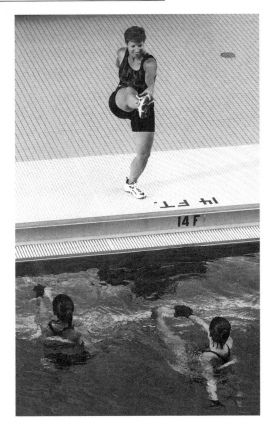

Additional Total-Body Moves

The following exercises use functional movements and work the total body. They are an important part of the conditioning segment because the core of the body (abdominals and low back) must support the torso while the upper- and lower-body movement patterns are performed.

SEATED V

The seated V position with arms and legs in deep water works the abdominals and low back, with assistance from the pectorals, rhomboids, middle trapezius, posterior deltoids, hip abductors and adductors. Flex at the hip with both legs and simultaneously cross the arms and the legs, keeping the shoulders over the hips and leaning slightly forward with the chin while keeping good posture with the torso.

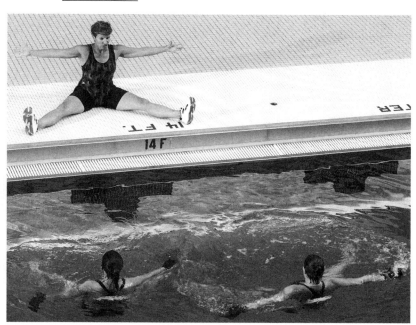

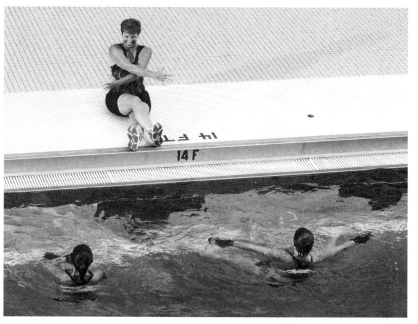

SEATED V WITH FORWARD MOVEMENT

This variation of the seated V position using the rhomboids and hip abductors along with the abdominals and low-back muscles produces forward movement. Simultaneously retract the shoulder blades with a long-lever arm and abduct the legs. Bend the knees, recover, and then repeat the movement.

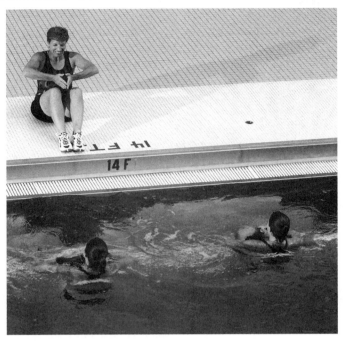

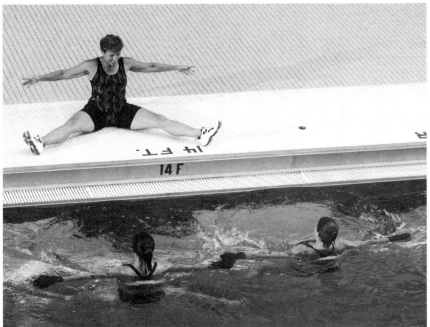

SEATED V WITH BACKWARD MOVEMENT

This seated V position using pectorals and hip adductors creates a backward motion in deep water. Some call this the torpedo move. When the hands and legs come together, flex the spine slightly forward to torpedo backward; then reset the position and repeat the movement.

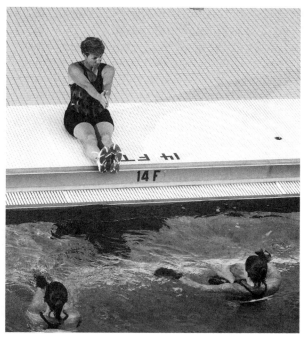

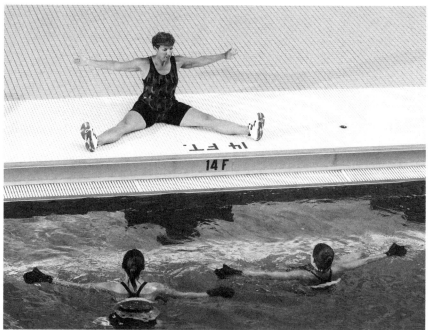

ALTERNATING SIT KICK

For the alternating sit kick movement, sit upright in the water with the hips bent at 90°. Perform knee flexion and extension with hands out of the water. This exercise works the quadriceps and hamstrings while at the same time challenging the abdominals and low back to stabilize the movement.

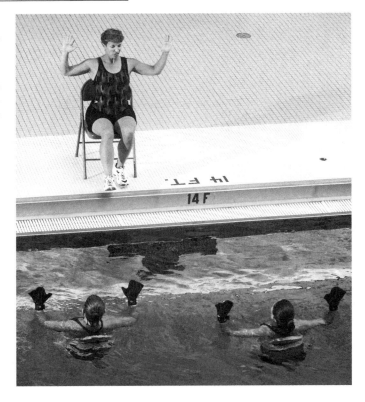

BICYCLING IN A CIRCLE

In deep water, lie on one side and make a bicycling motion with the legs. Keep one arm out to the side and the other straight up to challenge the abdominals and low back while turning in a circle (works the hamstrings, gluteal muscles, quadriceps, and deltoids). Switch directions every 3 or 4 revolutions to prevent dizziness.

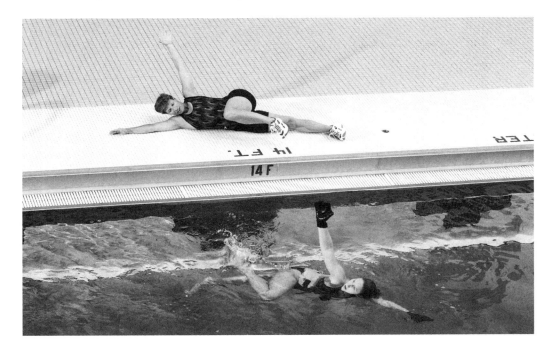

Muscle Isolating Moves

The next two exercises emphasize movements that are great to either warm up the core or to use in the conditioning segment of the workout. The reverse breast stroke, in addition to working the shoulder muscles, isometrically works the abdominal muscles while the rhomboids, posterior deltoids, quadriceps, and hamstrings propel the body into motion. The professional sitter isometrically works the abdominal muscles. Both of these exercises involve the core stabilizing the movement overall. These two movements are almost impossible to perform on the land and thus also challenge the neuromotor capacity of the body to perform the movements.

REVERSE BREASTSTROKE

The reverse breaststroke works the rhomboid, middle trapezius, and posterior deltoid muscle group. Retract the scapula in the horizontal plane with extended arms and contract the abdominals to hold the legs out in front. At first the body is moved forward to assist the movement (figure 14.20, a), and then a flutter kick with the legs is added to resist the scapular retraction movement (figure 14.20, b). The body will stay in one place if the movement is performed correctly. Participants should move their arms in different planes while working the pectorals or the upper back because multiplanar resistance is one of the advantages of water exercise. In the water, the body can move against resistance in more natural patterns, and the direction of resistance is less important than it is in land-based exercises.

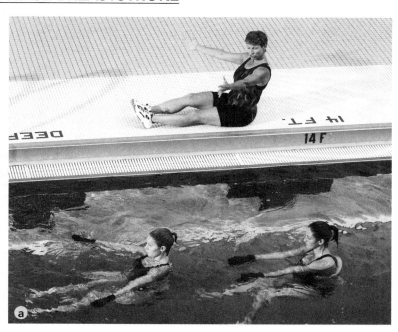

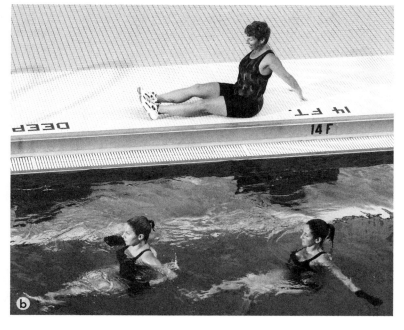

PROFESSIONAL SITTER

This exercise is a functional movement that trains the body for sitting, which most people do a lot of in their daily lives. With hands above the water and shoulders over the hips, flex and extend from the knee joints alternating right and left knee. Meanwhile contract the low-back and abdominal muscles as if sitting suspended in a chair. Lengthen the lower-body lever by straightening out the legs to turn this movement into a mall walk movement for added overload.

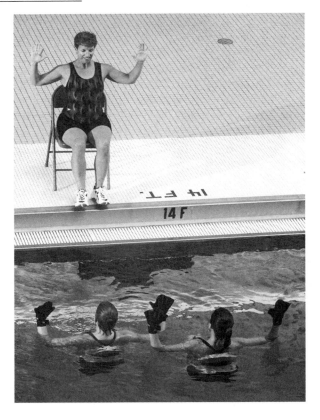

Chapter Wrap-Up

As fitness instructors, we need to broaden our concept of resistance training and use as many modalities as we can, especially as our participant population grows older and seeks more options for nonimpact exercise. Water exercise is an effective form of group exercise that minimizes impact. The perception that water exercise is for older adults or people with musculoskeletal injuries has been challenged. Many forms of land-based exercise, including Zumba, Pilates, and tai chi, are also finding success in the water. Water provides a sense of peace and relaxation that cannot be replicated on land. Plus, it can bring back fond memories of leisure time spent by the pool or on the beach. Connecting leisure and exercise helps enhance long-term adherence to exercise because it creates a sense of purpose and pleasure. As the instructor, you will be challenged teaching water exercise, particularly if your class is held outdoors. Being able to adapt the class format to the temperature of the air and water will enhance the experience for the participants. Seek input regularly by asking questions about comfort. Get in the water occasionally so you can keep a pulse on the comfort of the class. Use the principles specific to movement in the water, as well as Newton's laws of motion, when considering movement selection. Use the vast number of multiplanar movements made possible by the resistance of water in order to make your class a success. Add fun and enthusiasm, and you'll find that your participants repeatedly come back for more.

Group Exercise Class Evaluation Form: Key Points

- Include an appropriate amount of dynamic movement. Use total-body movements to get the body warmed up.

- Provide rehearsal moves. Perform 5 or 6 repetitions of the total-body moves focused on during the workout and work through the full ROM slowly and progressively.

- Stretch the major muscle groups in a biomechanically sound manner with appropriate instructions. In water exercise, there is no static stretching in the warm-up because participants get too cold. Dynamic, full-ROM movements provide for muscle lengthening and can replace static stretching because of the loss of gravity in water. Some static stretching can be performed at the end of the workout in shallow water or in deep water with a ledge but is not required since ROM is encouraged with each movement.

- Give clear cues and verbal directions. Use at least one posture cue when introducing a new movement. Because water speed needs to be one-half to one-third of land speed, slow down all demonstrations of movements on the deck so that they match participants' speed in the water.

- Use a variety of water exercise techniques. Use the properties of water and Newton's laws to evaluate the effectiveness of movements. For example, when wanting to increase intensity, use acceleration (Newton's second law) and have participants run more quickly against the water's resistance.

- Gradually decrease the intensity during the cool-down after the cardiorespiratory session. Once participants have relaxed and stretched, have them spend a few minutes performing total-body movements to rewarm the body before getting out of the pool—if the class is in cool water. If the water is warm, have participants concentrate on relaxation and visualization. Match the movements to the temperature of the land and water.

- Use music appropriately. Use motivating music that fits the segment and mood. Following the beat the entire time does not allow for individualization of exercises. Use the beat to challenge participants to move faster than the beat to increase intensity and slower than the beat to decrease intensity.

ASSIGNMENT

Attend a group water exercise class or view a water exercise video. Identify two properties of water and two of Newton's laws of motion you see at work in the class. Write down 10 motivational or instructional cues you observe being used in the class by the instructor. Type a one-page (double-spaced) paper with your observations.

Yoga

15

Chapter Objectives

By the end of this chapter, you will be able to

- understand the basic philosophy of yoga;
- investigate breathwork in yoga;
- understand how to begin a yoga class;
- apply appropriate yoga cues and music;
- understand technique and safety issues in yoga;
- teach basic yoga postures and make proper alignment, technique, and safety suggestions; and
- design a short yoga routine for beginners.

Background Check

Before working your way through this chapter, do the following:

Read

☐ chapter 8, "Muscular Conditioning and Flexibility Training."

Group Exercise Class Evaluation Form Essentials

Key Points for Warm-Up Segment

- Includes appropriate amount of dynamic movement
- Includes clear cues and verbal directions

- Uses movements that are at an appropriate tempo and intensity

Key Points for Conditioning Segment

- Uses a variety of muscle groups
- Minimizes repetitive movements
- Observes participants' form and provides constructive, nonintimidating feedback
- Continually offers modifications, regressions, progressions, or alternatives

- Provides alignment and technique cues
- Gives motivational cues
- Provides regular demonstrations and participation with good body mechanics
- Uses appropriate movement and music tempo

Key Points for Cool-Down, Stretch, and Relaxation Segment

- Appropriately emphasizes relaxation and visualization

- Ends class on a positive note and thanks class

The 5,000-year-old discipline of yoga continues to grow rapidly in popularity in most health and fitness settings. The 2013 IDEA Fitness Programs and Equipment Trends Report (IDEA 2013) found that 81% of program directors offer yoga classes in their facilities—a significant increase over previous years. Learning to teach yoga can be rewarding, increase your income and career opportunities, and contribute to your personal growth.

Since yoga is a unique and comprehensive philosophy of living, encompassing a system of physical movements that differs from systems used in traditional physical fitness, we recommend that you become trained and certified specifically to teach yoga before beginning to lead yoga classes. This chapter is intended to provide only an introduction to the basic philosophy, types, and styles of yoga, as well as present a basic yoga routine, complete with postures, alignment information, and breath work. Again, since yoga provides such an ancient, yet deep and profound approach to living and being, we strongly recommend extensive additional training. For information on yoga training and certification, see the "Yoga Websites" list.

Philosophy of Yoga

Yoga is not just a system of exercise or stretching, as is sometimes thought in the West. Rather, it is

Yoga Websites

- www.yogaresearchsociety.com
- www.iayt.org
- www.iynaus.org
- www.kripalu.org
- www.yogajournal.com
- www.yogateachersassoc.org
- www.sivananda.org
- www.anusara.com
- www.ashtanga.net
- www.yogafit.com
- www.yogaalliance.org
- www.yogilates.com

a complete system for living. Yoga can be an ideal way to improve quality of life since it enhances both physical and psychological well-being. The word *yoga* means to unite, or to yoke together, the mind, body, and spirit; ancient Indian sages (India is the land of yoga's origin) believed that to be whole and fully alive, a person must develop the most vital body, mind, and spirit possible. The practice of yoga encompasses a physical discipline (known as *hatha yoga*) as well as breathwork, meditation, positive thinking, healthy diet, and service to others.

Ultimately, yoga is intended to be a foundation for self-realization. Yoga is sometimes called the *discipline of conscious living* as it aims to teach its practitioners that every moment is an opportunity to be deeply present, real, kind, and true. Practicing yoga on a regular basis can help you experience a deep inner stillness and to know joy, bliss, and the truth of who you are. This is why in the Kripalu yoga tradition, yoga is called *the practice of being present* (Faulds 2006).

Five principles govern the practice of yoga:

1. Proper relaxation, which releases muscle tension, conserves energy, and helps release worries and fears.

2. Proper exercise, including the use of yoga postures (known as *asanas*), which systematically aligns and balances all parts of the body to promote strength and flexibility of the muscles and to improve the health of the internal organs.

3. Proper breathing (known as *Pranayama*), which increases the intake of oxygen, recharges the body, and improves mental and emotional well-being. Breathwork is said to be the link between mind and body.

4. Proper diet, which in yoga is based on natural, whole foods and is well balanced and nutritious. According to yogic wisdom, a proper diet keeps the body light and supple and the mind calm, increasing resistance to disease.

5. Positive thinking and meditation, which are essential in removing negative thoughts, quieting the mind, and promoting inner stillness.

Aside from the more familiar physical practice of yoga (hatha yoga), other branches of yoga exist and include the following:

- Raja (royal) yoga. Practitioners on this path focus on self-restraint, moral discipline, concentration, and meditation.

- Karma yoga. A person practicing karma yoga seeks self-transcendence and spiritual freedom by serving others.

- Jnana yoga. Jnana yoga encompasses the practice of discernment and wisdom and is said to be the path of the sage.

- Tantra yoga. Practitioners seek self-transcendence through tantra yoga, which is a more ceremonial form of yoga practice.

- Bhakti yoga. Bhakti yoga is said to be the path of love or of having an open heart.

In the West, hatha yoga is by far the most familiar form of yoga. See "Hatha Yoga Classes" in this chapter for descriptions of the types of classes commonly available in fitness and health facilities. This list of hatha yoga classes is organized on a continuum from the easiest to the most difficult in terms of physical difficulty.

Additionally, various styles, also known as *schools* or *traditions*, of yoga have evolved, often around the teachings of a particular guru, or teacher. Popular styles in the West include Iyengar, Bikram, viniyoga, Jivamukti, Kripalu, Sivananda, and Anusara.

A popular trend in the United States is the yoga fusion class. The most common fusion styles are fitness and yoga (check out www.yogafit.com) and Pilates and yoga (check out www.yogilates.com). Other creative instructors have combined yoga with Spinning, tai chi, and step. One of the main benefits of a fusion class is that it introduces yoga to participants who otherwise might not try yoga; on the other hand, yoga purists may be put off by such a class.

Breathwork in Yoga

Many yoga experts believe that breathwork is the single most important component of a yoga practice. It is thought that the breath carries *prana* (the Sanskrit word for *life force*), and so the term Pranayama, loosely translated as *breathwork*, may also be thought of as life force (life energy) work. Not only does physical life depend on breath, but breath is also associated with the emotions and mind. The breath speeds up when you are excited or nervous and grows shallow when you are experiencing stress. On the other hand, relaxation and peace can be created through deep, slow, relaxed breathing. Ancient yogis realized that by controlling the breath, they could affect their minds, emotions, and bodies, and thus breathwork remains a crucial component of yoga today.

Yoga Research Findings: Physical Fitness

Let's examine the scientific evidence on the benefits of yoga. Yoga's influence on physical and physiological fitness has been studied relatively thoroughly, especially in India. A number of large literature reviews are available, most notably the 2004 literature review conducted by the International Association of Yoga Therapists, which listed hundreds of studies (Lamb 2004). Here are some selected findings reported in these reviews:

- In a study commissioned by ACE, researchers Boehde and Porcari (2006) found that 50 minutes of power yoga burned approximately 237 calories and elevated participants' heart rates to 62% of maximal heart rate (MHR). Posttest measures showed that study participants increased flexibility, balance, and muscular strength and endurance (abdominal and chest).

- A study at Adelphi University found that the metabolic demand (energy cost) of Ashtanga yoga was similar to that of moderate-intensity aerobic dance or walking (Carroll et al. 2003).

- A study by Tran and colleagues (2001) measured improvements in muscle strength, endurance, flexibility, cardiorespiratory fitness, body composition, and lung function after an 8-week training study in which subjects participated in yoga classes 2 times per week.

- Kristal and coworkers (2005) found that practicing yoga on a regular basis helped study participants maintain or lose weight throughout the midlife years. Since yoga does not burn a high number of calories per session, researchers surmised that the benefit resulted from the increased mindfulness and body awareness of the participants, which led them to make better choices in food quality and quantity.

- Another review, published in 2010, examined yoga's health benefits relative to those documented from traditional exercise (Ross and Thomas 2010). Numerous studies reported in this review supported the idea that yoga may be as effective as or better than exercise at improving a variety of health-related outcome measures.

Yoga has been studied extensively as a therapeutic intervention for a variety of diseases and disorders. Numerous studies have examined yoga's effect on cardiovascular disease (including hypertension and regression of atherosclerosis); respiratory disorders (especially asthma), metabolic disorders (e.g., diabetes); and neurological, musculoskeletal, and psychological problems. Selected findings from a large literature review conducted by Khalsa (2004) include the following:

- Yoga has been found to be an effective modality for relieving low-back pain. For example, a 12-week therapeutically oriented viniyoga program was found to be more effective than conventional group exercise or a self-help program for improving back function and reducing chronic low-back pain (Sherman et al. 2005).

- Many other studies have also shown improvements in low-back pain with yoga (Galantino et al. 2004; Jacobs et al. 2004; Williams et al. 2003; Williams et al. 2005).

- Yogic breathing exercises improved asthma symptoms in study subjects (Cooper et al. 2003) and lung function in athletes (Rana 2011).

- An 8-day yoga program lowered low-density lipoprotein (LDL) cholesterol and reduced risk factors for coronary heart disease and diabetes (Bijlani 2005). A landmark study in 1990 showed that a program that included yoga and other lifestyle changes could reverse coronary heart disease (Ornish et al. 1990). Additionally, flexibility, arm strength, and endurance have improved in patients recovering from a stroke (Schmid et al. 2012). Anxiety, psychological stress, and circulating cortisol levels were decreased in patients with Type 2 diabetes (Vizcaino and King 2012). A study examining the effects of Ashtanga yoga found that bone density was increased in premenopausal women (Kim et al. 2011). Cancer fatigue was significantly reduced after 4 weeks of yoga training (Mustian et al. 2011).

- For older adults, yoga has been shown to improve dynamic balance, helping to reduce the risk of falls (Wang et al. 2012). For adolescents, yoga apparently improved mental health markers (mood, anxiety, resilience) (Khalsa et al. 2012).

Additionally, many studies have examined yoga's beneficial effects on psychological health (Arpita 1990; Lamb 2004; Khalsa 2004; Javnbakht, Hejazi Kenari, and Ghasemi 2009). Yoga has been repeatedly shown to improve not only important fitness parameters but also overall health and well-being.

Hatha Yoga Classes

Healing and Restorative

- Provides an excellent approach for those with special needs (e.g., colds, headaches, indigestion)
- Emphasizes a passive, soothing, nurturing approach
- Uses many resting postures
- Often incorporates props
- Involves practice of self-care
- Creates sensitivity to body's needs and inner wisdom
- Encourages participants to move in inwardly directed ways
- Is appropriate for all fitness levels

Gentle

- More pose (asana) driven than restorative yoga
- Involves relatively easy, basic postures
- Focuses more on flexibility than on muscular strength or endurance
- Provides many opportunities for rest between poses

Moderate

- Combines basic and moderate poses
- May be organized into a flow routine that participants are expected to follow together

- May require significant muscle strength and endurance as well as balance and flexibility
- Is more driven by form and alignment
- Provides less opportunity for resting between poses

Power

- Organizes poses into a more specific pattern, or flow
- Uses mostly continuous movement, with some holding of more difficult postures
- Requires muscle strength, endurance, flexibility, and balance
- Provides little rest until the final relaxation

Ashtanga

- Is vigorous and athletic
- Involves some jumping to transition between postures
- Uses many difficult, strenuous, and advanced poses
- Organizes poses into specific patterns, or forms, which all participants do together
- Provides no rest until the final relaxation

Most yoga classes begin with some focused breathwork, or Pranayama, and students are reminded to deepen the breath throughout class. Most yoga flows, or routines, are designed to flow with the natural rhythm of the breath, with each move consciously occurring on either an inhale or an exhale so that breath and movement become one. Staying mindful of the breath is a powerful way to stay focused on the present moment; if the mind projects into the future or rehashes experiences from the past, students can be instructed to gently bring it back to the present by concentrating on the sensations and sounds of their own breathing.

The *basic abdominal, or diaphragmatic, breath* is the foundation of all yogic breathing. Every-

one breathes abdominally during deep, restful sleep, but many people forget how to breathe abdominally during waking hours; instead, they habitually perform shallow chest breathing. One of the best things to do when teaching a yoga class (indeed, when teaching any class) is to help students relearn to breathe diaphragmatically. During the inhale, the diaphragm drops down to allow the lungs to inflate; this causes a displacement of the internal organs, which relax outward. Thus, the abdomen moves *out* on the inhale. During the exhale, the diaphragm pulls upward, forcing air out of the lungs, and the internal organs move back toward the spine. Thus the abdomen moves *in* on the exhale (see figure 15.1).

Yoga Research Findings: Psychological and Spiritual Well-Being

The benefits of yoga have long been promoted in ancient texts and today are touted by thousands of current authors and by even more yoga instructors. These benefits include enhanced physical and physiological fitness, improvements in psychological parameters such as decreased stress and depression, and increased spiritual well-being (this may include increased feelings of peacefulness, compassion, and a sense of oneness with all beings).

Another hallmark of yoga is its ability to induce the relaxation response. This relaxed mental state is helpful in therapeutic settings; in fact, yoga therapists specialize in helping patients recover from trauma, depression, anxiety, and other types of psychological stress.

Some researchers have even attempted to identify yoga's influence on spiritual health. Spiritual wellness has been described as a high level of faith, hope, and commitment in relation to a well-defined world view or belief system that provides a sense of meaning and purpose to existence in general and that offers an ethical path to personal connectedness with self, others, and a higher power or larger reality (Hawks et al. 1995). One study found that spirituality increased in cardiac patients who attended a yoga and meditation retreat (Kennedy, Abbott, and Rosenberg 2002). Questionnaires given before and after the retreat demonstrated that after the retreat participants experienced an increased sense of connection with others, increased awareness of an inner source of strength and guidance, increased desire to achieve higher consciousness, and increased confidence in their ability to handle problems.

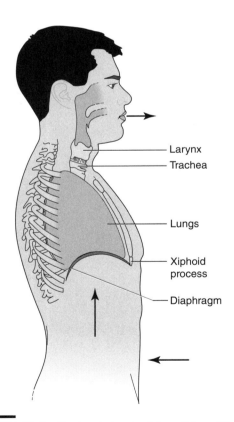

Larynx
Trachea

Lungs

Xiphoid process

Diaphragm

FIGURE 15.1 Basic abdominal breathing. The diaphragm relaxes downward and the abdomen relaxes out during inhalation; the diaphragm pulls upward and the abdomen pulls in during exhalation.

Another type of breath in yoga is the *ujjayi breath*, known variously as the *ocean-sounding breath* or the *victory breath*. While this breath is very similar to the abdominal breath described earlier, both the inhale and the exhale are accompanied by an audible sound even though the lips are closed. The sound made on the exhale is much like a soft, breathy, prolonged sigh; the same breathy sound is also produced while inhaling. The overall effect is somewhat like the sound of ocean waves going in and rushing out. Once this breath is mastered, most people find it very relaxing, deeply soothing, and peaceful. A primary purpose of this breath is to help focus the mind; it is hard for the mind to race all over if you are concentrating on making the ujjayi sound.

Integral to yoga is the concept of connecting the breath to various movements. Certain moves are always performed on an inhale, while others are done on an exhale. For example, exhaling while forward bending or flexing the spine feels natural since the abdomen pulls in during the exhale, facilitating spinal and trunk flexion. Likewise, spinal extension and backward bending work best while inhaling (see figure 15.2).

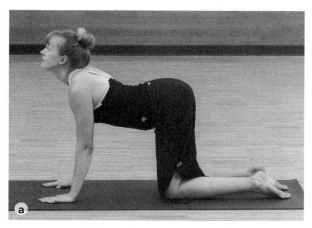

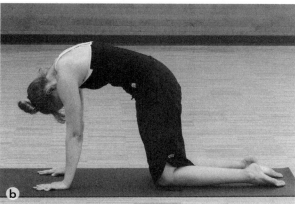

FIGURE 15.2 Breathing with movement in the all-fours position: (*a*) spinal flexion on the exhale and (*b*) spinal extension on the inhale.

Beginning a Yoga Class

The warm-up in yoga varies depending on the type of class being offered. Almost all yoga classes begin with breathing, Pranayama, centering, or meditation, generally in a seated position. In an Ashtanga, or a power-oriented yoga class, the initial breathing and centering is traditionally followed by a series of dynamic moves known as the Sun Salutation. This series may be repeated numerous times and serves to increase core temperature. In a restorative or gentle yoga class, the warm-up often starts with Pranayama or meditation and then continues with gentle limbering movements such as seated sun breaths, seated side bends, and cat tilts and dog tilts on hands and knees. Many yoga instructors blend techniques from the two types of classes so that the general warm-up flow may be as follows: breathing, Pranayama,

meditation, sun breaths, cat tilts and dog tilts, other limbering moves on hands and knees, downward dog and/or standing forward bend, and then sun salutations.

Practice Drill

Sit comfortably on the floor or in a chair; make sure your spine is straight. Place one hand on your chest and the other hand on your abdomen. Breathe normally in and out through your nose (keep your mouth closed) and notice which hand moves the most. Gradually deepen each inhale, allowing the hand on your abdomen to have the most movement, while exaggerating and lengthening each exhale.

The Sun Salutation (known as *Surya Namaskar* in Sanskrit) is a graceful flow of 12 postures. It is intended to be performed without stopping, alternating inhaling and exhaling on each posture. There are two main ways to perform the basic Sun Salutation (see table 15.1).

Both Sun Salutation variations involve a number of harder stretches (e.g., standing forward bend, downward-facing dog, upward-facing dog) as well as the plank and *Chaturanga dandasana*, which are strength moves. The fact that more difficult stretches and strength moves are part of the traditional Sun Salutation means that this flow may be problematic for beginners and for participants with special conditions such as low-back pain. When leading such participants, provide plenty of modifications for the poses of the Sun Salutation or substitute a gentler warm-up.

The following is a simple warm-up flow that does not incorporate the Sun Salutation:

1. Sit in cross-legged easy pose for deep breathing, Pranayama, and/or meditation.
2. Perform three sun breaths (inhale, arms up; exhale, arms down) in this position.
3. Continue with three side stretches. Lift the right arm up on the inhale and lower it on the exhale. Repeat the three stretches with the left arm.
4. Gently twist to the right on an exhale, keeping the spine straight. Inhale and return to center. Twist to the left, exhaling.

TABLE 15.1   Sun Salutation Variations

Step	Sun salutation #1	Sun salutation #2
1	Mountain pose, prayer position (exhale)	Mountain pose, arms overhead (inhale)
2	Mountain pose, arms overhead (inhale)	Forward bend (exhale)
3	Forward bend (exhale)	Monkey pose, head up (inhale)
4	Lunge, right foot back, head up (inhale)	Forward bend (exhale)
5	Plank position (retain the breath)	Plank (inhale)
6	Chaturanga dandasana (exhale)	Chaturanga dandasana (exhale)
7	Upward-facing dog (inhale)	Upward-facing dog (inhale)
8	Downward-facing dog (exhale)	Downward-facing dog (exhale)
9	Lunge, left foot back (inhale)	Monkey pose (inhale)
10	Forward bend (exhale)	Forward bend (exhale)
11	Mountain pose, arms overhead (inhale)	Mountain pose, arms overhead (inhale)
12	Mountain pose, arms at sides (exhale)	Mountain pose, prayer position (exhale)

5. Remain sitting and stretch the legs straight out in front. Circle the ankles 3 times in one direction followed by 3 times in the other. Dorsiflex the ankles, pressing heels away; then press the balls of the feet away. Finish by pointing the toes (plantar flexion). Repeat.

6. Move to hands and knees. Exhaling, flex the spine into the cat stretch, head and tailbone down. Gently and mindfully inhale and extend the spine into the dog tilt, head and tailbone up. Repeat 3 to 5 times, noticing all sensations.

7. Remain on hands and knees and place the spine in neutral, abdominal muscles lifted. Curve the spine to the right (lateral flexion), exhaling. Inhale and return to center. Exhale and curve the spine to the left. Repeat.

8. If comfortable, gently circle the pelvis, allowing the spine to move in all directions; allow the head to move freely.

9. Return to neutral spine and extend the right leg behind, toes curled under on the floor. Gently press the heel backward, feeling a comfortable stretch in the calf muscles. Breathe. Repeat with the left leg.

In this type of warm-up, a primary purpose is to connect mind, body, and spirit, or breath. Participants are encouraged to move in ways that feel best to their bodies in the moment; maintaining an ideal alignment is not the goal here. If students find a particular move uncomfortable, prompt them to avoid or modify that move. The goal is to find positions and movements that feel especially good and that help to relieve tension and stress.

 See online video 15.1 for a sample yoga warm-up.

Practice Drill

On hands and knees, gently and slowly move back and forth through spinal flexion and extension, synchronizing breath with movement. Exhale when your head and tailbone are down (spinal flexion) and inhale when your head and tailbone are up (spinal extension). Adjust the speed of your movements to your breathing rate.

Verbal Cues and Music

There are several types of cues that may be used when teaching yoga. Generally, yoga instructors try to speak in a soft, calm tone and use what may be called suggestions instead of direct commands. For example, instead of saying, "Stand tall, shoulders down, chest up, abdominals in, knees soft," a yoga teacher might say, "Lifting the crown of your head up, allow your shoulders to feel heavy. Expand and open your heart while scooping the abdominals in and softening your knees." Imagery cues help participants connect with their bodies, their environment, and their spiritual nature. For example, an instructor may guide participants through the Mountain Pose (*Tadasana*) by saying, "Feel the soles of your feet pressing down into the earth, and lengthen the crown of your head up to the heavens. Allow your body to be the connection between heaven and earth." Cues that create imagery and cues that help participants develop an inward meditative focus are hallmarks of the yogic style of teaching. Alignment cues are also used liberally, particularly with postures that require ideal alignment to help prevent injury. In the seated forward bend (*Paschimottanasana*), for instance, an instructor might pause to teach participants about hinging at the hips versus bending at the waist and explain that hinging from the hip when bending forward helps keep the spine in neutral and reduces the strain on the low back. Many other alignment cues could be given for the head, neck, shoulders, knees, and feet. The following are common types of yoga cues, with examples of each type.

- **Alignment cues.** Example (for the standing position): "Press your shoulders down, away from your ears."

- **Breathing cues.** Example (for the prone position): "Feel your back rising and falling and your ribs expanding with each breath."

- **Educational or informational cues.** Example (for the modified cobra pose): "This is a great posture for helping counter the force of gravity, which tends to pull us forward, creating rounded shoulders and a hunched back."

- **Safety cues.** Example (for *Utkatasana*, or chair pose): "Keep your hips level with your knees; dropping the hips below the knees increases the pressure on your kneecaps and can lead to knee injuries."

- **Visualization or image cues.** Example (for a standing or sitting position): "Feel a spiral of energy moving up the spine."

- **Affirmational cues.** Example (for a

seated forward bend): "I am releasing all tension; I am letting go."

- **Inward focus and spiritual transformation cues.** Example (for the resting, or corpse, pose): "Resting in the vastness of Being, I surrender to my Higher Self."

- **Visual cues.** Example: Instructor places a hand over the crown of the head and lifts it up, indicating that participants should lengthen the spine, stand tall, and elevate the crown of the head.

Music varies in a yoga class, depending on the style or particular class segment. During the rigorous, repetitive sequences of a power-type class, world ethnic music (often with drums) is frequently used as background, although there is no movement on the beat. During the more introspective opening and ending segments of class, music is soft, soothing, and meditative. Alternatively, some yoga instructors teach part or all of the class without music. The "Music Reference List" provides some good websites for finding yoga music.

Music Reference List

- www.gaiam.com
- www.powermusic.com
- www.shantiommusic.com
- www.spiritvoyage.com
- www.yoga.com

Technique and Safety Issues

Because yoga postures, or asanas, range from the very safe and gentle to the extremely difficult and controversial, a thorough understanding of common mechanisms of injury to the major joints is important so educated choices can be made about what to include in a class. Furthermore, a specific posture may have many modifications, ranging from easy to hard, from which instructors must choose when designing their class. We have developed a good model for the concept of progression: the progressive functional training continuum. This model is detailed in our book *Functional Exercise Progressions* (Yoke and Kennedy 2004) and shown with some variation in chapters 3, 5, 8, 9, and 13 of this text.

For an example of the functional exercise progression continuum at work in yoga, let's examine the Cobra pose, or *Bhujangasana*. You can see in figure 15.3 that as the variations of this pose progress across the continuum from easiest to hardest, spinal ROM increases dramatically, and greater amounts of strength are required of the spinal extensors and triceps. The more extreme versions of the cobra pose increase the risk of injury for all but the most advanced, flexible, strong, and adept practitioners of yoga. Therefore, it's best not to lead the majority of your students through the hardest versions of the Cobra; instead, be familiar with the easier and safer modifications.

The language, or vocabulary, of yoga includes many difficult postures and positions. In fact, the pretzel-type positions are probably what most people picture in their minds when they think of yoga. However, these more difficult postures are intended to be the result of years of diligent practice; they are at the end of the progression, not the beginning. Difficult postures are for long-term yoga practitioners who have high levels of muscle strength, endurance, flexibility, and balance. Table 15.2 lists some of the more problematic yoga postures and their potential mechanisms of injury.

All the postures listed in table 15.2 can be modified to minimize their injury potential. Before leading participants through these types of postures, provide safety information and cues for modification. For example, when teaching the standing forward bend (*Uttanasana*), suggest

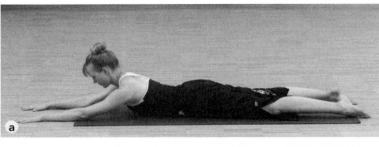
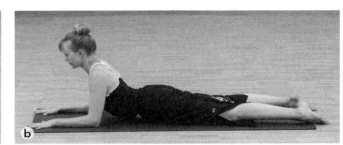
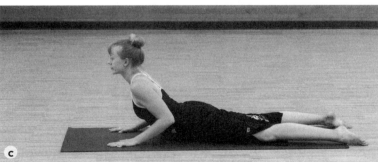
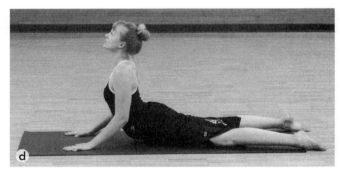
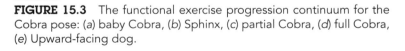
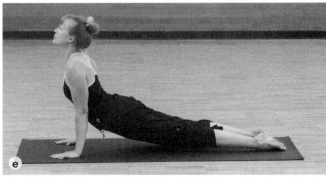

FIGURE 15.3 The functional exercise progression continuum for the Cobra pose: (*a*) baby Cobra, (*b*) Sphinx, (*c*) partial Cobra, (*d*) full Cobra, (*e*) Upward-facing dog.

TABLE 15.2 Problematic Yoga Postures and Their Potential Mechanisms of Injury

Joint	Posture (asana)	Mechanism of injury
Shoulder	Chaturanga dandasana	Hyperextension of shoulder in a weight-bearing position results in a dislocation force.
	Prayer position, hands behind back	Extreme shoulder internal rotation and overstretch of external rotator cuff muscles.
Cervical spine	Plow pose and shoulder stand	Weight bearing on hyperflexed cervical spine may cause vertebral fracture, nerve impingement, and occlusion of blood vessels; position increases cranial blood pressure and pressure in the eyes.
Lumbar spine	Standing forward bend (if participant is too inflexible to place hands on floor)	Unsupported spinal flexion overstretches the long ligaments of the spine, leading to spinal instability.
	Seated forward bend with hands in air (especially if participant is unable to hinge at the hips)	Unsupported spinal flexion overstretches the long ligaments of the spine, leading to spinal instability.
	Standing forward bend with twist (if participant is too inflexible to place hands on floor)	Unsupported spinal flexion with rotation my cause tearing in the annulus fibrosis of the disks, leading to disk herniation.
	Crescent moon pose	Unsupported lateral spinal flexion overstretches the long ligaments of the spine, leading to spinal instability.
	Upward-facing dog and full cobra pose	Extreme lumbar hyperextension overstretches that long ligaments of the spine, leading to spinal instability.
	Boat pose (V-sit)	Long-lever traction creates a shearing force on the vertebrae of the lumbar spine.
Knee	Deep squats (e.g., malasana)	Hyperflexion in a weight-bearing position places large shearing forces in the knee joint, leading to knee instability and excess compression of the knee cartilage.
	Hero pose, Lotus pose, Pigeon pose	Knee torque overstretches the ligaments of the knee, leading to knee instability.

that participants start with a yoga block, which shortens the distance between the hands and the floor. By using a yoga block, participants who are too inflexible to place hands on the floor are still supported (with hands on the block), and the back is therefore protected. A yoga block can be placed vertically, on its side, or flat to match the participant's flexibility. You can suggest that participants keep the block nearby so they can use it whenever they are performing a standing forward bend. If several inflexible participants are in your class, it is helpful to use a yoga block in your demonstration of standing forward bends.

Note that during the Sun Salutation, the spine is at increased risk whenever the practitioner moves back and forth between the standing Mountain Pose (Tadasana) and the standing forward bend (Uttanasana). A teacher concerned about safety might instruct participants to keep the hands at the sides (as opposed to overhead) while moving between the two postures or to place the hands on the thighs for support while lowering into or lifting out of the forward bend. We strongly recommend that you get competent instruction in yoga safety before becoming a yoga instructor.

Technique and Safety Check

To help keep your yoga classes safe, observe the following recommendations:

- Provide an appropriate warm-up.
- Encourage participants to listen to their bodies and only do postures in ways that feel appropriate.
- Provide plenty of modifications and show ways to make a pose easier.
- Avoid high-risk, advanced, or controversial postures.
- Give plenty of alignment cues in traditional postures and in classes that are alignment driven.
- Help participants integrate mind, body, and spirit by giving frequent reminders about breathing.

Equipment and Class Setting

A yoga class can be taught with a minimum of equipment. All that is needed is a yoga mat (most yoga mats are relatively thin, allowing a sense of contact with the floor or earth below). However, there are many props that can enhance the yoga experience or help students attain proper alignment. These include straps, belts, ties, yoga blocks, towels, eye pillows, sandbags, and blankets.

Creating the proper environment is crucial for the practice of yoga. The yoga room needs to be quiet, private, and somewhat warm so that it facilitates stretching and relaxation. Many instructors like to set the mood for peace and introspection by burning candles or incense.

BASIC ASANAS (POSTURES)

Yoga postures, or asanas, can be divided into the following categories: standing postures, backward-bending postures, forward-bending postures, twisting postures, and inverted postures. Also, a relaxation pose is always provided at the end of class. In the following sections, we will discuss a few of these postures; for more instruction, please attend a yoga teacher-training course.

 See online video 15.2 for a brief demonstration of common standing and back-bending yoga postures.

Standing Postures

Standing postures are ideal for teaching proper alignment. They also help develop balance and lower-body strength.

MOUNTAIN POSE

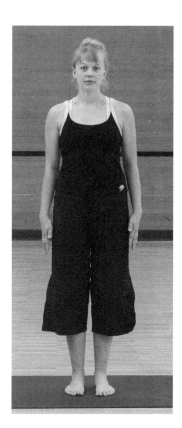

The Mountain pose is the classic standing posture from which all other standing postures are derived. It has several arm variations, including arms at the sides with fingertips actively pointing down, arms reaching straight overhead with fingertips pointing up and shoulder blades down, and hands pressed together in front of the heart in the prayer (*Namaste*) position. In all cases, cue participants to feel the oppositional energy of the pose: Parts of the body are pressing down, while parts of the body are pressing up. The Mountain pose is an active, energetic posture; it is much more than mere standing in place.

CUES Stand with feet pressed firmly into the ground, weight evenly distributed. Feet may be hip-width apart for increased stability or may be placed together, big toes touching, for an increased balance challenge. Lift the kneecaps and the thigh muscles; feel the pubic bone lifting upward while the tailbone presses downward. Lift the abdominal muscles and the rib cage. Simultaneously, feel the shoulder blades pressing down. Lengthen the neck and lift the crown of the head. Breathe deeply and fully.

MODIFIED CRESCENT MOON POSE

When teaching beginners or students with back pain, start with the modified version of the Crescent Moon pose. In the modified version (*a*), one hand remains down, pressed into the side of the body for support. Performing lateral spinal flexion in this way is safer for the low back.

CUES Stand in mountain pose and stretch both arms overhead. Press the palms together or interlace the fingers with the index fingers pointing up (so that hands are in steeple or temple position). Inhale and lengthen the spine, the crown of the head, and the fingers upward. Exhale and arc to one side (*b*). Imagine your body is between two panes of glass and is unable to lean forward or backward—only to the side. Inhale and lengthen to straighten up; exhale and repeat to the other side.

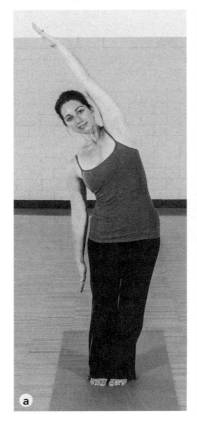
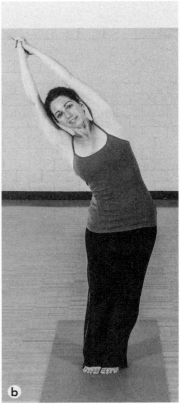

WARRIOR II POSE

This beautiful pose, also known as Peaceful Warrior or *Virabhadrasana II*, requires lower-body strength and endurance, particularly if it is held for any length of time. Because of its requirements, the Warrior II pose can heat and energize the body; even so, the upper body should feel calm, balanced, and at peace. This dynamic of work (lower body) and peace (upper body) helps practitioners learn to stay calm and relaxed under pressure.

Proper alignment of the front knee is critical in the Warrior II pose; remind students not to torque, or rotate, the knee. The knee should flex no more than 90°. Participants who wish to progress the warrior II pose should step the feet farther apart and bend the front knee to the full 90°. Novice practitioners may keep the feet closer together and bend the front knee less.

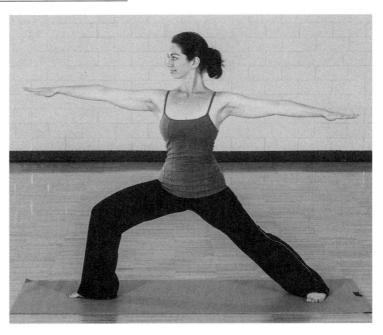

CUES   Step your feet wide apart and turn the left foot 90° toward the side of the room. Angle your back (right) foot slightly inward, keeping the entire foot on the floor. Bend your left knee in the direction of your second toe, and check to see that it stays straight ahead, twisting neither to the right or the left. Square your hips and torso toward the front of the room, keeping your torso perfectly upright. Straighten your arms out to the sides at shoulder height (parallel to the earth) and reach your fingertips to the sides of the room. Turn your head to the left and gaze out over your left fingers. Feel your abdominal muscles lift and contract, and lift the muscles between the legs. Feel the lines of energy radiating out from the center of the body. Hold the posture and continue to breathe comfortably.

TREE POSE

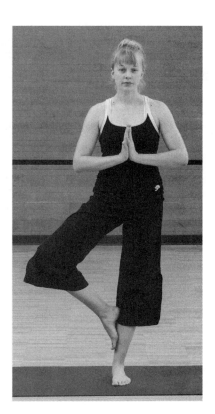

The Tree pose (*Vriksasana*) is one of the many balance postures found in yoga. It not only promotes physical balance but it is said to help create a deep sense of peace and inner balance. Many variations exist for the Tree pose; they can be arranged from easiest to hardest along the progressive functional training continuum. A low-to-intermediate version is shown in the photo. To make the Tree pose easier, simply keep the toes of the nonsupporting leg on or near the ground and stand near a wall or bar for support. To make the posture more difficult, place the foot of the nonsupporting leg high up on the inner thigh of the supporting leg, or place the nonsupporting leg in a half-lotus position. Arm variations for the tree pose include holding the hands in prayer (Namaste) position in front of the heart, holding the hands in prayer position overhead, and stretching the arms up and opened out overhead.

CUES   Stand on one foot with the sole of the foot firmly rooted into the earth. Feel the line of energy from the earth lifting up and through the supporting leg. Bend the knee of the nonsupporting leg and place the foot against your calf, turning the knee out. Engage the abdominal muscles and breathe comfortably, placing the hands in prayer (Namaste) position in front of the heart. Lift the crown of the head and feel energy spiral upward through the spine. To maintain your balance, focus your gaze on a spot directly in front of you or on the floor about 8 feet (2.4 m) in front of the body.

Backward-Bending Postures

Postures involving spinal extension and hip extension fall under the category of backward-bending postures. Backward bending is helpful in counteracting the forward pull of gravity experienced in daily living. When done regularly, backward-bending poses improve posture and help maintain a supple, youthful spine. Encourage your students to listen carefully to their bodies when performing these postures; spinal extension, particularly through a large ROM, may not be appropriate for everyone.

COBRA POSE

Perhaps the most famous of the backward-bending postures, the Cobra pose (Bhujangasana) is considered controversial for the general population due to its overstretching of the anterior longitudinal ligament of the spine and its potential for excessive vertebral and disk compression. As discussed earlier, several variations of the Cobra pose exist, including safer and easier modifications (see figure 15.3).

Even though we give cues for the traditional Cobra pose in the following paragraph, it's important to know the basic modifications, including the modified Cobra, or Sphinx pose, and the baby Cobra. In the Sphinx pose, the forearms are placed on the floor so that the torso is propped up on the elbows; the fingertips are spread wide. In the baby Cobra, the spine is only slightly extended, with the arms either straight out in front or splayed wide with the elbows bent. Instructors should make certain to teach and demonstrate these easier modifications if novices or participants with back pain are present in the class.

CUES   Lie facedown on the mat with your hands under your shoulders and your elbows bent. Before lifting up into the Cobra pose, energize your body, feeling a line of energy running from your toes, up through your legs, up your spine, and all the way to the top of your head. Lengthen and engage the leg muscles and point the toes. Press your sacrum down and slide your shoulder blades down away from your ears. Using your back muscles, raise your torso to a comfortable height, lifting and pressing the chest and heart forward. Allow your head and neck to continue the line of the spine (no cranking, or hyperextending, of the cervical spine). Spread the fingers wide, slightly bend the elbows, and move the shoulders away from the ears.

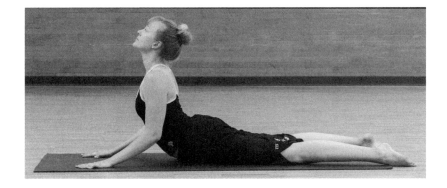

PRONE BOAT POSE

The Prone Boat pose (*Navasana*), like many other prone postures, is said to help tone the internal organs as well as strengthen the spinal and hip extensors. We provide cues for an easy version of the prone boat pose in the following paragraph. For an even easier version, have students lift only one leg and the opposite arm. To progress the pose, students simply extend both arms overhead and lift both arms and legs.

CUES   Lie facedown on your mat with your arms at your sides and your palms facing down. Lengthen your entire body from head to toes, energizing your muscles. Keeping your head and neck in line with your spine, inhale and lift your upper body and legs off the floor to a comfortable height. Hold for three or more breaths, feeling the body rise and fall with each inhalation and exhalation.

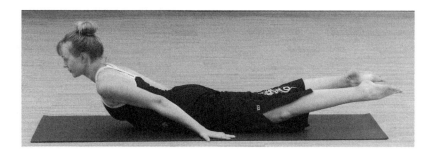

Forward-Bending Postures

Commonplace in yoga, forward-bending postures can feel incredibly wonderful to advanced yoga practitioners, who find that hinging at the hips is easy due to flexible hamstring muscles. For participants with less flexibility, however, forward bending can be extremely uncomfortable and potentially injurious to the spine. For this reason, it's important to provide plenty of modifications to make forward bending safer and more enjoyable for all.

Props can be helpful in forward bending; you can suggest to your students that they use a strap or belt around the outstretched foot and/or a blanket or rolled towel under the edge of the buttocks. Both devices facilitate flexing at the hips, an important aspect of proper alignment in forward bending. When the hips are able to flex to 90° or more, it is much more likely that the spine will remain in neutral as the practitioner fully enters the head-to-knee pose. A spine kept in or near neutral is in a safer position than one that is fully flexed (especially unsupported) due to overstretching of the posterior longitudinal ligament. When props are unavailable, participants who are unable to flex the hips at 90° and thus exhibit a hunched, flexed spine should be instructed to place their hands behind the hips to help prop the spine into a more upright and neutral position.

 See online video 15.3 for a brief demonstration of common forward-bending, twisting, and relaxation yoga postures.

HEAD-TO-KNEE POSE

The Head-to-Knee pose (also known as *Janusirshasana*, or the seated unilateral forward bend) is generally easier than bilateral (both legs) forward bending. It provides a deep stretch for the hamstrings as well as for the gluteus maximus, erector spinae, and calves.

CUES   Sit on your mat with your right leg extended out in front and your left knee bent with the sole of the left foot pressed against the right inner thigh. Lengthen through your right leg, feeling the line of energy pressing out through the heel (the foot is dorsiflexed). Start by sitting tall with your spine lengthened in neutral and your hips squared (a). Feel your weight directly above the sitting bones; your tailbone should be off the floor. Hinging from the hips, keep the waist long and lower your torso over the thigh (b). Place the hands wherever it feels comfortable: Place them under the calf or ankle, grasp the toes, or (if flexible enough) clasp the hands around the bottom of the foot. Alternatively, hold a strap placed around the bottom of the foot. Hold this pose for several breaths, inhaling and exhaling deeply. When exhaling, feel your abdominal muscles lift up against the spine; imagine letting go with each exhale.

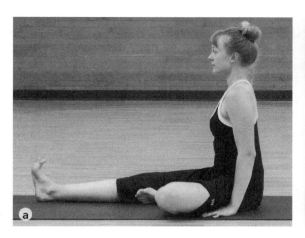
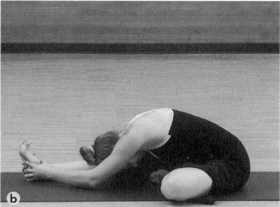

CHILD'S POSE

The Child's pose (*Garbasana* or *Balasana*) is a healing posture often regarded as a blissful resting pose; it also provides a relaxing stretch for the erector spinae and gluteus maximus muscles. While most practitioners find the Child's pose to be very comfortable, those with knee problems may not be able to relax fully due to the deep hyperflexion at the knee joint. Fortunately, there are modifications and props that can make the pose enjoyable for almost everyone. Allow your participants to choose whether they prefer to have the knees closer together or farther apart, depending on comfort. Placing a blanket or doubled-up mat under the knees can keep them from grinding into the floor. If deep knee hyperflexion is a problem, place a blanket or rolled-up towel behind the knee joints to decrease the knee flexion. If knee pain still persists, have the participant try placing a yoga block under the sitting bones to minimize weight bearing on the knees. Ankle pain can be eased with a rolled-up towel under the ankle joints. Several upper-body variations exist, for example, extending the arms overhead on the floor (a great latissimus dorsi stretch), resting the arms alongside the body with palms up (let the shoulder blades protract and relax), folding the arms across the low back, and cupping the sides of the face with the hands.

CUES   Sit back in a kneeling position with your hips resting toward your heels. Your knees can be closer together or farther apart, based on what your body prefers at the time. Allow your arms to rest alongside your body with your hands near your feet, palms up. Let your forehead rest on the mat and close your eyes. Allow your shoulder blades to feel heavy; feel them separating and relaxing toward the floor on each side. Breathe deeply and feel your back rising and falling and your ribs expanding and releasing. Let your whole body sink toward the earth. Rest in the pose for 5 to 10 breaths.

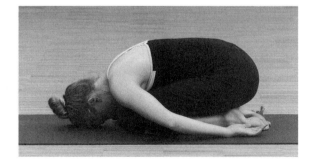

Twisting Postures

Twisting poses are asymmetrical; a spinal twist pulls one side of the body in the opposite direction from the other side of the body. To keep the spine safe, it's best to lengthen it before twisting. Twisting while the spine is in flexion or extension increases the risk of disk injury. On the other hand, twisting is a natural motion of the spine; moving the spine through a rotational ROM on a regular basis promotes lifelong suppleness and flexibility of the spine.

SEATED SPINAL TWIST

The Seated Spinal Twist (*Ardha Matsyendrasana*) is a multimuscle stretch. It is also said to provide a gentle massage and stimulation to the digestive system. The Seated Spinal Twist can be modified by placing a blanket or rolled-up towel under the edge of the buttocks; it can be progressed by bending the extended knee around and under the body. An advanced progression involves wrapping the top arm around and through the top knee and binding the hands together behind the back.

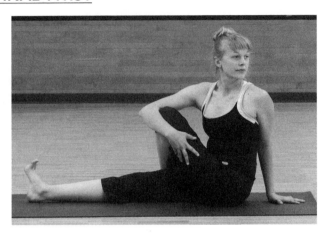

CUES Sit upright on your sitting bones with your right leg extended in front, foot flexed. Cross your left leg over the right; bend your left knee and place the left foot on the floor next to your right thigh. Press your left leg in toward your torso; sit tall with your pelvis grounded and shoulder blades pressed down. Rotate your spine to the left, crossing your right arm over the left knee (alternatively, you can hug the left knee with your right arm). Allow your left arm to travel behind the body; press your left palm down into the mat. Smoothly turn your head to the left and gaze over your left shoulder at the horizon, chin level. On each inhale, lift your spine higher; on each exhale, gently rotate a bit farther.

SUPINE SPINAL TWIST

The Supine Spinal twist (*Suptaikapadaparivrttasana*) is easier than the Seated Spinal Twist. When leading this pose, let your students decide which variation they want to use for the most healing effect. Variations include bending both knees to one side (knees can be close to the armpits or far away, depending on individual comfort), crossing the top knee over the bottom knee and rolling to one side, bending the top knee to the side and keeping the bottom leg straight in line with the body, abducting the arms perpendicular to the body, placing the arms overhead, and placing one hand on the top knee. The Supine Spinal Twist is a multimuscle

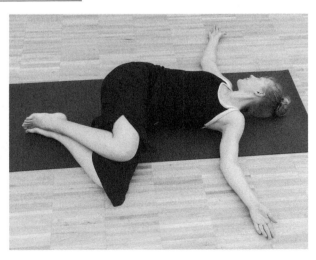

stretch and is also helpful for sciatic pain: It opens up the space between the vertebrae where the sciatic nerve passes through, helping to minimize nerve impingement.

CUES   Lie on your back and bring both knees to your chest. Gently roll both knees to the left and onto the mat. Allow your arms to open out into a T, perpendicular to your body, with palms facing up. If you like, hold your top knee with your left hand. If comfortable, turn your head to the right, feeling a stretch in your hips, waist, back, and chest. Relax, breathe deeply, and allow your body to sink into the earth.

Inverted Postures

Many inverted postures exist in yoga. In fact, some experts consider a Standing Forward Bend or a Downward Dog to be a mild inversion. Others consider the Legs-up-the-Wall pose to be a gentle modification of the Shoulder Stand and therefore a mild inversion. However, an inverted posture more commonly refers to poses such as the Headstand, Shoulder Stand, Plow, or Handstand. Most of these postures are advanced and are beyond the scope of this text. If you want to learn more about these postures and about yoga, please seek a qualified yoga teacher-training program.

Relaxation Pose and Ending the Class

A yoga class always ends with a few moments of deep relaxation. This is the time to completely let go of all muscular tension and all cares and concerns. Yogic texts tell us that when we lie in total relaxation, the benefits of the yoga class are fully integrated into the body. The traditional relaxation pose is called *Savasana*.

Encourage participants to get as comfortable as possible. Since they'll be lying in relaxation pose for 5 minutes or more, they may want to put socks and sweaters back on or cover themselves with a blanket. Some facilities provide eye pillows, which are small, sand-filled, scented silk pillows especially designed to rest over closed eyes and enhance relaxation. If extra blankets are available, you may suggest that participants with back issues place a rolled-up blanket under the knees for additional comfort.

After several moments in the Relaxation pose, have participants roll to one side and rest for a few more breaths, and then gradually return to an easy cross-legged sitting pose. It is traditional to finish a yoga class with sitting in meditation, although in many classes the instructor may read an inspirational poem or saying. Finally, the instructor may finish by

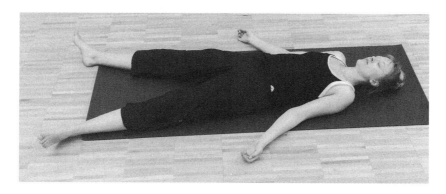

saying, "Namaste," hands pressed together in prayer position over the heart. Namaste is a Sanskrit word meaning "the light within me honors the light within you." Alternatively, yoga classes may end with chanting *Om*, the sound of the universe, one, or peace.

CUES After covering yourself for warmth, lie on your back with your legs slightly apart and rolled out. Allow your arms to lie a slight distance away from your body; let your palms face up. Gently press your shoulders back and down, feeling the earth below. Let your neck lengthen and continue the line of your spine. Slightly tuck your chin. Breathing deeply and slowly, sense your muscles letting go and falling toward the earth. Let your joints relax and open and feel your breath expanding into each cell of your body. With each exhale, let go a little more, feeling a profound peace come over your body.

Practice Drill

Using yoga music that is soft, amorphous, and relaxing, or that has a gentle world beat, put together your own short combination of yoga moves, starting with an appropriate warm-up and concluding with the relaxation pose. Practice cueing the basic moves and postures in a way suitable for yoga.

Chapter Wrap-Up

Yoga has been called a discipline for living. It is a holistic practice that unites body, mind, and spirit. This chapter covered some basic yoga philosophy, styles and types of yoga, fundamentals of breathwork, yoga research findings, verbal cues, music, props, technique and safety, appropriate environment, the warm-up, basic yoga postures, and the final relaxation. We hope this chapter will inspire you to explore yoga more fully and take a yoga teacher-training course. You will find many personal benefits from the practice of yoga as well as increase your ability to help others.

Group Exercise Class Evaluation Form: Key Points

- Connect the breath to the mind and body by performing breathing exercises.
- Give verbal cues on posture and alignment. Every yoga movement requires correct posture and alignment, and such cues are critical to leading participants in yoga.
- Encourage and demonstrate good body mechanics. Yoga movements generally require visual demonstration by the instructor. Make sure all your demonstrations are appropriate and emphasize proper progressions.
- Observe participants' form and suggest modifications for participants with injuries or special needs as well as progressions for advanced participants. Walk around the room after giving a visual demonstration of the movement to observe participants and make sure they are performing the postures correctly.
- Use appropriate music. Usually light background instrumental music is the most appropriate for yoga classes. Keep the volume low so you can also keep your voice low, calm, and soothing.
- Emphasize relaxation. The last 5 to 8 minutes of a yoga class often include a relaxation and visualization segment. This segment is essential to allow participants to relax fully and integrate the yoga postures.

ASSIGNMENTS

1. Write a 100-word paragraph describing the elements of yogic philosophy. Research one of the yoga styles and write a 250-word summary of your findings. Look up a recent yoga study and write a 100-word paragraph describing the study and its results.

2. Be prepared to teach a small group and cue a short yoga warm-up, a standing posture, a backward-bending posture, a forward-bending posture, a twisting posture, and a relaxation pose. Write out your plan.

Pilates

Chapter Objectives

By the end of this chapter, you will be able to

- understand the basic principles of Pilates,
- understand how to begin a Pilates class,
- create appropriate verbal and visual cues,
- apply safety and technique guidelines to Pilates exercises,
- teach basic Pilates mat exercises, and
- design a short Pilates mat routine appropriate for beginners.

Background Check

Before working your way through this chapter, do the following:

Read

☐ chapter 8, "Muscular Conditioning and Flexibility Training."

Group Exercise Class Evaluation Form Essentials

Key Points for Warm-Up Segment

- Includes appropriate amount of dynamic movement
- Gives clear cues and verbal directions

- Uses movements that are at an appropriate tempo and intensity

Key Points for Conditioning Segment

- Minimizes repetitive movements
- Observes participants' form and provides constructive, nonintimidating feedback
- Continually offers modifications, regressions, progressions, or alternatives
- Provides alignment and technique cues

- Gives motivational cues
- Provides regular demonstrations and participation with good body mechanics
- Uses appropriate movement or music tempo

The Pilates system of movement was developed by Joseph H. Pilates (1880-1967) in the first half of the 20th century. At first known to only a small group of dancers and elite athletes in New York City, the Pilates method gradually spread, and since 1990 it has become widely popularized in many cities around the world. According to the 2013 IDEA Fitness Programs and Equipment Trends Report (IDEA 2013), 74 % of program directors at fitness facilities offer Pilates mat classes on their group exercise class schedules, with 50 % offering a fusion-type class combining Pilates and yoga. Learning to teach Pilates will grow your career opportunities!

The Pilates Method: Basic Principles

The Pilates method of body conditioning is quite comprehensive, encompassing more than 2,000 exercises. This chapter introduces the major concepts underlying the Pilates method; describes the most familiar mat exercises; and discusses basic alignment, technique, and safety concerns. We strongly recommend that you seek additional training and certification in Pilates before teaching a mat class or working with Pilates equipment. For help with training and certification, see "Pilates Resources" later in this chapter.

In his 1945 book, *Pilates' Return to Life Through Contrology,* Joseph Pilates outlined the guiding principles of the Pilates method and detailed 34 mat exercises. We will discuss several of these mat exercises in this chapter. However, many more Pilates exercises can be done on special Pilates equipment. Standard apparatus includes the Pilates reformer, cadillac, barrel, and chair as well as small pieces such as the Pilates circle, arc trainer, half barrel, and spine supporter. Currently, you can find the larger pieces of equipment in Pilates studios, although more fitness facilities are investing in specially equipped Pilates rooms that are staffed with teachers specifically trained and certified in Pilates. Generally, training on the Pilates apparatus is done one on one with a Pilates trainer, although some studios offer small-group training if enough equipment is available. For example, if a studio has four reformers, a group of four clients may practice Pilates together while being led by a qualified Pilates instructor.

The Pilates system of exercise improves muscle strength, endurance, flexibility, balance, and coordination. It is often listed as a mind–body discipline and an ideal way to promote core stability. According to the 2006 position statement of the Pilates Method Alliance, "Pilates exercise focuses on postural symmetry, breath control, abdominal strength, spine, pelvis, and shoulder stabilization, muscular flexibility, joint mobility and strengthening through the complete range of motion of all joints. Instead of isolating muscle groups, the whole body is trained, integrating the upper and lower extremities with the trunk" (2006, p. 2).

TABLE 16.1 Core Muscles and Joint Actions

Joint	Muscle	Joint action
Pelvis	Iliopsoas	Hip flexion, anterior pelvic tilt
	Gluteus maximus	Hip extension, posterior pelvic tilt
	Rectus abdominis	Posterior pelvic tilt
	Quadratus lumborum	Lateral pelvic tilt
Spine	Rectus abdominis	Spinal flexion
	Obliques	Spinal flexion with rotation
	Transverse abdominis	Abdominal compression
	Erector spinae	Spinal extension, spinal rotation
	Multifidi	Spinal extension, spinal rotation
	Quadratus lumborum	Spinal lateral flexion
Shoulder girdle	Trapezius	Scapular retraction, depression, upward rotation, elevation
	Levator scapulae	Scapular elevation
	Rhomboids	Scapular retraction, downward rotation
	Pectoralis minor	Scapular depression, protraction
	Serratus anterior	Scapular protraction, upward rotation
Neck	Trapezius	Cervical spinal lateral flexion, extension
	Erector spinae	Cervical spinal extension
	Sternocleidmastoid	Cervical spinal rotation, flexion

The Powerhouse

Joseph Pilates' idea was that the body's core is the powerhouse of strength from which all movements emanate. Most Pilates experts agree that core stability is the ability to keep the pelvis, spine, neck, and shoulder girdle stable while performing various activities. See table 16.1 for a list of key core muscles and their actions.

Many, if not most, of the exercises in the Pilates repertoire challenge the core muscles to contract isometrically against resistance and stabilize the core joints while the extremities move. Such exercises include the hundred, the leg circle, the single straight-leg stretch, swimming, the seated spinal twist, the side kick, and the leg pull-up.

Mobility Versus Stability

Joseph Pilates believed that a fit body is both strong and flexible and that a healthy spine is both stable and mobile. Accordingly, many Pilates exercises promote spinal suppleness (along with fluidity of motion). Practitioners are taught to articulate the vertebrae of the spine, which means to move one vertebra at a time. Exercises that articulate the spine include the roll-up and roll-down, rollover, and spine stretch. If the spine is supple, it is able to flex fully, which is important for optimal performance of exercises such as rolling like a ball.

Abdominal Hollowing

Abdominal hollowing (also known as *scooping* or the *drawing-in maneuver*) is a hallmark of Pilates exercise. The muscle responsible for abdominal hollowing is the transverse abdominis, which performs abdominal compression. You can use many images to help participants perform abdominal hollowing; for example, you might cue participants to pull the navel to the spine or to pretend they're zipping up a pair of jeans that are a size too small. The ability to draw in the abdominal muscles may help prevent low-back pain, since conscious abdominal contraction can support the spine anteriorly during tasks that involve bending over and lifting heavy objects. Abdominal

Pilates Research Findings

Although Pilates research is relatively new, several studies have attempted to verify the efficacy of Pilates exercise. A review by Bernardo (2007) found that over 277 studies and abstracts had been published but pointed out that the methodology used in many of these studies was not rigorous. However, Bernardo did state that there is "cautious support" for improvements in flexibility, core stability, and muscle strength and endurance due to Pilates training.

For example, a 12-week training study using a series of 25 mat Pilates exercises found that participants improved abdominal and upper-body endurance as well as hamstring flexibility (Kloubec 2010), whereas another training study measured improvements in muscle strength (Amorim et al. 2011). Neither study found any change in balance measurements. However, a study by Johnson and coworkers (2007) did find positive changes in dynamic balance after 10 Pilates sessions. An interesting study evaluated the ability of Pilates-trained subjects compared with traditional abdominal crunch–trained subjects to activate the transverse abdominis and maintain lumbopelvic control (stability); Pilates training resulted in a significantly greater improvement versus the results for those who had trained with standard abdominal exercises (Herrington and Davies, 2005). Otto and Yoke (2004) conducted a 12-week training study comparing the efficacy of Pilates apparatus exercise with traditional resistance training; no significant difference was found between the two muscular conditioning modalities in terms of body composition, muscle strength, or muscle endurance measurements. That is, both groups improved equally in the measured components of fitness—Pilates apparatus training apparently works as well as traditional weight room training. Olson and colleagues measured caloric expenditure in 12 subjects who performed beginner, intermediate, and advanced mat Pilates workouts (2004). She concluded that in order to make significant changes in body composition, a person would have to perform the intermediate or advanced workouts 4 days per week for 45 to 60 minutes. Olson and Smith also performed EMG studies (2005), finding that Pilates exercises provide a significant challenge to abdominal muscles. Several studies have found improvements in flexibility from mat Pilates practice (Otto et al. 2004; Schroeder et al. 2002; Rogers and Gibson 2005; Segal, Hein, and Basford 2004). Additionally, a few studies have examined the effects of Pilates training on low-back pain relief, and, in the words of one author, have found it "superior to minimal intervention for pain relief" (Lim et al. 2011; Anderson and Spector 2000). Most literature review authors (Bernardo 2007; Shedden and Kravitz 2006; Lim et al. 2011) agree that better-controlled studies are needed in Pilates research in order to validate the many claims that are publicized.

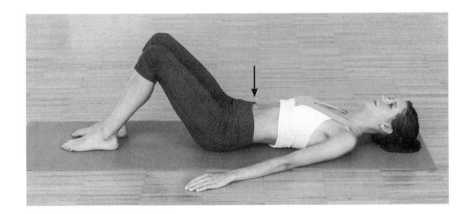

FIGURE 16.1 Abdominal hollowing in the supine neutral position.

Pilates Resources

Books

M. Clark and C. Romani-Ruby. 2001. *The Pilates Reformer: A Manual for Instructors.* Tarentum, PA: Word Association.

S. Gallagher and R. Kryzanowska. 2000. *The Joseph H. Pilates Archive Collection: Photographs, Writings and Designs.* Philadelphia: Bainbridge Books.

R. Isacowitz. 2006. *Pilates.* Champaign, IL: Human Kinetics.

D. Lessen. 2005. *The PMA Pilates Certification Exam Study Guide.* Miami, FL: Pilates Method Alliance.

J.H. Pilates. 1945. *Pilates' Return to Life Through Contrology.* (Original publisher: J.J. Augustin).

B. Siler. 2000. *The Pilates Body.* New York, NY: Broadway Books.

Web Sites

Balanced Body, www.pilates.com

Bodies in Balance, www.bibpilates.net

Peak Pilates, www.peakpilates.com

PHI Pilates, www.phipilates.com

Physicalmind Institute, www.themethod pilates.com

Pilates Method Alliance (PMA), www. pilatesmethodalliance.org

Polestar Pilates, www.polestarpilates.com

Stott Pilates, www.stottpilates.com

hollowing has also been advocated as a means of stabilizing the spine (Hodges et al. 1996) and increasing the action of the pelvic floor muscles. Abdominal hollowing may be performed in all positions, including standing, sitting, side lying, all fours, supine imprinted, and supine neutral (see figure 16.1).

Practice Drill

Inhale and exhale using the abdominal breathing technique described in chapter 15. On the exhale, when your abdomen naturally pulls in, consciously draw it in, attempting to press your navel even further toward the spine. Feel your abdomen hollow, or scoop inward. See if you can do this move when standing, sitting, lying supine, and lying prone.

Imprinting

An imprinted spine is one that is consciously pressed into the mat when a person is lying in the supine position. An imprinted spine is no longer in neutral since the lumbar curve is flattened against the floor, and the pelvis is tilted posteriorly. The imprinted position may be optimal for beginners or participants with low-back pain because it provides more spinal stability than does a neutral position; in addition, the imprinted position enables more tactile reinforcement since the participant can feel the spine contacting the mat. Ideally, the imprint and posterior pelvic tilt should be performed by contracting the rectus abdominis and not by tensing the gluteals (see figure 16.2). The imprinted position, while safe and effective for most people, is not comfortable for everyone. Participants who find the imprinted spine uncomfortable should be encouraged to work in a neutral spinal position.

Neutral Spine

While Joseph Pilates did not discuss the concept of a neutral spine, believing instead that the back should be kept flat (forming a plumb line), most contemporary Pilates practitioners have updated his original ideas to match what we now know about the body, including the benefits of the neutral spine. A neutral spine is one that is in ideal alignment, with its four natural curves assuming their ideal relationship to each other. The spine is not meant to be flat like a wall; rather, it is designed to have an inward curve at the cervical spine, an outward curve at the thoracic spine, another inward curve at the lumbar spine, and another outward curve at the sacrum

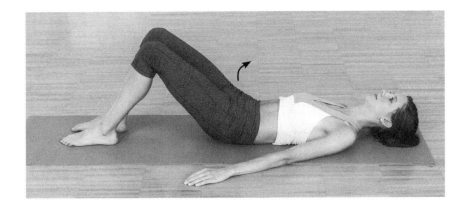

FIGURE 16.2   The imprinted spine.

(see figure 16.3). When the spine is in neutral, the neck and the pelvis are also in neutral. Most experts maintain that a neutral spine distributes stress, shock, and impact forces in the safest way possible (Norris 2000; Cholewicki et al. 1997; McGill 2002). A Pilates class is an ideal medium for teaching students about neutral alignment because the purpose of many of the exercises is to keep the spine in neutral against a resistance or against the movement of the extremities. Such exercises include the leg circle, corkscrew, spine twist, side kick, leg pull-down, leg pull-up, kneeling side kick, and push-up.

Breathing

Joseph Pilates was emphatic that full inhalations and exhalations are essential to oxygenate the body; each breath cleanses and replenishes the

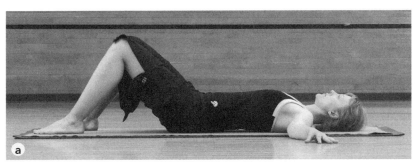

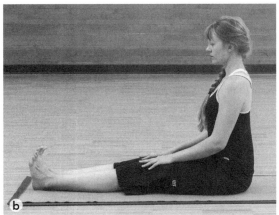

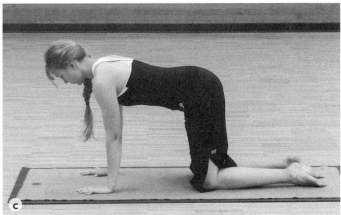

FIGURE 16.3   The neutral spine in the (a) supine, (b) seated, and (c) all-fours positions.

body. He recommended inhaling and exhaling on specific parts of each exercise, as shown later in this chapter. In general, a full exhale is recommended during spinal flexion movements since this is more anatomically correct, while an inhalation is often more natural when extending the spine or opening the body. Many experts recommend maintaining abdominal hollowing for the duration of any exercise in which the spine is stabilized (hollowing helps maintain stability); therefore, lateral rib cage expansion is encouraged during breathing. This is in contrast to moving the abdomen out and in as is done in relaxed abdominal breathing (discussed in chapter 15). Allowing the abdomen to relax out and in may have the undesirable result of destabilizing the spine when a person is holding certain positions, such as the plank position, or is carrying heavy objects.

Practice Drill

Sit in a comfortable position, either in a chair or on the floor. Your spine should be long and in neutral. Take a full diaphragmatic inhale, allowing your abdomen to expand slightly. Exhale, consciously pulling your abdomen in, imagining that your navel is touching your spine. Then, keeping your abdomen hollowed and as far in as possible, continue to breathe for several breaths. Do not allow your abdomen to move with your breathing; maintain abdominal hollowing. Feel as if your rib cage were expanding laterally with each breath and allow your upper back to move with each inhale and exhale. Feel your abdominal wall remaining firm and inwardly contracted during the entire practice.

Setup and Maintenance of Proper Alignment

Many Pilates instructors begin each exercise with a setup. This is simply a teaching technique in which participants are asked to place their bodies in the ideal alignment, or setup, for the upcoming exercise. For example, when teaching side kicks, take a moment to fully detail and place students in the optimal starting position, fully describing the alignment of each major joint, the neutral position of the spine,

and the hollowing of the abdominal muscles. Only after being satisfied that all students are in the proper starting position do you actually cue the exercise. Executing all moves with proper alignment is a central concept in Pilates. Moving with concentration, control, and precision at all times is critical. Joseph Pilates himself wrote that performing one precise and perfect movement is better than completing many half-hearted ones.

Lengthening

Most Pilates exercises are designed to promote a lengthening sensation throughout the body: One part of the body energetically reaches in one direction, while another part of the body reaches in the opposite direction. Elongation is felt through the joints and the muscles. Toes, fingertips, and the crown of the head are often cued to reach as far from center as possible. In many exercises, there is a sensation of stretch even though the working muscles are contracting concentrically. Such exercises include leg circles, rollover, single straight-leg stretch, corkscrew, double-leg kick, spine twist, and teaser.

Creating a Warm-Up

In Joseph Pilates' original method for mat exercise, there is no warm-up, at least not according to the standard definition given in chapter 6. The first exercise in his authentic series is the hundred, which he intended to serve as a warm-up exercise. While the hundred does involve vigorous pumping of the arms (100 times) and is intended to be performed with strong, rhythmic inhalations and exhalations, the rest of the body remains stable, lying supine on the floor in sustained spinal and hip flexion. We believe (along with a number of Pilates experts) that more dynamic movement is needed before beginning the hundred in order to safely prepare the body for the Pilates mat exercises that follow.

Since the majority of a Pilates mat class is on the floor, warm-ups, when provided, are also generally on the floor or mat. The warm-up is an ideal time to introduce key concepts such as proper breathing, neutral spine, spinal mobility, abdominal hollowing, imprinting, lengthening, control, precision, and mindfulness. The following are cues for a sample warm-up appropriate for a Pilates class:

1. **Seated breathing practice.** Sit on your mat with your knees bent, legs together, and feet flat on the floor. Wrap your arms and hands around your legs and let your spine round. Rest your torso on your thighs and relax your head and neck. Breathe deeply and feel your back and posterior and lateral rib cage expand and release with each inhale and exhale. Take 3 to 5 deep breaths.

2. **Round and release.** Sit on the mat with your legs crossed, spine straight, and hands on knees or shins. Exhale, rounding and flexing your spine, allowing your pelvis to tilt posteriorly; coordinate the exhale with abdominal hollowing (pull your navel toward your spine). Inhale and lift and lengthen your spine back up to neutral; return your pelvis to neutral as well, sitting well up on your sitting bones. Repeat this limbering move 3 to 5 times, connecting your breath to the movement and emphasizing abdominal hollowing with each exhale.

3. **Side bend and twist.** Remaining in the cross-legged position, place your left hand on the floor and reach your right hand up to the ceiling, inhaling and flexing the spine laterally (to the side). Exhale as you return the right hand to the floor. Repeat three times to the right before repeating the entire move on the left side. Then, sitting quite tall, rotate your spine to the right on an exhale. Inhale as you return to center; exhale as you twist to the left. Repeat 3 times.

4. **Supine imprint and release.** Lie on your back with your knees bent, feet flat on the floor and arms at your sides. Place the pelvis, spine, shoulder blades, and neck in neutral. Exhale and gently press your low back into the mat, pulling the abdominal muscles into your spine (drawing in, or hollowing, maneuver). Remember to use the abdominal and not the gluteal muscles for hollowing. Inhale and allow your pelvis and spine to return to neutral (do not overextend your spine past neutral). Repeat 3 to 5 times.

5. **Supine articulated bridge.** Lie on your back with your knees bent, feet flat on the floor, arms at your sides, and your pelvis, spine, shoulder blades, and neck in neutral. Exhale and posteriorly tilt your pelvis, tipping your tailbone upward. Still exhaling, peel your spine off the floor, tailbone first, keeping your head and shoulders down. Inhale at the top of the motion. Exhale and—one by one—articulate the spine, lowering the vertebrae back down onto the mat. Inhale to rest. Repeat 3 to 5 times.

6. **Supine rib cage placement.** Lie on your back with your knees bent, feet flat on the floor, arms at your sides, and your pelvis, spine, shoulder blades, and neck in neutral. Inhale and slide your shoulder blades up toward your ears; exhale and press them away from your ears, keeping your scapulae on the mat at all times. Repeat 3 to 5 times. Then inhale and protract your shoulder blades up and away from the mat; exhale and press them firmly down into the mat, retracting them toward each other if possible. Your chest will lift, and a space may form under the thoracic spine when the shoulder blades are fully retracted. Repeat 3 to 5 times. Finally, allow your shoulder blades to rest on the mat in neutral (neither protracted nor retracted).

7. **All-fours cat tilt and dog tilt.** On your hands and knees, exhale and flex your spine up into the angry cat stretch, head and tailbone down, abdominal muscles drawn up and in. Inhale and gently extend your spine, head and hips up. Move back and forth through these two positions 3 to 5 times, allowing your spine to become more supple and limber.

 See online video 16.1 for a demonstration of a Pilates warm-up.

Verbal Cues and Music

Cueing in Pilates is perhaps more alignment driven than it is in other forms of group exercise. Remember that two of the underlying principles of Pilates are control and precision. Ideally, each exercise is executed with concentration and flawless alignment, every time. Skilled Pilates instructors have a well-developed eye for subtle alignment issues in their students. By knowing the common alignment and technique errors in the standard Pilates repertoire and in their students, competent instructors are ready with effective cues, ideally preventing the errors before they occur. To that end, it is common to *detail*, that is, to give many specific alignment cues for each major joint during an exercise, as well as to remind students about breathing, abdominal hollowing, and lengthening. Additionally, instructors need to be able to say the same cue in multiple ways since each student will respond differently to a cue. For example, if the exercise requires a flexed spine, some participants will flex it immediately upon hearing, "Round your back," whereas others will not respond at all. To reach these students, the instructor might try other cues such as, "Curve your spine," "Make your spine into a C curve," "Pull your ribs and hips toward each other," "Curl your spine into a half-moon shape," and so on. An adept instructor needs a large vocabulary of alignment words and ideas to describe each exercise.

Practice Drill

Using a piece of paper to record your responses, come up with as many ways as you can to cue the following:

- Neutral spine
- Head high
- Shoulders down
- Abdominal muscles in
- Neutral pelvis
- Spinal articulation

Did you come up with any image cues in the practice drill? Image cues are commonly used to detail Pilates exercises. A common image cue for guiding students to curl up or flex the spine, for example, is to ask them to curve into a half-moon shape or to form the letter *C* with the spine. Can you think of other image cues? Some instructors are quite creative, humorous, or fanciful with their cues. Remember that each student is unique. Some participants will respond better to image cues than to more straightforward cues. A skilled instructor is able to cue in a variety of ways in order to most effectively reach all participants.

The majority of participants learn best with visual cues. Be sure to demonstrate each exercise

at least once before getting up and moving around your class so that your students know what the exercise is supposed to look like. Alternatively, ask a skilled participant to model the exercise. When detailing an exercise, it is helpful if you provide visual cues using your own body. For example, practice giving head to toe alignment cues while pointing to various joints on your own body. When you say, "Shoulders down and back," point to your own shoulders as you exaggerate pressing them down and back. When you say, "Abdominal muscles in," exaggerate pulling your own abdominal wall in, pressing inward with your hand. This type of cue is quite effective in helping your class perform an exercise correctly.

It's important to include educational or informational cues throughout your class. Especially in Pilates, the rationale for doing a particular exercise is not always immediately obvious. Many students will want to know why they should do a move in a certain way or where they should feel their muscles working. Explaining the purpose of an exercise or the principles behind Pilates can enhance adherence and keep your class motivated. For example, when teaching single-leg circles you might explain, "The purpose of this exercise is to promote core stability, so keep your abdominal muscles hollowed, your shoulder blades grounded, and your core very still while limbering your hip joint and allowing your leg to move freely." You could even go on to explain why core stability work is important. With these cues, your students will become more educated and enthusiastic about Pilates.

A tactile cue is a hands-on touch cue. While tactile cueing is common among Pilates instructors, it is not without controversy. Since some participants are uncomfortable being touched and may feel that touch violates their personal space, it's critical to always ask permission before touching someone. Even if your student grants you permission, it's probably best to avoid touching if you detect any discomfort (such as drawing away or cringing from your touch). This is especially important for male instructors cueing female participants. However, when participants are comfortable with being touched, there are benefits to tactile cueing. These include improving your student's alignment to make Pilates exercises safer and more effective.

Generally, a student will be much more focused and concentrated on the exercise, without letting the mind wander, when an instructor is providing tactile cueing. This student is more likely to get the optimal benefit from the exercise.

Using music in Pilates classes is a matter of instructor choice. Many instructors opt to teach their Pilates classes without music, believing that silence allows participants to be more mindful and have better concentration and focus. When music is used, it is usually amorphous, meaning that it lacks a strong, rhythmic beat. Some instructors prefer mellow classical or jazz; others choose new age or soft world music. If you choose to use music when teaching Pilates, make sure it is in the background.

Technique and Safety Issues

Like the yoga postures (discussed in chapter 15), Pilates exercises run the gamut from easy to hard, from extremely basic and safe to advanced and potentially risky. It's important for Pilates instructors to understand the potential mechanisms of injury to each joint—and especially to the spine since so much of Pilates concerns the core. Table 16.2 briefly reviews the common mechanisms of injury to the spine.

Since several Pilates exercises place the student in potentially injury-producing positions, it's best to provide appropriate modifications, carefully detail each exercise in such a way that

participants perform it completely correctly, or entirely avoid leading the class in the high-risk Pilates exercises. Table 16.3 lists some of the more problematic Pilates exercises and their mechanisms of injury.

TABLE 16.3 Mechanisms of Injury in Pilates Exercises

Exercise	Mechanism of injury
Hundred, roll-up, double-leg stretch, teaser	Long-lever traction
Spine stretch forward, rolling down the wall	Unsupported spinal flexion
Full swan dive, rocking	Extreme lumbar hyperextension
Rollover, jackknife, bicycle	Weight bearing on cervical spine

Once again, let's revisit the progressive functional training continuum, which is discussed in our book *Functional Exercise Progressions* (Yoke and Kennedy 2004) and shown in chapters 3, 5, 8, 9, and 13 of this text. Remember that the continuum can be used to organize a variety of exercises or to organize variations of one exercise from easiest to hardest. Figure 16.4 shows an example of the progressive functional training continuum for the hundred. When teaching Pilates to a mixed-level class, it is best to start with the easiest and most conservative variation of an exercise, such as

TABLE 16.2 Common Mechanisms of Injury to the Spine

Cause	Effect
Unsupported spinal flexion	Overstretches the long posterior ligaments of the spine, which can lead to a loss of spinal stability
Unsupported spinal flexion with rotation	Overstretches the long posterior ligaments of the spine, which can lead to a loss of spinal stability; also carries an additional risk of disk herniation
Unsupported lateral flexion	Overstretches the long ligaments of the spine, leading to a loss of spinal stability
Extreme lumbar hyperextension	Overstretches the long anterior ligaments of the spine, leading to a loss of spinal stability
Long-lever traction	May produce a shearing force on the spine, leading to ligament overstretch or protruding (bulging) disks
Weight bearing on the cervical spine	Causes undue stress on the small cervical vertebrae and may impinge nerves and blood vessels

the variation shown in figure 16.4a. We strongly recommend that you get competent safety and technique instruction as well as certification if you decide to become a Pilates instructor.

Ending a Pilates Class

Traditionally, a Pilates class ends with a plank or a push-up followed by walking the hands back to the feet to form a standing forward bend and rolling up to a standing finish. We recommend incorporating a flexibility and cooldown segment as discussed in chapter 8 under "Cueing Flexibility Exercises and Ending a Class Appropriately". Since the chest muscles, erector spinae, hip flexors, hamstrings, and calves are commonly tight, it's always a good idea to stretch these muscles.

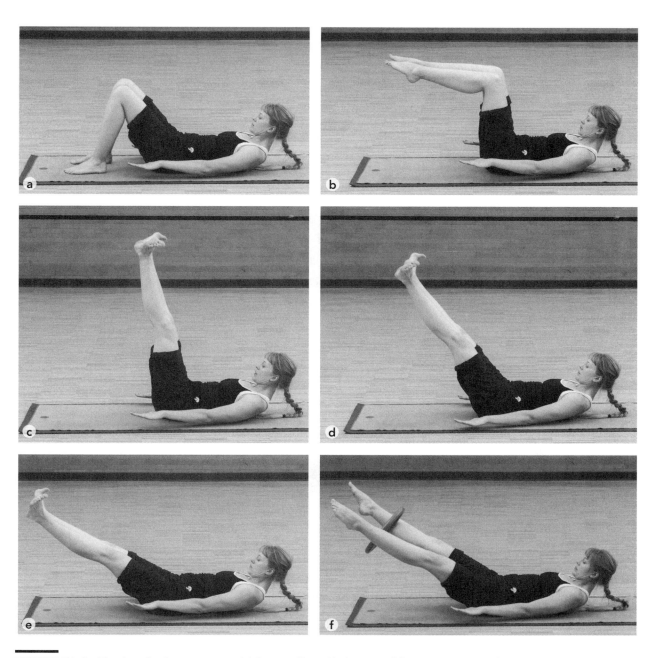

FIGURE 16.4 The hundred progression: (a) feet on floor, (b) legs in tabletop position, (c) legs straight up, (d) legs at 45°, (e) legs close to ground, and (f) legs close to ground with circle.

Technique and Safety Check

To help keep your classes safe, observe the following recommendations:

- Provide an appropriate warm-up.
- Provide plenty of modifications for each exercise, always starting with the easiest variation (unless you are teaching a class only for advanced students).
- Avoid high-risk or controversial exercises unless teaching an advanced class (even then, offer modifications).
- Provide plenty of alignment cues and detail each exercise carefully.
- Keep reminding participants to breathe.

BASIC MOVES

Joseph Pilates specified that his mat exercises be performed in a particular order, and there are still some Pilates organizations that scrupulously adhere to his original method. Other organizations tout a more contemporary approach, modifying Joseph Pilates' work when necessary for reflecting a more scientifically correct practice. In this chapter we present a few Pilates mat exercises that are either more basic or that can be easily modified to enhance safety.

 See online video 16.2 for a demonstration of the hundred, roll-up, single-leg circle, and rolling like a ball.

 See online video 16.3 for a demonstration of the leg pull front, one leg kick, breast-stroke, spine stretch forward, and seated twist.

THE HUNDRED

This classic Pilates exercise is intended to promote core stability while the body is in resisted spinal flexion. It is also meant to oxygenate the body and increase circulation through a vigorous and rhythmic breathing pattern. The traditional version of the hundred exerts a long-lever traction force on the spine and should be done only by participants who are able to fully stabilize the spine in flexion; the traditional version is *not* for beginners! Modify the traditional version by keeping the feet on the floor or by lifting the legs into the tabletop position (see figure 16.4).

CUES   Lie supine with the spine imprinted and the abdominal muscles hollowed. Flex the hips and knees to 90°, placing the legs in tabletop position. Curl the spine into flexion, lifting the shoulder blades off the floor and allowing the head and neck to continue the line of the curved spine. Raise long, straight arms off the ground, keeping them parallel to the floor. Reach the fingers straight ahead. Inhale for 5 counts and exhale for 5 counts; continue this pattern 10 times (for a total of 100 counts). Keep pressing the abdominal muscles down and relaxing the neck and shoulders for the duration of the exercise.

ROLL-UP

Both core stability and core mobility are challenged in the roll-up. The goal is to flex the spine as much as possible throughout the exercise, a feat that requires spinal suppleness. The rounder the spine, the more even and smooth the roll-up and roll-down; if the spine is rigid and inflexible in places, rolling up or down smoothly will be impossible. Rectus abdominis strength and endurance are required to maintain a full contraction throughout the entire range of motion (ROM) of the exercise. If the abdominal muscles are weak and unable to maintain spinal flexion, the hip flexors may take over and create a long-lever traction force on the spine, causing the exercise to become unsafe. It is recommended that beginners practice a half roll-up (crunch) first, preferably with the knees bent, in order to develop a foundation of abdominal strength. A half roll-back (start in the seated position, round the spine and roll back halfway, and then return to sitting) can also prepare the beginner for the traditional roll-up. Yet another modification is to hold both ends of a strap secured around the feet; the strap allows participants (depending on body segment lengths) to roll up and down more smoothly and safely.

CUES Lie supine with the spine imprinted and abdominal muscles hollowed. Your legs are straight and long, toes are pointed, shoulders are flexed, and fingers are reaching toward the ceiling. Inhale and lift your head and neck off the floor. Exhale and continue to curl up the rest of the spine, lifting it from the floor vertebra by vertebra (*a*). Keep your shoulder blades down and away from your ears throughout the movement. At the end of the exhale, your spine should be fully flexed as you reach your arms forward, keeping them parallel to your legs (*b*). Make certain your abdominal muscles are fully drawn in and your ribs are lifted up and over the belly. Inhale and begin to roll down, staying in flexion. Exhale and continue rolling down, letting each vertebra independently lower onto the floor until the body is supine again, with arms reaching toward the ceiling. Repeat 3 to 5 times.

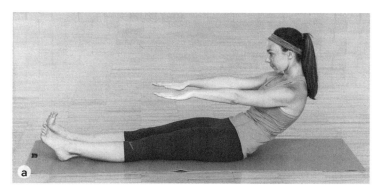

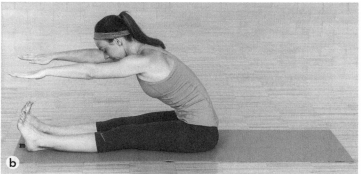

SINGLE-LEG CIRCLE

The single-leg circle requires maintaining spinal and pelvic stability in the neutral position while moving an extremity (the leg). When performing this exercise, you should feel as if the hip is moving effortlessly in its socket while the core is stable. The single-leg circle may be troublesome for participants with tight hamstrings: Because these students are unable to lift the leg to 90°, they may experience unnecessary hip flexor tension that pulls on the lumbar spine. Modifications include bending the bottom (supporting) leg and placing the foot on the floor; this will help relieve tension in the low back. Additionally, novice exercisers can be encouraged to make small circles instead of large ones or can even use a strap around the foot (holding the ends with the hands) to help the leg move in circles.

CUES Lie supine with the spine imprinted and the abdominals hollowed. Your arms should be at your sides, your palms should face down, and your scapulae should be stabilized. Stretch the left leg out along the floor, ideally with toes pointed. Reach the right leg up toward the ceiling, keeping the toes pointed. Start the leg circle by bringing the leg across the midline of the body (*a*). Inhale. Move the leg down and around (*b-c*) and then back up to 90°. Exhale. Your torso and pelvis should remain motionless throughout the movement. The size of the leg circle will be determined by your ability to stabilize the torso. Beginners should start with small circles; the circle circumference can be increased as you become more adept. Repeat the circle 3 to 5 times in each direction. Then switch legs and repeat with the left leg circling.

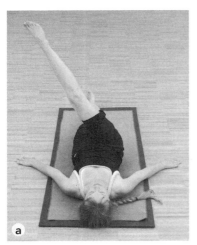 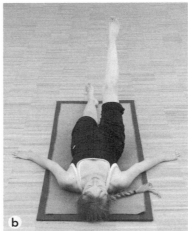 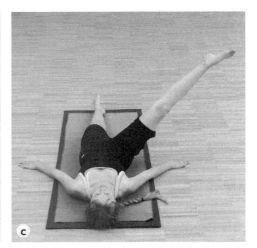

ROLLING LIKE A BALL

Rolling like a ball is similar to the roll-up in that the more supple and flexible the spine, the rounder the back and the easier it is to roll back and forth without any thumping or uneven movement. When performing rolling like a ball, you should maintain the spine in the finest *C* curve possible; this is best accomplished by firmly hollowing the abdominal muscles throughout the exercise and maintaining core stability. In addition, rolling like a ball requires you to exert control when returning to the starting or balance point, a feat that is difficult without abdominal hollowing and mental focus. Rolling like a ball is a beginner exercise that can progress to a harder exercise such as the open-leg rocker.

CUES   Start in the up position, finding the balance point on your sitting bones. Your spine should be fully flexed and rounded into a *C* curve and your abdominal muscles should be drawn in. Hold the lower legs with your hands; your legs should be together and your toes should be pointed with the feet off the floor (*a*). Hollow the abdomen even further and allow yourself to roll back while you inhale (*b*). Be sure to maintain the distance between the abdomen and the thighs (in other words, do not change the angle of hip flexion). While exhaling, rock back up to the starting position. Avoid rolling so far back that you place weight onto the neck or head; keep your head off the floor. Roll back and forth 5 to 6 times.

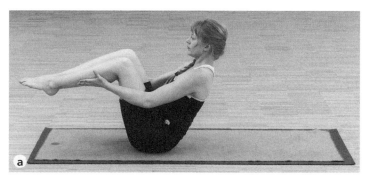

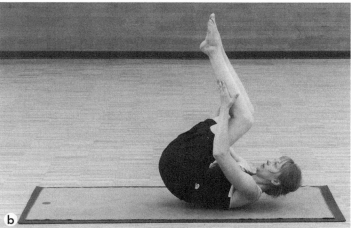

SINGLE-HEEL KICK

The single-heel kick requires the spine to be maintained in slight extension, making this exercise a good counterbalance to all the flexion exercises found in Pilates. Throughout the kick the abdominal muscles are drawn up and in for support, which means this exercise helps promote core stability in spinal extension. Additionally, this exercise challenges the scapular depressors (lower trapezius and pectoralis minor) because without concentration, gravity pulls the thoracic and cervical spine down, and the scapulae ride up the back of the rib cage toward the ears. To prevent these effects, participants must develop stamina and endurance in the upper body to maintain scapular depression against gravity for the duration of the exercise. A note of caution: Some participants may not be comfortable with the degree of spinal extension required by this exercise. If participants report back discomfort, modify the exercise by allowing them to lie completely prone and rest the forehead on the hands. Then they can maintain spinal stability in the prone position throughout the exercise.

CUES   Start in the prone position and prop up the upper torso on the elbows. Rest the forearms on the floor. Press the shoulders down and away from the ears, lengthening the neck. Minimize spinal extension as much as possible by contracting the abdominal muscles to prevent the low back from sagging toward the floor (*a*). Ideally, the belly is up and off the floor. Stabilize the shoulder blades, neck, torso, and pelvis while performing the leg movement. Energize and lengthen your legs and point your toes. Bend the right knee and exhale as you pulse the heel toward the body two times, attempting to kick the buttock (*b*). Inhale as you straighten the knee and return it to the mat. Switch sides and kick with the opposite leg. Repeat 5 to 10 times.

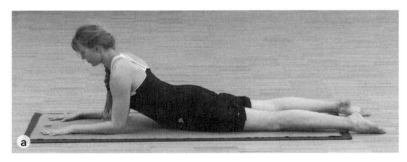

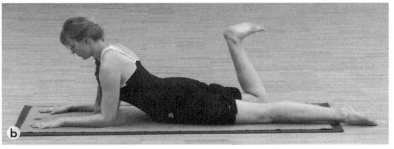

BREASTSTROKE

The breaststroke emphasizes spinal extension and can serve as a preparatory exercise for harder Pilates extension moves such as swimming and the swan. If bringing the arms into full flexion overhead is too challenging or causes back or shoulder discomfort, modify the exercise by simply abducting the arms into a T position (90° angle to the torso) instead.

CUES   Start in the prone position with the elbows bent, the hands under the shoulders, and the forearms on the floor (*a*). The spine, pelvis, and neck are all in neutral alignment; the legs are together, and the toes are pointed. Keep the lower body energized by anchoring it to the floor throughout the exercise. Exhale and send the arms overhead and forward, hovering off the floor (*b*). Inhale and sweep the arms around to the sides while you simultaneously lift the chest and extend the spine, keeping the head and neck in line with the spine (*c*). Exhale and send the arms overhead again, as if performing a breaststroke; inhale and repeat the sweeping arm movement and spinal extension. Repeat 5 to 10 times.

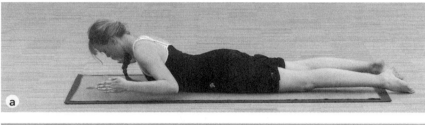

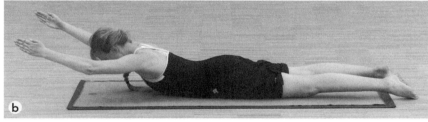

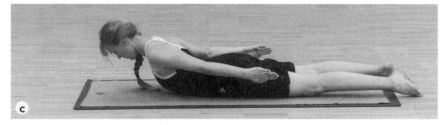

SIDE-LYING POSITION

The side-lying position is slightly more challenging than the supine or prone position because in this position the body makes less contact with the floor, and therefore the stabilizers must work harder to maintain good alignment. Some Pilates texts show more challenging variations, such as resting the head on the hand or placing both hands behind the ears while propping the upper body up on the elbow; however, we suggest using the more basic and stable variation of resting the head on the arm with the cervical spine in neutral. The goal is to keep the pelvis, spine, scapulae, neck, and head in neutral and maintain abdominal hollowing throughout the exercise. To achieve this goal you must be particularly focused when bringing the leg back into extension because during this motion the spine naturally tends to extend.

CUES   Lie on your side with your hips and shoulders stacked; keep spine and pelvis in neutral and your abdominal muscles contracted. Your bottom arm is stretched out under your head; your head and neck are in neutral. Bend your top arm and place your hand on the floor for stability. Dorsiflex your top ankle. Inhale and bring your top leg forward, flexing at the hip; pulse twice (a). Stay in control with abdominals securely contracted, as you exhale and bring the leg behind the body, pointing your toes (b). Be sure to keep the moving leg parallel to the floor. Repeat 8 to 10 times and then switch sides.

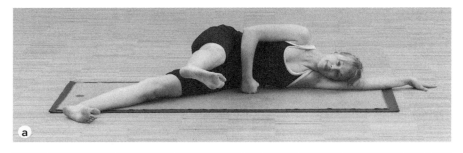

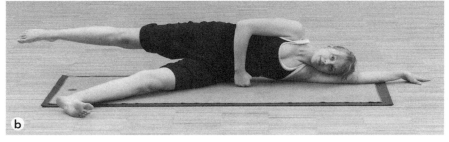

SPINE STRETCH FORWARD

The spine stretch forward is useful for improving sitting posture. Additionally, it teaches participants to automatically contract the abdominal muscles whenever the spine is rounded so that the spine is protected during unsupported forward flexion (technically, if the abdominal muscles are securely lifted and contracted, the spine is no longer unsupported). The ability to articulate the spine and keep the spine supple is a further benefit of this exercise.

CUES   Sit with your legs straight out in front, your feet hip-width apart, and your ankles dorsiflexed. Lengthen your legs through your heels. Start with ideal, neutral sitting alignment, with your pelvis, spine, scapulae, and neck all in neutral. Your weight should be directly on the sitting bones (your tailbone should be slightly off the floor), and your hips should form a 90° angle. The shoulders are flexed, also at a 90° angle, and parallel to the floor (*a*). Reach long in front with the fingers. Exhaling, start to move into spinal flexion, head and neck first, articulating the spine from the top down. While forcing the air out of the lungs, keep pulling in with the abdominal muscles, feeling as if they are lifting in and up behind the rib cage and as if you are curving over a bar without allowing your belly to touch it (*b*). Inhale and sequentially return the spine back to neutral, once again finding ideal sitting alignment. Repeat 5 to 8 times.

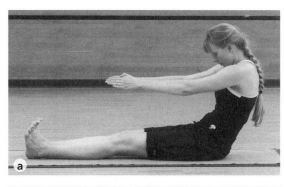

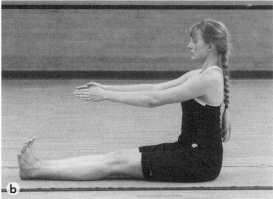

SEATED SPINE TWIST

Most people in developed countries are sedentary, and it is ironic that few actually sit correctly. The seated spine twist can help correct improper sitting because it develops core stability and stamina in the seated position as well as promotes mobility in spinal rotation. Since this exercise requires a person to have adequate hamstring flexibility in order to sit in 90° of hip flexion, it will be difficult for some participants. Modifications include sitting on a pillow, a blanket, or the edge of a mat, or simply sitting cross-legged or bending the knees.

CUES Sit with the legs together and straight out in front and the ankles dorsiflexed. Lengthen the legs through the heels. Start with ideal sitting alignment, with the pelvis, spine, scapulae, and neck all in neutral. Your weight should be directly on your sitting bones (your tailbone should be slightly off the floor) and your hips should form a 90° angle. Lift up through the crown of the head and maintain the longest spine possible throughout the exercise. Abduct the shoulders out to the sides at a 90° angle so that your chest is open and lifted and your shoulder blades are down and back (*a*). Exhale and rotate your spine to the right (*b*); pulse to the right 3 times (perform a short exhale on each), sitting taller and taller with each pulse. Inhale and return to center. Exhale and repeat the twist with pulse to the left. Perform 3 to 5 repetitions per side.

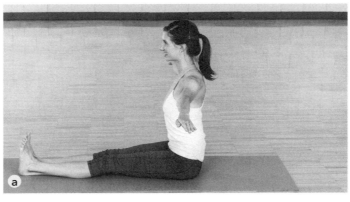

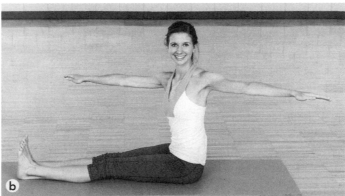

PLANK AND LEG-PULL FRONT

Participants may be familiar with the plank from traditional muscle conditioning because a full plank is required in order to do a proper push-up. The plank, push-up, and variations of the two, such as the leg-pull front, are also part of Joseph Pilates' original repertoire of exercises. These exercises require a considerable amount of core stability because gravity tends to pull the spine, pelvis, and scapulae out of alignment. Dozens of variations of the plank and push-up exist. Two of the most common variations of the plank are the forearm plank (weight is on forearms and toes) and the knee-down plank (weight is on knees and hands). Both are good variations for novice exercisers since they are generally easier to perform correctly.

CUES Start on your hands and knees. Place your pelvis, spine, scapulae, and neck in neutral and your hands directly below your shoulders. Maintaining the neutral position, extend the legs back into a full plank position (*a*); hollow the abdomen. Hold the position and take several even breaths (breathe with the rib cage) without letting the abdomen release. To perform the leg-pull front, maintain the plank position while extending the right leg (keep knee straight and ankle dorsiflexed) up and away from the floor (*b*). Exhale, point the toes, and slowly lower the leg to the floor. Repeat with the opposite leg, alternating legs 3 to 5 times.

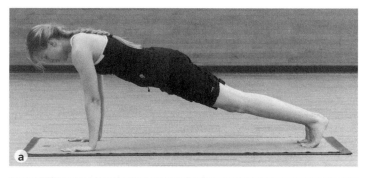

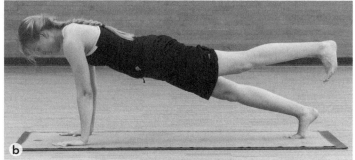

Practice Drill

Start by performing a warm-up appropriate for a Pilates class. Then practice demonstrating and cueing five of the exercises described in this chapter. Pay special attention to incorporating the many alignment and image cues that are so important in teaching Pilates.

Chapter Wrap-Up

The Pilates method of exercise has become popular for both group exercise and personal training. This chapter covered the basic principles of Pilates exercise, such as the powerhouse and the neutral spine, as well as control, concentration, precision, proper breathing, imprinting, and abdominal hollowing. We also reviewed the major research findings on Pilates, provided suggestions for a warm-up, covered major technique and safety issues, and discussed elements of cueing that are unique to Pilates. We detailed 10 basic Pilates exercises and suggested drills for Pilates practice. It is our hope that this chapter motivates you to learn more about this valid method of exercise and to go on to become a certified Pilates instructor.

Group Exercise Class Evaluation Form: Key Points

Pilates does not have a cardiorespiratory component.

- Provide rehearsal moves. Focus on postural symmetry; breath control; abdominal strength; and stabilization of the spine, pelvis, and shoulder. Rehearse any movements that you might introduce in class that day. Rather than warming up and stretching individual muscle groups, review and perform specific Pilates movements for the first 5 to 8 minutes of class. Concentrate on joint mobility and imprinting the spine. Teach neutral spine and breathing throughout the class and not just during the warm-up segment.
- Give verbal cues on posture and alignment. Every movement in Pilates requires appropriate cues on posture and alignment. Focus on lengthening the movements to increase flexibility.
- Encourage and demonstrate good body mechanics. Pilates movements require visual demonstration by the instructor. Make sure all your demonstrations are appropriate and emphasize proper progressions.
- Observe participants' form and suggest modifications for participants with injuries or special needs as well as progressions for advanced participants. Walk around the room after giving a visual demonstration of the movement to observe participants and make sure they are performing the exercise appropriately with correct posture and alignment.
- Use music appropriately. Light background instrumental music or no music at all is appropriate for Pilates classes. Keep the volume low so you can also keep your voice low, calm, and soothing.
- Emphasize relaxation and stretching in the last few minutes of class. Stretch individual muscle groups and focus on relaxation at the end of a Pilates class.

ASSIGNMENTS

1. Look up 3 to 4 Pilates certifications and training programs. Write a 1-page paper on which certification you prefer. Justify your opinion with research and practice methods outlined in this chapter.
2. Prepare to teach a short warm-up and five or more basic Pilates exercises to a small group of participants. Be prepared to use as many cues as possible.

Alternative Modalities in Group Exercise

Chapter Objectives

By the end of this chapter, you will be able to

- create client-centered group exercise classes;
- design classes for niche markets;
- develop lifestyle-based physical activity classes, such as walking, in-line skating, and pedometer programs;
- investigate dance-style classes, such as ballet barre, NIA, Zumba, and hip-hop classes;
- design equipment-based classes such as rebounding, trekking, circuit style, TRX training, and BOSU balance training;
- understand how to develop fusion and mind–body group fitness classes; and
- apply ethical practice guidelines for group fitness instructors.

Background Check

Before working your way through this chapter, do the following:

Read

- ☐ Chapter 3, Review "The Group Exercise Class Evaluation" section.
- ☐ Chapter 6, the sections titled "Designing a Warm-Up" and "Evaluating Stretching in the Warm-Up,"
- ☐ Chapter 7, "Cardiorespiratory Training," and
- ☐ Chapter 8, "Muscular Conditioning and Flexibility Training."

Group Exercise Class Evaluation Form Essentials

Key Points for Warm-Up Segment

- Includes appropriate amount of dynamic movement or rehearsal moves
- Provides dynamic or static stretches for at least two major muscle groups
- Provides intensity guidelines for warm-up
- Uses movements that are at an appropriate tempo and intensity

Key Points for Conditioning Segment

- Gradually increases intensity
- Uses a variety of muscle groups
- Minimizes repetitive movements
- Observes participants' form and provides constructive, nonintimidating feedback
- Continually offers modifications, regressions, progressions, and alternatives
- Provides alignment and technique cues
- Gives motivational cues
- Educates participants about intensity; pro-
- vides HR or RPE check 1 or 2 times during the workout stimulus
- Promotes participant interaction and encourages fun
- Provides regular demonstrations and participation with good body mechanics
- Uses appropriate music volume and tempo that encourage proper movement patterns and progressions
- Gradually decreases impact and intensity during cool-down

Key Points for Cool-Down, Stretch, and Relaxation Segment

- Includes static stretching for major muscles worked
- Demonstrates using proper alignment and technique
- Observes participants' form and offers modifications, regressions, progressions, and alternatives
- Provides alignment cues
- Appropriately emphasizes relaxation and visualization
- Ends class on a positive note and thanks class

The group exercise field is constantly changing. Having the skills to update class formats both safely and effectively is essential for group exercise leaders. In this chapter we detail how to create new formats for group exercise; then we close with an overview of the ethical guidelines and standards for group fitness instructors. Group exercise is a diverse field with many teaching options. We recommend that you become skilled in teaching at least one of the mainstream modalities, such as basic cardio training, boot camp, step, kickboxing, sport conditioning, functional training, yoga, Pilates, indoor cycling, or water exercise, as well as be competent at instructing muscular conditioning and flexibility training classes. After you have achieved a secure foundation in these formats, you may want to expand your employment opportunities and increase your marketability

by developing the skills to create and teach additional exercise modes, such as some of the specialty classes that are described in this chapter. To lead specialty classes, you may need further training and education, or you may just need some creative energy to put a few class segments together. We refer to the Group Exercise Class Evaluation Form both at the beginning and at the end of this chapter to remind you of the basic principles for teaching a safe and effective class.

Creating a Client-Centered Group Exercise Class

As discussed in chapter 1, group exercise has evolved from just a few formats to weekly offerings of 20 to 30 different classes on some program schedules. What started out as aerobic dance has turned into an enjoyable movement experience involving group dynamics, music, and fun. Given the continual rise in obesity, intentional exercise is here to stay. As fitness professionals, it is our job to keep people excited about moving and help them gain much more than fitness when they work out. People who have a sense of purpose for their movement are much more likely to continue being physically active. People are often busy, and movement experiences can provide them with a way to connect with others and create a sense of community. Sallis and colleagues (2006) believe that multilevel interventions, which they refer to as an ecological model, must be achieved in order to make population-based changes in physical activity levels.

Over the years, we have witnessed group exercise activities broaden outside the four walls of a gym or facility. Creating client-centered group exercise classes has assisted with this growth. People want to get outside more, dance more, and have more fun in their lives. Many of the modalities we discuss in this chapter do not require a fitness center; they are actually community outreach efforts similar to the ecological model Sallis and colleagues (2006) describe in the public health approach to improving physical activity patterns. Everyone needs and seeks more fulfilling movement experiences in their lives. Group exercise classes that help participants meet others with similar interests, and that enable participants to discuss their lives and health, create a unique exercise experience. For example, a group exercise class for breast cancer survivors has much more going on than just exercise. It allows participants to connect with others who have experienced a life change due to breast cancer. Holmes and colleagues (2005) studied breast cancer survivors and found that walking 3 to 5 hours per week reduced death rates from the disease by almost 50%. Their study did not find that increasing the energy expenditure (i.e., increasing the exercise intensity) provided any additional benefits. It appeared to be the regular adherence to exercise that helped these participants survive cancer. Now that is a sense of purpose for exercise! This type of client-centered exercise program is simple to create but makes a huge difference

in the lives of those who attend. Forming focus groups to discover the needs of your clients, as well as keeping up on the research literature on the benefits of physical activity, will help you get ideas for client-centered exercise groups you might like to form.

Group Exercise for Niche Markets

Let's look at some other potential niche markets for group exercise. For example, many fitness professionals are targeting new mothers as exercise participants who could use camaraderie and support during their life transition into motherhood. Until 2000, classes for new moms were hard to find, but today stroller-based exercise programs are on the rise (Asp 2006). Baby Boot Camp, StrollerFit, and Stroller Strides are only a few of the new group exercise classes that promote engaging in outdoor activity with babies. These classes are held either indoors or outdoors in neighborhoods and provide a 60- to 75-minute workout combining all the health-related components of fitness. These classes average from 5 to 15 participants and are held in more than 150 locations in many U.S. states. They are a wonderful way to get new mothers to interact with one another and enjoy a movement experience together. Most participants stay in the program until their children are around 3 years old. These mother-and-child programs, which are franchises that can be started by any fitness professional, are included in the "Key Internet Search Phrases for Other Modalities" list toward the end of this chapter.

Another niche class that has gained popularity is a postpartum class in which babies are involved directly with the exercise experience. Davies (2006) described a class called *Baby Steps* in which the mother and baby work out together. This type of class is often called a *mommy and me* program (for more information, see the "Key Internet Search Phrases for Other Modalities" list later in this chapter). The format is usually strength based, with the new moms using their babies as weights, rather than holding a dumbbell or a resistance tube. A class such as this can be a rich experience in so many ways. Mothers avoid the guilt of leaving their children in order to go exercise, and families don't have to pay for day care. Babies seem to love the interaction and attention, while the moms get a wonderful experience with their children and simultaneously get a good workout. And this form of exercise is definitely functional training since the mothers become fit using the weight they carry around all day—their babies.

Another creative example of a niche market program is a class that combines the enjoyment of music with physical movement. This class, which is based on basic conducting techniques, is called *Conductorcise*. The inventor is a retired conductor, David Dworkin, who played clarinet for the American Symphony Orchestra. He suggests that Conductorcise is a good workout, especially for the upper body (Gerard 2006). He also believes the class improves the listening skills of participants and teaches them about the lives and works of great composers. Many musicians are sedentary due to the nature of their activity. Yet they love listening to and learning about music. Thus, this mode of exercise can bring a whole new group of participants— musicians—to the exercise experience.

As exercise instructors, we know there are clients out there whom we are missing, and so we need to be creative when coming up with new movement experiences. Keller (2008) outlines several ideas that have brought energy to group exercise. There's drop-in dodgeball, a game that is held on a basketball court and resembles the dodgeball game played by children. Or there's stadium stompers, a class whose participants use the stairs of an outdoor football stadium to enhance their fitness. Finally, there is the breakfast club, a senior fitness class that combines all the components of fitness with an opportunity to eat breakfast and socialize at the facility's café. All of these programs are client centered and involve not only a fitness component but also a meaningful life experience. This is what creating niche markets in group exercise is all about.

Lifestyle-Based Physical Activity Classes

Aside from the outdoor classes just discussed (StrollerFit, stadium stompers, and so on), there are several lifestyle group exercise opportunities

that focus on getting exercise into daily life as a means to help people accomplish their physical activity goals. Many experts believe that public health and fitness professionals need to work together to get people to be more active in their general lives and not just in fitness facilities. Church and coworkers (2011) showed that during the last 50 years in the United States, there has been a progressive decrease in the percent of individuals employed in occupations that require moderate intensity physical activity. Van der Ploeg and colleagues (2012) demonstrated a dose-response association between sitting time and mortality from all causes and between sitting time and cardiovascular disease , independent of leisure-time physical activity. It is clear that we can no longer assume people are active outside the typical group exercise experience. As Hooker (2003 p. 10) states, "Collaboration between public health experts and fitness professionals is not new, but the opportunities for such collaboration are expanding, especially at the community level, and are essential to stem the rising tide of sedentary living and its associated risks for many chronic diseases and conditions."

Pedometer Walking Programs

Several fitness professionals have started group pedometer training classes. A pedometer is a device that is worn on the hip and measures how many steps are taken in a day; it helps give the user an idea of daily activity levels. Some facilities give pedometers to all members, especially those members who are interested in moving outside the organized exercise session. Working out in a facility builds fitness, but a workout a few times a week does not necessarily expend enough energy to create a large caloric deficit. Everyday movement is also needed to reach and maintain a healthy weight.

This is an important concept for fitness professionals to model for our class participants. Increasing movement in our own activities of daily living, as well as providing programs that help participants measure their activity levels outside the fitness facility, is key to reducing sedentary living. Online pedometer recording and a 6-week pedometer competition program are group activities that allow participants to have more movement experiences throughout the day but still support and talk to one another if desired. An online lifestyle-based physical activity program can provide a means for participants to record activity, communicate with others, set up walking meetings, or just chat about walking opportunities and issues. Technology devices such as the Fitbit (www.fitbit.com) or the Jawbone (www.jawbone.com) are computerized devices that contain accelerometers that access movement and sleep patterns. They also contain a way to log food choices. These technology devices are more expensive than pedometers but are becoming more common for monitoring lifestyle choices. Programs that allow participants to monitor their lifestyle habits in a group setting may be added to a group exercise offerings in the future. More group exercise programs involve going to the person versus having the person come to a facility. Consider having your program reach out to local communities and perform a pedometer or lifestyle interactive group program using movement tracking devices as an outreach activity to remove the participant barrier of having to drive to a specified place for a movement experience.

An example of a lifestyle-based physical activity program in the United States is the President's Challenge (www.presidentschallenge.org), which includes the Presidential Active Lifestyle Award that recognizes children for their regular participation in physical activity; they can receive a presidential emblem and a certificate signed by the U.S. president. For this program, participants engage in physical activity for at least 60 minutes or take 10,000 steps each day, 5 days per week, for 6 weeks. Creating a similar program allows fitness instructors to demonstrate concern for participants by educating them that physical activity happens not just in a facility or in a group exercise class, but also in daily life.

Outdoor Walking and In-Line Skating

People often rank walking as their number one sport and recreational activity, and so leading a walking class can be a great way to expand your teaching options. A walking class ought to include a warm-up and cool-down with plenty of stretching. Many instructors also include

drills such as walking backward or sideways, or incorporate interval training. Some even provide strength training stations along the walking route for circuit-type muscular conditioning (this is also known as a parcourse). It's ideal to lead a walking class with two instructors, one as the leader in front and one as the shepherd in back. In this way the class can accommodate participants of varying fitness levels, and participants can walk at the appropriate speed. Various walking devices may be used to increase the intensity (Porcari 1999). These include weighted vests, hand weights or weighted gloves, trekking poles, and power belts (a belt worn around the waist that provides resistance cords with handles). Another way to increase intensity is power walking, or power striding, a high-intensity version of walking that uses more vigorous upper-body movements and some hip rotation (see figure 17.1). Regardless of participants' walking speed, encourage your class members to walk with good technique: head and neck in neutral, eyes looking ahead, arms and hands relaxed, each step rolling from heel to toe, knees soft, pelvis in neutral. Having class meetings at a park or walking trail to help participants experience a new setting also allows participants to understand that exercise doesn't necessarily have to occur in a gym. Our goal as fitness educators is to introduce participants to as many experiences for movement as possible; ultimately, we want them to be successful at creating movement opportunities on their own. Having your class meet at various places can introduce community resources to participants and thus broaden their scope of physical activity opportunities.

 See online video 17.1 for a demonstration of a group walking class.

In-line skating is another lifestyle-based group exercise option. It has been shown to be an appropriate form of exercise for improving cardiorespiratory fitness (Melanson et al. 1996). However, instructors who want to lead in-line skating classes need to have proper training, use appropriate locations (e.g., an empty parking lot), require proper equipment (e.g., skates, helmets, wrist guards, elbow and knee pads), and promote safety and fun!

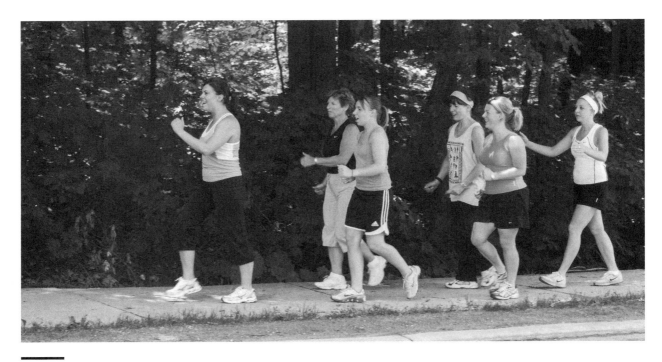

FIGURE 17.1   An outdoor walking class, showing a power walking variation.

Dance-Based Classes

Several dance-based classes have found their way into the group exercise setting. Many people who once danced on a high school dance team or took dance lessons as children find that moving to music is what they enjoy doing most for their daily physical activity. An example of such a program is a cheer–dance class offered on a college campus. For this class, a college cheerleader or dance group member taught all the routines performed during the school fight song and movements used during the half-time show. Participants came to the cheer-dance class wanting to learn these movements. They enjoyed the movement experiences and often commented that it did not feel like exercise because they were enjoying the dance routines. Tharrett and Peterson (2012) discussed how the Los Angeles Sports Club offered a class based on the dance movements and routines of the Los Angeles Lakers cheerleaders. Such a class is an example of using the client-centered approach to reach individuals who enjoy dance. There are several other dance formats used for dance-style group exercise that we will review in this chapter, including NIA, Latin dance, hip-hop,

disco, country dancing, Zumba, and ballet barre. Williams (2012) predicts that any group exercise class with a dance component will continue to be popular.

NIA (neuromuscular integrative action) is a group exercise modality that incorporates freestyle modern and ethnic dance, tai chi, martial arts, and yoga. It combines a cardiorespiratory stimulus with increased mind–body awareness, blending elements of Eastern and Western philosophies. According to Rosas and Rosas (2006), a typical NIA class is part choreographed movement, with students following the instructor's lead, and part freestyle movement, with participants dancing as if no one were watching. Dancing with partners or dancing in lines, circles, and rows may be used to vary the group dynamics. A variety of music styles are included—new age, funk, Latin, rock, rhythm and blues, and jazz—and the music tempo varies from song to song, depending on the instructor's plan. Shoes are off, impact is reduced, and participants are encouraged to express themselves. A major objective of NIA is to help participants become more internally directed in their physical expressions, listen to their bodies, and move in ways that are holistic, pleasurable, and joyful.

Zumba classes have become especially popular around the world; the 2013 American College of Sports Medicine (ACSM) "Worldwide Survey of Fitness Trends" listed Zumba twelfth on a list of the top 20 fitness trends (Thompson 2012). Zumba is a Latin-inspired, dance-fitness class—also known as a Zumba Fitness-Party (Perez, Robinson, and Herlong 2011). Since it is a branded, copyrighted program, instructors must obtain a license from Zumba Fitness in order to use the Zumba name. Part of the reason Zumba appeals to so many participants is because every effort is made to create a party-like atmosphere that is fun, easy, and effective. Interestingly, Zumba instructors are not taught anticipatory cueing and are encouraged to keep all verbal cueing at a minimum in order to promote the dance-party vibe. Unfortunately, this may lead to some participants feeling less successful since new moves are shown without warning and feelings of clumsiness may result, not to mention that participants may run into each other with the sudden changes of direction. We would like to see more Zumba instructors master the skill of anticipatory cueing. Little research has been done on Zumba, despite claims of extremely high caloric expenditures. One study has shown the energy cost to be approximately 7 kilocalories per minute, or about 350 to 400 kilocalories per hour, depending on the length of the warm-up and cool-down and on the sequencing of the moves (Otto et al. 2011). Another study reported caloric expenditures of approximately 9.5 kilocalories per minute (Luettgen et al. 2012). In any event, Zumba purports to be "exercise in disguise," and the organization states that over 6 million people take Zumba classes each week—it is definitely a phenomenon that we recommend you experience.

 See online video 17.2 for a demonstration of a Zumba class.

Many clubs also offer specialty classes in other dance styles such as generic Latin dance, funk, hip-hop, or country. Kahn (2008) states that people are growing bored with traditional fitness classes and enjoy dancing and learning new movements they can use when they go out

dancing for fun. Many of the dance styles used in group exercise classes come with specific moves or dance steps. Latin moves, for example, include those of the samba, rumba, merengue, cha-cha, lambada, cumbia, salsa, calypso, and mambo. Country moves include the swivel, hip bump, tush push, and boot scoot; these moves are frequently arranged into line dances and can be readily adapted for cardiorespiratory classes (Lane 2000). Funk and hip-hop styles are performed to downbeat-centered music and combine upper-body isolations and many familiar dance moves such as the step touch, march, jazz square, and plié with African and street stylizations and complex rhythmic patterns.

 See online video 17.3 for a demonstration of a hip-hop class.

 See online video 17.4 for a demonstration of a Latin dance class.

A few clubs offer ballet barre or other dance-based classes fused with traditional fitness elements. Class content varies depending on the instructor's background and skills and can include muscular conditioning exercises performed at the barre, traditional cardio or jazz dance in the center of the room, Pilates exercises, and dance-based stretches. Barre work can consist of traditional fitness moves, such as standing hip abduction, hip adduction, extension work, lunges, and squats, or ballet moves, including the plié, relevé, tendu, battement, frappé, rond de jambe, and port de bras. Center work might include traditional high-low impact moves or ballet moves such as turns, pirouettes, jumps, and choreographed routines. In these types of classes, care should be taken to modify the high-risk dance moves to make them appropriate for the general population. Moves such as the full port de bras, grand plié, and cervical hyperextension are risky for the neck, back, and knees and are not appropriate for deconditioned adults desiring health-related fitness. As always, a dance-based class should provide a proper warm-up and a sufficient cool-down, including flexibility work.

Equipment-Based Cardiorespiratory and Strength Training

Equipment-based cardio and strength training in group exercise classes involves the use of cardiorespiratory equipment such as treadmills, rowing machines, Krankcycles, or mobile strength equipment such as a cable-column machine or TRX suspension devices. Popular programs using one or more of these modalities have been developed by innovative instructors at several facilities (Nichols, Sherman, & Abbott 2000; Pillarella 1997). Williams (2012) reviews strength training in prechoreographed programs such as Les Mils BodyPump or programs such as BODYVIVE and Zumba Toning. Strength-training freestyle programs may include TRX suspension training, ViPR (Vitality, Performance & Reconditioning) training, and metabolic conditioning—which can be a combination of cardio and strength. The steps involved in instructing an equipment-based cardio- and strength-conditioning class are fairly simple:

1. Make certain you understand how to set up the machines, including how to use the instrument panel (if any) and how to adjust the machine to each individual.

2. Learn how to demonstrate and teach proper biomechanics, alignment, and technique on the machines.

3. Design a physiologically sound class format.

An appropriate class format adheres to the points outlined in the group exercise class evaluation form and includes a warm-up (usually performed on the machine), a cardio conditioning segment, and a cool-down after the cardio segment. Some instructors move the class into another room for muscular conditioning or stretching after the cardio segment, although this is not necessary. Many equipment-based classes incorporate interval training, which can be adjusted to match all fitness levels (see table 17.1). Remember that participants will need instruction regarding appropriate intensity levels during the intervals. In general, you can encourage your class to work at an RPE that is moderate to somewhat hard during the easier intervals, and hard during the harder intervals (see chapter 7 for more on using RPE to monitor intensity).

In a treadmill (trekking) class, participants can walk or run, depending on their fitness levels. If participants want to increase the intensity, they can increase the treadmill speed, elevation, or both. You might play motivating music in the background using a song with an appropriate beat for movement, offering your class the option of walking or running on the beat (see figure 17.2).

 See online video 17.5 for a demonstration of a treadmill class.

TABLE 17.1   Sample Equipment-Based Class

Workout segment	Duration (min)	Intensity
Dynamic warm-up and stretching	5-8	Light
Introduction to modality	3	Light
Practice modality use	5	Moderate
Cardio or strength interval training	5	Moderate to hard
Recovery	2	Light
Cardio or strength steady work	5	Moderate
Cardio or strength interval training	5	Hard
Cardio or strength steady work	5	Moderate
Cardio or strength interval training	5	Moderate to hard
Cool-down and stretching	5	Light

Slide and Glider Training

Another cardiorespiratory modality for group exercise is slide training, also known as *lateral-movement training.* The slide workout provides an aerobic workout that compares with high-low impact, step, and cycling in terms of caloric expenditure (Ludwig et al. 1994; Williford et al. 1993). Slide training involves lateral (side-to-side) motion and trains the body's systems in the frontal plane, which can be useful in many sports. Tennis, skating, skiing, basketball, and football all require the ability to move laterally and maintain lateral stability around the joints. Slide training is low impact, enhances balance and agility, and injects variety into group exercise.

Specially designed boards, known as *slide-boards,* and special booties that fit over the shoes are required for slide training. Most slideboards used in the fitness setting are 6 feet (1.8 m) long and have end ramps that stop the participant from sliding off the ends. The workouts can resemble athletic training (performed without

music or without following the beat) or can be choreographed to music with combinations and the 32-count phrase discussed in chapter 4. There are two basic stances on the slideboard: the upright stance and the athletic ready stance (which is more difficult and resembles the position of a speed skater). Possible moves on the slideboard include cross-country skiing and speed skating as well as the basic slide, slide touch, knee lift, hamstring curl, fencing slide, lunge, and slide squat. All of these can be accompanied by a variety of arm movements (see figure 17.3*a*). Appropriate music speeds for slide training are 124 to 140 beats per minute. A warm-up that includes rehearsal moves on the slideboard and a cool-down that stretches the muscles used in lateral training (especially the hip abductors and adductors) are essential.

Another form of slide training that may be easier to incorporate into a group exercise class (because the equipment is less expensive and less bulky) is gliding, using a device called the *gliding disc.* Gliding discs are slippery, flat, round devices that are placed under the feet to

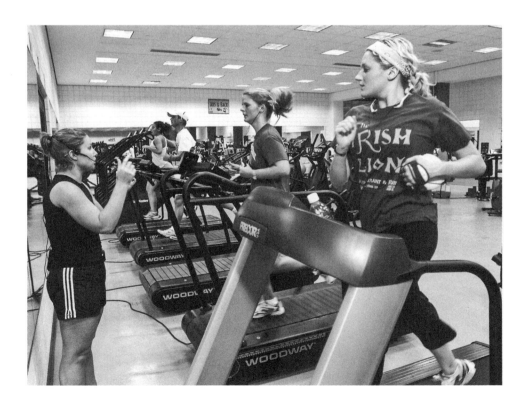

FIGURE 17.2 A group treadmill class.

destabilize the lower body. The movements performed on gliding discs can be similar to those performed on a slideboard; the discs can also be placed under the feet or hands for push-up or plank work, for example (see figure 17.3*b*). Gliding discs are portable and cost around US$10.00 per pair. If slideboards are not in the budget, gliding discs or even paper plates can be used to accomplish some of the same fun, fitness, and core-stabilization exercises possible on a slideboard.

 See online video 17.6 for a demonstration of slide training.

Rebounding

In rebounding, participants exercise on a rebounder, a device that looks like a mini-trampoline. At least one study has shown that rebounding and treadmill exercise produce comparable cardiorespiratory results (McGlone, Kravitz, and Janot 2002). This finding indicates that rebounding meets ACSM criteria for the achievement of aerobic fitness. Rebounding is classified as a low-impact activity and appears to place minimal stress on the joints and connective tissues. Routines choreographed to music (~126 beats per minute) can be created with a

variety of moves such as jumping jacks, twists, and alternating strides (all double-leg moves in which both feet contact the rebounder at the same time) and jogging, knee lifts, and kicks (single-leg moves in which only one foot contacts the rebounder at a time). Rebounding is fun and playful and can provide a challenging workout.

BOSU Balance and Core Board Training

In chapter 8 we discuss the appropriate use of the stability ball in the group exercise setting. Stability balls are a staple in most fitness facilities. They are so popular that many facilities place them in the weight room so participants can use them when working out on their own. Two other destabilizing products are available, as well. They are the core board made by Reebok and the BOSU balance trainer. The core board is sold for around US$150.00 and is a bit more expensive than a stability ball, which generally sells for around US$40.00. Still, some facilities have invested in core boards for their group exercise classes. The idea behind a core board is that it destabilizes the body, so the core experiences a greater challenge. Some instructors use the board for a combination cardio and strength class, while others use it in a strength-oriented class.

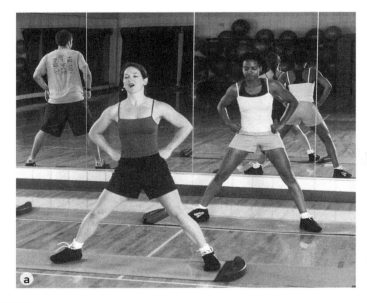 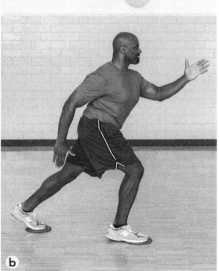

FIGURE 17.3 (*a*) Slideboard basic slide movement and (*b*) cross-country movement using gliding discs.

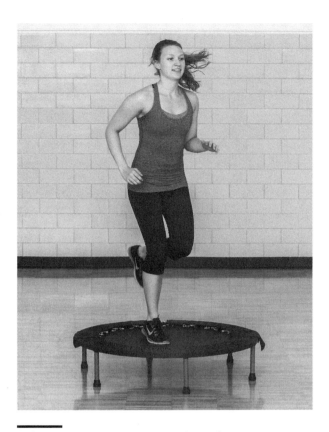

FIGURE 17.4 Jogging on a rebounder.

Webb (2006) states that the board is designed to respond dynamically to a user's movements. The core board may have been ahead of its time, as balance and proprioception (neuromotor fitness) have recently been added to the health-related fitness components of the ACSM guidelines.

The BOSU balance trainer is similar to the core board, costing US$120.00 to US$150.00, and has a rounded, pliable, rubber dome with a solid, flat base. Newcomers may find the BOSU intimidating because staying on it does require a great deal of balance (Webb 2005), and having to balance and move the body as a unit can be overwhelming at first. However, many exercises are possible on a BOSU balance trainer, including cardio movements such as jumps, hops, and traditional step aerobic moves, as well as muscular conditioning moves such as squats, lunges, push-ups, bridges, quadrupeds, and abdominal curl-ups. The fitness industry continually invents products that help the fit get fitter, and the BOSU balance trainer and

core board are examples of such products. It's important to note that the BOSU and core board equipment pieces are not recommended for the beginning exerciser.

Hooping

Body hooping is yet another new fitness trend using weighted hoops. These hoops are larger and heavier than the familiar toy hula hoop; at least one study has shown this low-impact modality to have a significant caloric expenditure—approximately 210 calories per 30 minutes of hooping (Holthusen et al. 2011). Fitness hoops can weigh 1 to 4 pounds and therefore can rotate around the body more slowly that the hula hoop, making them easier to control. Hooping is touted as a total-body workout and, according to researchers, is effective at providing a mid- to high-level workout stimulus—besides, it's fun and feels a bit like child's play!

TRX and RIP Training

TRX is a popular body-weight exercise system that uses suspension equipment to promote total-body stability and muscle fitness, mobility, spinal stability, explosive power, and rotational movements. Developed as a way to build and maintain fitness in almost any setting, the TRX device is lightweight, portable, and can be anchored to walls, ceilings, and even tree limbs! Many facilities are designating entire rooms for group TRX programs; multiple TRX devices are generally either anchored into the ceiling or are suspended from a large steel S-frame (the S-frame can hold up to 22 TRX devices). Resistance is provided by the participant's body weight and can be adjusted for most fitness levels by varying the body position to be more or less horizontal or vertical, depending on the exercise. One study (Scheett et al. 2010) found that suspension training elicited lactate and heart rate responses indicative of a moderate-intensity stimulus.

Rip Training, also developed by the TRX company, is a new exercise system that provides a variable, asymmetric load to familiar strength exercises. A special elastic resistance cord is attached to only one end of a bar, exerting a one-sided, unbalanced pull on the bar. To compensate, the participant must use core stabilizer muscles to maintain proper form and alignment. A special free-standing anchoring device can be purchased for use in the group exercise setting; up to 10 Rip Trainers can be attached for challenging group workouts (figure 17.5).

Mind–Body Classes

Tai chi (figure 17.6) and Qigong are practices that promote movement and meditation based on ancient Chinese philosophies. These philosophies are purported to promote mental and physical health, vitality, and functional well-being and are said to cultivate social and spiritual values. Several versions of tai chi exist, but the Yang style is perhaps the most popular and accessible. It encompasses 24 forms, or series of movements. These forms are meant to be practiced daily and can be performed anywhere. In terms of the health-related components of fitness, both Tai Chi and Qigong promote flexibility, balance, muscle endurance, and coordination. They have been advocated as ideal exercises for lifelong well-being, and they may especially appeal to seniors due to their gentle, nonimpact nature. In fact, several studies have shown that tai chi improves balance and reduces falls in the elderly (Lan et al. 1998; Li et al. 2005). The dramatic increase in literature on mind–body movement experiences has yielded information showing that mind–body programs can be effective for treating fibromyalgia (Wang et al. 2010) and migraine headaches (Wahbeh, Elsas, and Oken 2008), reducing anxiety (Hoffmann-Smith et al. 2009), and decreasing stress in the workplace (Wolever et al. 2012); these programs can also be an accepted form of integrative medicine (Walach et al. 2012). Another study (Young et al. 1999) found that aerobic exercise and tai chi had similar effects on reducing blood pressure in older people. Tai chi and qigong encourage the integration of mind, body, and spirit, and, like yoga, focus on bringing the practitioner's attention into the present moment. This principle of mindfulness, as well as the focus on performing slow movements with complete awareness, is a concept that can be applied to other forms of group exercise. Chodzko-Zajko and colleagues (2006) published recommendations that can assist agencies and facilities seeking to develop and implement successful mind–body programs for their clients. These recommendations are worth reviewing before setting up such programs. We predict that as our culture continues to be faster paced and use more types of technology, we will twitter more, answer more e-mails, create more apps,

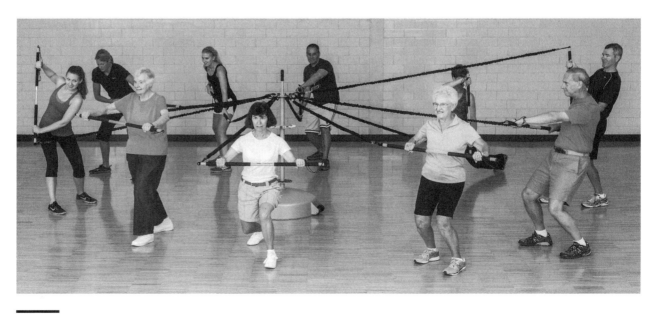

FIGURE 17.5   Group Rip Training.

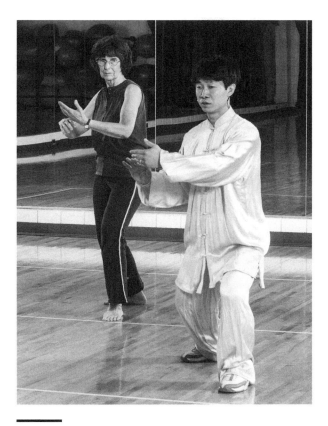

FIGURE 17.6 A group tai chi class.

and be inundated with more information than ever before. Stress relief through mind–body classes will become not only a staple in the group exercise environment but also a necessity for healthy living.

 See online video 17.7 for a demonstration of a Tai Chi class.

Fusion Classes

A continuing buzzword in group exercise classes is *fusion*. A fusion class blends components of exercise. For example, a cardio and core class could be a fusion class in which 20 minutes of cardio is followed by 20 minutes of core strength training. Because people are busy, lack time, and bore easily, fusion classes have been created to provide exercise formats that are more entertaining and efficient. The numbers and types of possible fusion classes are limited only by an instructor's imagination. Popular combi-

nations include Yogilates (yoga plus Pilates); PiYo; yoga tai chi; Spinning plus yoga, ballet and Pilates; outdoor walking followed by muscular conditioning on a stability ball; step intervals interspersed with intervals of Latin dance; and rebounding followed by 20 minutes of stretching. Some group exercise programs offer jump and pump: intervals of jumping rope interspersed with intervals of muscular conditioning. One organization (AFAA [Aerobics and Fitness Association of America] FuzeCraze) is promoting a dance-fusion continuing education workshop in which Bollywood, Irish, African, Latin, and other world dance styles are taught. Freestyle strength circuits are another great way to accomplish a lot of work in a short amount of time. To devise a circuit, set up muscular conditioning stations around the room and have participants rotate through the stations, either individually or in small groups (or pods). When designing fusion classes, be creative; you have an unlimited number of options and people like to have choices!

The word fusion can have different interpretations for fitness professionals. For example, budokon is a blend of yoga, martial arts, and meditation that combines both the mental and the physical aspects of wellness into one group exercise offering. The inventor of budokon does not talk about the health benefits of exercise but rather the human potential and the art of movement (Anders 2006). The word *fusion* does not always mean the combining of two modes of exercise; it can also be used to describe a combination of mind and body movements. This type of fusion brings us closer to calling our profession a *wellness or health profession* rather than an *exercise* or a *fitness profession*.

Ethical Practice Guidelines for Group Fitness Instructors

We want to take a moment to thank the IDEA Health and Fitness Association and the AFAA for providing us with so much of the information collected in this book. Both organizations have led the way in setting practice guidelines and ethical standards for the field of group exercise.

IDEA has outlined ethical practices for group fitness instructors (IDEA 2011), and AFAA has developed basic exercise standards and guidelines for group exercise (AFAA 2010). If you keep these in mind along with the group exercise class evaluation form presented in this book, you will be well on your way to making a difference in the health and wellness of your participants.

Following are IDEA's ethical practice guidelines for group fitness instructors:

1. Always be guided by the best interests of the group while still acknowledging individuals.
2. Provide a safe exercise environment.
3. Obtain the education and training necessary to lead group exercise.
4. Use truth, fairness, and integrity to guide all professional decisions and relationships.
5. Maintain appropriate professional boundaries.
6. Uphold a professional image through conduct and appearance.

AFAA's basic exercise standards and guidelines are presented in chapter 17 of AFAA's *Fitness Theory and Practice* (AFAA 2010). First formulated in 1983, these basic standards and guidelines have been updated periodically based on new research findings. They include basic fitness terminology; the AFAA 5 Questions (an excellent system of exercise analysis); lists and photographs of high-risk exercises and appropriate modifications; detailed descriptions and photographs of proper body alignment; and specific standards and guidelines for warm-up, cardiorespiratory training, muscle strength and endurance training, flexibility training, and the final class segment.

Chapter Wrap-Up

This chapter covered practical techniques for leading a wide variety of group exercise classes. When developing your own class, check yourself against the key points of the Group Exercise Class Evaluation Form provided in this chapter and the IDEA and AFAA practice guidelines and ethical standards to be sure your class meets the basic criteria for each segment. Using the combination of an effective class format, plus information from professional organizations that make it their business to help you be a better group exercise professional, is a good way to become the best professional you can be. Being the finest group exercise professional you can be is important to the health and well-being of your participants. We must all do our best to help participants improve the quality of their lives through a safe, effective group exercise experience based on scientific research, sound principles of instruction, and FUN! For more class content ideas, see the "Key Internet Search Phrases for Other Modalities" for specific exercise formats.

Key Internet Search Phrases for Other Modalities

- Concept Two Rowing
- American Institute of Reboundology
- Urban Rebounding
- Balletone
- International In-Line Skating Association
- Baby Boot Camp
- StrollerFit

- Stroller Strides
- Conductorcise
- Zumba
- Budokon
- Hooping
- National Qigong Association
- NIA
- Tai Chi Network

- Gliding
- TRX training
- Rip Training
- Tabata training
- ViPR Fit
- Krankcycle
- PiYo
- Yogilates

Group Exercise Class Evaluation Form: Key Points

Key Points for Warm-Up Segment

- Includes appropriate amount of dynamic movement and rehearsal moves
- Provides dynamic or static stretches for at least two major muscle groups
- Gives intensity guidelines for warm-up
- Uses movements that are at an appropriate tempo and intensity

Key Points for Conditioning Segment

- Gradually increases intensity
- Uses a variety of muscle groups
- Minimizes repetitive movements
- Observes participants' form and provides constructive, nonintimidating feedback
- Continually offers modifications, regressions, progressions, or alternatives
- Provides alignment and technique cues
- Gives motivational cues
- Educates participants about intensity; provides HR or RPE check at least 1 or 2 times during the workout stimulus
- Promotes participant interaction and encourages fun
- Provides regular demonstrations and participation with good body mechanics
- Uses appropriate movement or music speed
- Gradually decreases impact and intensity during cool-down

Key Points for Cool-Down, Stretch, and Relaxation Segment

- Includes static stretching for major muscles worked
- Demonstrates with good alignment and technique
- Observes participants' form and offers modifications, regressions, progressions, or alternatives
- Gives alignment cues
- Appropriately emphasizes relaxation and visualization
- Ends class on a positive note and thanks class

ASSIGNMENT

Using the Group Exercise Class Evaluation Form in appendix A to record your observations, evaluate (but do not participate in) a unique group exercise class that uses any of the modalities mentioned in this chapter. See yourself as the supervisor of the class instructor and fill in the group exercise evaluation form providing corrective feedback you would give this instructor to help improve the class. After recording what you observe on the form, attach a bullet-point list of the top three things you thought went well and the top three things you felt could use improvement.

Appendix A

Group Exercise Class Evaluation Form

Instructor: _____   Evaluator: _____

Date: _____   Class: _____

Time: _____

Scoring system: 2 = proficient, 1 = adequate, 0 = inadequate

Pre-Class Procedures

- ☐ Begins class on time
- ☐ Introduces self
- ☐ States class format
- ☐ Has equipment and music ready for use
- ☐ Acknowledges class
- ☐ Orients new participants
- ☐ Creates positive atmosphere
- ☐ Dresses appropriately

Comments:

_____

_____

_____

Warm-Up

- ☐ Includes appropriate amount of dynamic movement
- ☐ Provides rehearsal moves
- ☐ Provides dynamic or static stretches for at least two major muscle groups
- ☐ Includes clear cues and verbal directions
- ☐ Uses an appropriate music tempo (120-136 beats per minute) or music that inspires movement

Comments:

_____

_____

_____

Warm-Up

Muscle groups	Warm-up	Stretch
Quadriceps and hip flexors		
Hamstrings		
Calves		
Shoulder joint muscles		
Low-back muscles		

Conditioning Segment

- ☐ Gradually increases intensity
- ☐ Uses a variety of muscle groups (especially hamstrings and abductors)
- ☐ Minimizes repetitive movements
- ☐ Observes participants' form and provides constructive, nonintimidating feedback
- ☐ Continually offers modifications, regressions, progressions, and/or alternatives
- ☐ Provides alignment and technique cues
- ☐ Gives motivational cues
- ☐ Educates participants about intensity; provides HR (heart rate) and/or RPE (rate of perceived exertion) check at least 1 or 2 times during workout stimulus
- ☐ Promotes participant interaction and encourages fun
- ☐ Provides regular demonstrations and participation with good body mechanics
- ☐ Gradually decreases impact and intensity during cool-down after the cardiorespiratory session
- ☐ Uses appropriate volume and music tempo (118-128 beats per minute)

Comments:

_____

_____

_____

Flexibility Training

- ☐ Includes static stretching for major muscles worked and for commonly tight muscles (hip flexors, hamstrings, calves, erector spinae, pectorals, anterior deltoids, upper trapezius)
- ☐ Demonstrates using proper alignment and technique
- ☐ Observes participants' form and offers modifications, regression, progressions, and/or alternatives
- ☐ Provides alignment cues

☐ Appropriately emphasizes relaxation and/or visualization

☐ Uses appropriate movement and/or music tempo

☐ Ends class on a positive note and thanks class

Comments:

_____

_____

_____

Muscle group worked	Strengthening or flexibility exercise	Comments
Upper body		
Lower body		
Torso		

Overall Summary:

_____

_____

_____

_____

_____

_____

_____

_____

_____

_____

_____

_____

_____

_____

_____

_____

Appendix B

Short Health History Form

Name: _____ Date: _____

The following information will be kept strictly confidential and will be utilized only to help make your workout safe. Please check any conditions that may apply to you.

Have you ever been told by a physician that you have or have had any of the following?

YES	NO	
☐	☐	Heart attack
☐	☐	Seizure
☐	☐	Stroke
☐	☐	High Cholesterol levels (>200)
☐	☐	High blood pressure
☐	☐	Abnormal electrocardiogram (EKG)
☐	☐	Cancer
☐	☐	Diabetes
☐	☐	Lung problems
☐	☐	Arthritis
☐	☐	Osteoporosis
☐	☐	Gout

If you are currently taking any prescription or over-the-counter medications, please list them here:

_____

_____

_____

YES	NO	
☐	☐	Do you smoke?
☐	☐	Can you swim?
☐	☐	Do you exercise aerobically three to four times per week?

Do you have any past or current injuries or problems

YES	NO	
☐	☐	Irregular heart beat
☐	☐	Cramping
☐	☐	Low back
☐	☐	Chest pain
☐	☐	Shin splints
☐	☐	Midback
☐	☐	Loss of coordination
☐	☐	Neck
☐	☐	Shoulders
☐	☐	Heat intolerance
☐	☐	Hands
☐	☐	Feet
☐	☐	Dizziness
☐	☐	Hips
☐	☐	Ankles
☐	☐	Fainting
☐	☐	Calves
☐	☐	Knees

I realize that there are risks, including injury and possible death, to all exercise. While every effort will be made to decrease any risk of injury, I take full responsibility for my participation in this class. Knowing that I may participate at my own pace and that I am free to discontinue participation at any time, I will inform the instructor of any problems immediately.

Signature: _____   Date: _____

From Carol Kennedy-Armbruster and Mary M. Yoke, 2014, *Methods of Group Exercise Instruction, 3rd ed.* (Champaign, IL: Human Kinetics).

Appendix C

Long Health History Form

Name: _____

Street address: _____

City, state, zip code: _____

Home and work phone numbers: _____

Date of birth and age: _____

Physicians: _____

Date of last physical: _____

Date of last surgery: _____

Date of last electrocardiogram (EKG): _____

Please list any physician-prescribed drugs or dietary supplements you are taking now.

Drug: _____

Dosage: _____

For: _____

Reactions: _____

Drug: _____

Dosage: _____

For: _____

Reactions: _____

Please list any self-prescribed drugs or dietary supplements you are taking now.

Drug: _____

Dosage: _____

For: _____

Reactions: _____

Drug: _____

Dosage: _____

For: _____

Reactions: _____

If necessary, please list other medications on the back of this page.

Please indicate a yes response to the following questions by placing a check in the space provided.

Have you ever been told by a doctor that you have or have had the following?

YES	NO	
☐	☐	Rheumatic fever
☐	☐	Diabetes
☐	☐	Heart murmur
☐	☐	Lung or pulmonary conditions
☐	☐	Heart or vascular problems
☐	☐	Arthritis
☐	☐	Heart attack
☐	☐	Osteoporosis
☐	☐	Seizure or epilepsy
☐	☐	Gout orhyperuricemia
☐	☐	Stroke
☐	☐	Thyroid disorder
☐	☐	High cholesterol (>200)
☐	☐	Allergies
☐	☐	High blood pressure
☐	☐	Neck problems
☐	☐	High blood triglycerides
☐	☐	Midback problems
☐	☐	Abnormal electrocardiogram (EKG)
☐	☐	Low-back problems
☐	☐	Blood clots or thrombophlebitis
☐	☐	Varicose veins
☐	☐	Cancer

Has anyone in your immediate family (grandparents, parents, brothers, or sisters) had any of the following?

YES	NO	
☐	☐	Heart attack or stroke before the age of 55
☐	☐	High blood pressure
☐	☐	Heart surgery
☐	☐	High blood triglycerides
☐	☐	High cholesterol (>200)
☐	☐	Diabetes

Do you smoke?

☐ Yes

☐ No

If you smoke, how much?

☐ Half a pack or less a day

☐ One pack a day

☐ Two or more packs a day

If you smoke, for how long?

☐ Less than 5 years

☐ Between 5 and 15 years

☐ More than 15 years

What type of exercise do you participate in regularly?

☐ None

☐ Competitive sports

☐ Walking

☐ Outdoor cycling

☐ Jogging

☐ Weightlifting

☐ Running

☐ Dancing

☐ Group exercise (step, kickboxing, indoor cycling)

☐ Rebounding

☐ Swimming or water exercise

☐ Stationary cycling

Other: _____

How many times per week do you participate in the previously listed activities?

- ☐ 1
- ☐ 2
- ☐ 3
- ☐ 4
- ☐ 5
- ☐ 6
- ☐ 7

How much time do you spend at each session?

- ☐ Less than 15 minutes
- ☐ 15 to 20 minutes
- ☐ 20 to 30 minutes
- ☐ 30 to 45 minutes
- ☐ 45 to 60 minutes
- ☐ More than 60 minutes

What word best describes the intensity of your average workout?

- ☐ Very light
- ☐ Light
- ☐ Moderate
- ☐ Hard
- ☐ Very hard
- ☐ Extremely hard

During or after exertion, do you experience any of the following?

YES	NO	
☐	☐	Shortness of breath or wheezing
☐	☐	Vomiting
☐	☐	Side aches or side stitches
☐	☐	Swelling of ankles or hands
☐	☐	Extremely high heart rate
☐	☐	Cramping
☐	☐	Irregular heartbeat
☐	☐	Shin splints
☐	☐	Sharp chest pain

YES	NO	
☐	☐	Arm or neck pain
☐	☐	Dull, aching chest pain
☐	☐	Hip pain
☐	☐	Overall or one-sided weakness
☐	☐	Calf pain
☐	☐	Loss of coordination
☐	☐	Low-back pain
☐	☐	Heat intolerance
☐	☐	Midback pain
☐	☐	Dizziness
☐	☐	Shoulder pain
☐	☐	Mental confusion
☐	☐	Foot or ankle pain
☐	☐	Fainting
☐	☐	Knee pain

What would you like to accomplish through exercise?

_____

_____

_____

I acknowledge that my answers to these questions are true and complete. I will immediately inform the exercise instructor of any changes in my health.

Signature: _____ Date: _____

Appendix D

Informed Consent and Agreement Form

I desire to engage voluntarily at _____ (name of program, club, or agency) to improve my physical fitness.

I know that I am required to fill out a health and lifestyle questionnaire before I begin to exercise. The information obtained from the questionnaire will be used in the following ways:

- To indicate any cardiac risk or other reason why I should not exercise based on the ACSM guidelines
- To determine the need for a physician's evaluation and written approval before I enter the exercise program
- To recommend the types of exercise I should concentrate on to reach my fitness goals and the types of exercises I should avoid

I understand that my participation in the program may not benefit me directly in any way. I realize that the program may help me evaluate my lifestyle, choose the activities I may safely carry out, and increase my quality of life.

I also understand that the reaction of the body to activity cannot always be predicted with complete accuracy. The changes that may occur and are associated with physical activity include, but are not limited to, the following signs and symptoms:

- Abnormal blood pressure or heart rate responses
- Breathlessness
- Chest discomfort
- Muscular or skeletal injury
- Heart attack and death, in very rare instances

I realize my responsibility in recognizing these potential hazards; monitoring myself before, during, and after exercise; and seeking help in the event of injury, if possible. I will attend the orientation session and talk to my personal trainer or exercise instructor to learn how to minimize these potential hazards and what I should do in an emergency. I understand that I can minimize my risk during exercise by following these steps:

- I will give priority to regular attendance.
- I will not withhold any information pertinent to my health from the instructor or supervisor in charge of the program, and I will immediately update my health and lifestyle questionnaire if changes in my medication or status occur.
- I will report any unusual symptoms or problems that I experience before, during, or after exercise.
- I will follow the amounts and types of activities recommended during the orientation session.
- I will not exceed my target heart rate.
- I will not exercise when not feeling well or for 2 hours after eating a large meal, smoking a cigarette, drinking alcohol, or taking over-the-counter medications or street drugs.
- I will cool down slowly after exercise and will not take an extremely hot shower after exercise.
- I will not undertake exercises that I know by my experience or my physician's or therapist's recommendation to be painful or detrimental to me.

I realize that unsupervised exercise done on my own is performed at my own risk, even though I may be following guidelines or recommendations established during this program.

The information obtained from this exercise program will be treated as privileged and confidential and will not be released to any person without my written consent. Information regarding my health and program may be shared with instructors involved in my instruction or physical training. The information obtained also may be used for statistical or scientific purposes, with my right to privacy retained.

I, the undersigned, waive and release _____ (name of program, club, or agency) and its employees, officers, or directors from any and all claims in any way connected with my participation in this program. This agreement is binding on my heirs and executors.

I acknowledge that I have read or heard this document in its entirety and that I fully understand it. I have asked any questions that may have occurred to me and have been answered to my satisfaction.

Signature: _____   Date: _____

Witness: _____   Date: _____

From Carol Kennedy-Armbruster and Mary M. Yoke, 2014, *Methods of Group Exercise Instruction, 3rd ed.* (Champaign, IL: Human Kinetics).

Appendix E

Physical Activity Readiness
Questionnaire - PAR-Q
(revised 2002)

PAR-Q & YOU

(A Questionnaire for People Aged 15 to 69)

Regular physical activity is fun and healthy, and increasingly more people are starting to become more active every day. Being more active is very safe for most people. However, some people should check with their doctor before they start becoming much more physically active.

If you are planning to become much more physically active than you are now, start by answering the seven questions in the box below. If you are between the ages of 15 and 69, the PAR-Q will tell you if you should check with your doctor before you start. If you are over 69 years of age, and you are not used to being very active, check with your doctor.

Common sense is your best guide when you answer these questions. Please read the questions carefully and answer each one honestly: check YES or NO.

YES	NO		
☐	☐	1.	**Has your doctor ever said that you have a heart condition <u>and</u> that you should only do physical activity recommended by a doctor?**
☐	☐	2.	**Do you feel pain in your chest when you do physical activity?**
☐	☐	3.	**In the past month, have you had chest pain when you were not doing physical activity?**
☐	☐	4.	**Do you lose your balance because of dizziness or do you ever lose consciousness?**
☐	☐	5.	**Do you have a bone or joint problem (for example, back, knee or hip) that could be made worse by a change in your physical activity?**
☐	☐	6.	**Is your doctor currently prescribing drugs (for example, water pills) for your blood pressure or heart condition?**
☐	☐	7.	**Do you know of <u>any other reason</u> why you should not do physical activity?**

If you answered

YES to one or more questions

Talk with your doctor by phone or in person BEFORE you start becoming much more physically active or BEFORE you have a fitness appraisal. Tell your doctor about the PAR-Q and which questions you answered YES.

- You may be able to do any activity you want — as long as you start slowly and build up gradually. Or, you may need to restrict your activities to those which are safe for you. Talk with your doctor about the kinds of activities you wish to participate in and follow his/her advice.
- Find out which community programs are safe and helpful for you.

NO to all questions

If you answered NO honestly to <u>all</u> PAR-Q questions, you can be reasonably sure that you can:
- start becoming much more physically active – begin slowly and build up gradually. This is the safest and easiest way to go.
- take part in a fitness appraisal – this is an excellent way to determine your basic fitness so that you can plan the best way for you to live actively. It is also highly recommended that you have your blood pressure evaluated. If your reading is over 144/94, talk with your doctor before you start becoming much more physically active.

DELAY BECOMING MUCH MORE ACTIVE:
- if you are not feeling well because of a temporary illness such as a cold or a fever – wait until you feel better; or
- if you are or may be pregnant – talk to your doctor before you start becoming more active.

PLEASE NOTE: If your health changes so that you then answer YES to any of the above questions, tell your fitness or health professional. Ask whether you should change your physical activity plan.

<u>Informed Use of the PAR-Q</u>: The Canadian Society for Exercise Physiology, Health Canada, and their agents assume no liability for persons who undertake physical activity, and if in doubt after completing this questionnaire, consult your doctor prior to physical activity.

No changes permitted. You are encouraged to photocopy the PAR-Q but only if you use the entire form.

NOTE: If the PAR-Q is being given to a person before he or she participates in a physical activity program or a fitness appraisal, this section may be used for legal or administrative purposes.

"I have read, understood and completed this questionnaire. Any questions I had were answered to my full satisfaction."

NAME _____

SIGNATURE _____ DATE _____

SIGNATURE OF PARENT _____ WITNESS _____
or GUARDIAN (for participants under the age of majority)

Note: This physical activity clearance is valid for a maximum of 12 months from the date it is completed and becomes invalid if your condition changes so that you would answer YES to any of the seven questions.

 © Canadian Society for Exercise Physiology   Supported by: Health Santé Canada Canada

continued on other side...

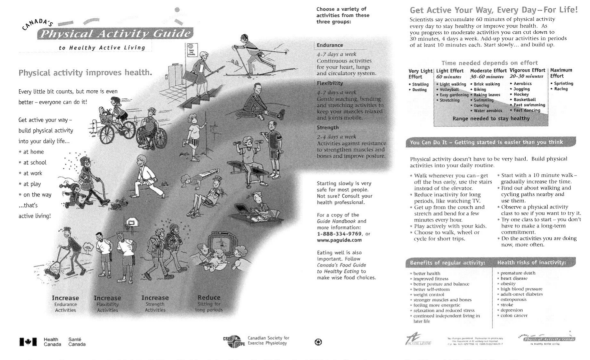

PAR-Q & YOU

Physical Activity Readiness
Questionnaire - PAR-Q
(revised 2002)

Source: *Canada's Physical Activity Guide to Healthy Active Living*, Health Canada, 1998 http://www.hc-sc.gc.ca/hppb/paguide/pdf/guideEng.pdf

© Reproduced with permission from the Minister of Public Works and Government Services Canada, 2002.

FITNESS AND HEALTH PROFESSIONALS MAY BE INTERESTED IN THE INFORMATION BELOW:

The following companion forms are available for doctors' use by contacting the Canadian Society for Exercise Physiology (address below):

The **Physical Activity Readiness Medical Examination (PARmed-X)** — to be used by doctors with people who answer YES to one or more questions on the PAR-Q.

The **Physical Activity Readiness Medical Examination for Pregnancy (PARmed-X for Pregnancy)** — to be used by doctors with pregnant patients who wish to become more active.

References:
Arraix, G.A., Wigle, D.T., Mao, Y. (1992). Risk Assessment of Physical Activity and Physical Fitness in the Canada Health Survey
    Follow-Up Study. **J. Clin. Epidemiol.** 45:4 419-428.
Mottola, M., Wolfe, L.A. (1994). Active Living and Pregnancy, In: A. Quinney, L. Gauvin, T. Wall (eds.), **Toward Active Living: Proceedings of the International
    Conference on Physical Activity, Fitness and Health**. Champaign, IL: Human Kinetics.
PAR-Q Validation Report, British Columbia Ministry of Health, 1978.
Thomas, S., Reading, J., Shephard, R.J. (1992). Revision of the Physical Activity Readiness Questionnaire (PAR-Q). **Can. J. Spt. Sci.** 17:4 338-345.

To order multiple printed copies of the PAR-Q, please contact the:

Canadian Society for Exercise Physiology
202-185 Somerset Street West
Ottawa, ON K2P 0J2
Tel. 1-877-651-3755 • FAX (613) 234-3565
Online: www.csep.ca

The original PAR-Q was developed by the British Columbia Ministry of Health. It has been revised by an Expert Advisory Committee of the Canadian Society for Exercise Physiology chaired by Dr. N. Gledhill (2002).

Disponible en français sous le titre «Questionnaire sur l'aptitude à l'activité physique - Q-AAP (revisé 2002)».

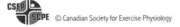 © Canadian Society for Exercise Physiology   Supported by: Health Canada / Santé Canada

Appendix F

Sample Step Warm-Up

The following is an outline of the sample step warm-up found on the accompanying online video. This routine demonstrates

- the appropriate amount of dynamic movement for a step warm-up,
- appropriate rehearsal moves for step, and
- methods to limber and stretch the erector spinae, hamstrings, calves, hip flexors, chest muscles, and anterior shoulder muscles.

TABLE F.1   Teach Block 1

Move	Foot pattern	Number of counts
Grapevine	R, L, R, tap	4
Tap-up, tap-down	Up, tap, down, tap[a]	4
Grapevine	L, R, L, tap	4
Tap-up, tap-down	Up, tap, down, tap[b]	4
Repeat combination		16

R = right; L = left. Keep drilling the combination until participants know it. [a]Lead L off R end of step; [b]lead R off L end of step.

TABLE F.2   Teach Block 2

Move	Foot pattern	Number of counts
March on floor	R, L, R, L	4
March on step	R, L, R, L	4
March on floor	R, L, R, L	4
March on step	R, L, R, L	4

R = right; L = left. Repeat block, adding arms: Pump or shake hands down when marching on floor. Pump hands up, shaking R, L, R, L, when marching on step. Keep drilling this combination until participants know it.

TABLE F.3   Teach Block 3

Move	Foot pattern	Number of counts
Step touch on floor	R, tap, L, tap (repeat)	8
Step touch on step	R, tap, L, tap (repeat)	8
Step touch on floor	R, tap, L, tap (repeat)	8
Step touch on step	R, tap, L, tap (repeat)	8

R = right; L = left. Keep drilling this combination as necessary.

TABLE F.4   Combine Elements of the Blocks to Create a Total Combination

Move	Foot pattern	Number of counts
March on floor	R, L, R, L	4
March on step	R, L, R, L	4
March on floor	R, L, R, L	4
March on step	R, L, R, L	4
Step touch on floor	R, tap, L, tap	4
Step touch on floor	R, tap, L, tap	4
Grapevine R	R, L, R, tap	4
Tap-up, tap-down on step	L, tap, R, tap	4

R = right; L = left.

TABLE F.5   Repeat All Leading Left

Move	Foot pattern	Number of counts
March on floor	L, R, L, R	4
March on step	L, R, L, R	4
March on floor	L, R, L, R	4
March on step	L, R, L, R	4
Step touch on floor	L, tap, R, tap	4
Step touch on floor	L, tap, R, tap	4
Grapevine L	L, R, L, tap	4
Tap-up, tap-down on step	R, tap, L, tap	4

R = right; L = left. Entire combination can be repeated with arms.

TABLE F.6 Incorporate Joint-Specific Limbering and Static Stretches Near Left Corner

Move	Foot pattern	Number of counts
Tap-up, tap-down on step	R, tap, L, tap	4
Wide squat on floor, hands on thighs	Wide for 2, together for 2	4
Tap-up, tap-down on step	R, tap, L, tap	4
Wide squat on floor, hands on thighs	Wide for 2, together for 2	4
Stay in squat position with hands on thighs and rhythmically move in and out of spinal flexion (e.g., neutral spine, spinal flexion, neutral spine, spinal flexion)		16+
Hold in spinal flexion for erector spinae static stretch		8+
Move to L corner of bench; place R heel on bench and hinge at hips for R hamstring stretch; perform ankle dorsiflexion and plantar flexion		8+
Hold static R hamstring stretch		8+
Place R foot completely on step and move into calf-stretch position; perform L ankle limbering with dorsiflexion and plantar flexion (add arms reaching up and down)		8
Hold L calf stretch		8+
Bending L knee, roll L heel up and down, adding rhythmic pelvic tilting (add biceps curls)		8+
Hold L hip flexor stretch (pelvis is posteriorly tilted); simultaneously perform a static chest stretch		8+

R = right; L = left.

TABLE F.7 Transition to Other Side by Performing Initial Combo One Time

Move	Foot pattern	Number of counts
March on floor	R, L, R, L	4
March on step	R, L, R, L	4
March on floor	R, L, R, L	4
March on step	R, L, R, L	4
Step touch on floor	R, tap, L, tap	4
Step touch on floor	R, tap, L, tap	4
Grapevine R	R, L, R, tap	4
Tap-up, tap-down on step	L, tap, R, tap	4

R = right; L = left.

TABLE F.8   Incorporate Joint-Specific Limbering and Static Stretches Near Right Corner

Move	Foot pattern	Number of counts
Tap-up, tap-down on step	L, tap, R, tap	4
Wide squat on floor, hands on thighs	Wide for 2, together for 2	4
Tap-up, tap-down on step	L, tap, R, tap	4
Wide squat on floor, hands on thighs	Wide for 2, together for 2	4
Stay in squat position, alternately press shoulders down toward floor, rotating the upper spine		16
Hold R shoulder down for static stretch, turn head to L		8
Hold L shoulder down for static stretch, turn head to R		8
Move to R corner of bench; place L heel on bench and hinge at hips for L hamstring stretch; perform ankle dorsiflexion and plantar flexion		8+
Hold static L hamstring stretch		8+
Place L foot completely on step and move into calf-stretch position. Perform R ankle limbering with dorsiflexion and plantar flexion (add arms reaching up and down)		8
Move to R corner of bench; place L heel on bench and hinge at hips for L hamstring stretch; perform ankle dorsiflexion and plantar flexion		8+
Hold R calf stretch		8+
Bending R knee, roll R heel up and down, adding rhythmic pelvic tilting (add biceps curls)		8+
Hold R hip flexor stretch (pelvis is posteriorly tilted); simultaneously perform a static chest stretch		8+

R = right; L = left.

From Carol Kennedy-Armbruster and Mary M. Yoke, 2014, *Methods of Group Exercise Instruction, 3rd ed.* (Champaign, IL: Human Kinetics).

Appendix G

Sample Water Exercise Plan

Warm-Up—8 Minutes

- Play "Brilliant Disguise" and "Sneaker Pumps."
- Teach proper posture for using buoyancy belts.
- Review basic total-body movements such as the jog, mall walk, cross-country skier, and rock climber.
- Review the muscle groups and perform movements through full ROM.
- To work the upper back, lift hands in front, thumbs up.
- To work the chest, lift hands out to the sides and horizontally adduct toward the front; use different planes.
- To work the abdominal muscles, move side-to-side and perform the superman or lie in the sun.
- To work the latissimi dorsi, lift the arms out to the sides and adduct them toward the body, action and reaction, move up.
- To work the biceps and triceps, review movement.
- To work the abductors and adductors, perform jumping jacks with full ROM.
- To work the hamstrings and quadriceps, perform the sit kick and the straight-leg raise with the opposite hand and foot for hip flexion or extension.

Hip Joint Exercises—5 to 7 Minutes

- Play Afro Celtic music.
- To work the pectorals and adductors, move into the seated V-position with arms and legs; power the move.
- To work the rhomboids and abductors, stay in the seated V-position and work the arms and legs together.
- To work the pectorals and abductors, stay in the seated V-position (do little traveling).
- To work the rhomboids and adductors, stay in the seated V-position (do little traveling).
- To work the rhomboids and abductors, sit and scissor the arms, legs starting with arms, legs in front.
- To work the adductors and abdominal stabilizers, keep the legs straight and crisscross them with a small ROM.

Upper-Body Segment—7 Minutes

- Play "I Can See Clearly Now" and "Mixica."
- To work the pectorals, mark the movement, move backward, and run against the water resistance.
- To work the upper back, mark the movement, move forward, and flutter kick against the water resistance.
- To work the latissimi dorsi, take advantage of action and reaction and then overload the muscles by not moving the legs at all.

Quadriceps and Hamstrings Knee Flexion and Extension—8 Minutes

- Play "Beautiful Life" and "Born to Run."
- To work the quadriceps and hamstrings, perform sit kicks using knee flexion and extension.
- Lead the participants in the frustrated dolphin by performing upright double-leg curls.
- To work the hamstrings and gluteal muscles, bicycle in a circle and slice the arms out to the side.
- Bicycle in a circle and add overload by opening the hand while circling.
- To work the hamstrings and deltoids, sit in the V-position and flex the heel to the seat.

Interval Training Using Total-Body Movements and Abdominal Work—6 to 8 Minutes

- Perform 30 seconds work followed by 30 seconds rest—watch the big clock. Suggested movements include jogging, the mall walk, the cross-country skier, the rock climber, the latissimi dorsi leap frog, the straight-leg raise with opposite hand and foot, and the jumping jack. Perform all abdominal movements first.
- Depending on participants' feedback, perform 6 to 8 different intervals.

Inertia Current Work—4 Minutes

- Play "Turn Turn Turn."
- Form a circle and jog into the circle.
- Turn around and run against the inertia current.
- Use all four corners to move. Change the movement to a rock climber.

Wall Movements to Cool-Down—4 Minutes

- Play "Secret Garden."
- Perform standing hip rotation exercises.
- Perform standing stretches to stretch the total body.
- Put the feet on the wall for a hamstring and calf stretch.
- Hold the legs in a V-shape and walk side to side on the wall.
- Face into the pool and stretch the shoulders (Titanic move).

Thermal Rewarming—3 Minutes

- Play "Streets of Philadelphia."
- Perform flutter kick using belts on stomach and in front.
- Stand on the belt for balance training.
- Perform your favorite move and then put the equipment away.

From Carol Kennedy-Armbruster and Mary M. Yoke, 2014, *Methods of Group Exercise Instruction, 3rd ed.* (Champaign, IL: Human Kinetics).

References

Chapter 1

American College of Sports Medicine [ACSM]. (2014). *ACSM's guidelines for exercise testing and prescription*. 9th edition. Chapters 7 and 34. Baltimore, MD: Wolters Kluwer/Lippincott Williams & Wilkins.

American Council on Exercise. (2005). What every fitness professional needs to know about the accreditation of certification programs. *Ace Certified News* October-November 20-21.

American Council on Exercise [ACE]. (2010) *Salary survey results*. www.acefitness.org/salary/default. aspx

Astrand, O. 1992. Why exercise? *Medicine Science Sports Exercise,* 24(2): 153-62.

Baicker, K., Cutler, D., Song, Z. (2010). Workplace wellness programs can generate savings. *Health Affairs,* 29(2): 1-8.

Bergeron, M., Nindl, B., Deuster, P., Baumgartner, N., Kane, S., Kreamer, W., Sexauer, L., Thompson, W., O'Connor, F. (2011). Consortium for Health and Military Performance and American College of Sports Medicine consensus paper on extreme conditioning programs in military personnel. *Current Sports Medicine Reports,* 10(6): 383-89.

Blair, S. (2009). Physical inactivity, the biggest public health problem of the 21st century. *British Journal of Sports Medicine,* 43:1-2.

Brathwaite, A., D. Davidson, and J. Eickhoff-Shemek. (2006). Recruiting, training, and retaining qualified group exercise leaders: Part 1. *ACSM Health and Fitness Journal* 10(2): 14-8.

Brown, P., and O'Neill, M. (1990). A retrospective survey of the incidence and pattern of aerobics-related injuries in Victoria, 1987-1988. *Aust J Sci Med Sport* 22(3): 77-81.

Brown, W., Bauman, A., Owen, N. (2009). Stand up, sit down, keep moving: Turning circles in physical activity research? *British Journal of Sports Medicine,* 43: 86-88.

Centers for Disease Control and Prevention [CDC]. (2012). How much physical activity do adults need? www.cdc.gov/physicalactivity/everyone/guidelines/adults.html

Church, T., Thomas, D., Tudor-Locke, C., Katzmarzyk, P., Earnest, C., Rodarte, R., Martin, C. Blair, S., Bouchard, C. (2011). Trends over the 5 decades in U.S. occupation-related physical activity and their associations with obesity. *PLoS ONE* 6(5): e19657. doi:10.1371/journal.pone.0019657

Davidson, D., Brathwaite, A. and Eickhoff-Shemek, J. (2006). Recruiting, training, and retaining qualified group exercise leaders: Part II. *ACSM Health and Fitness Journal* 10(3): 22-26.

DuToit, V., Smith, R., (2001). Survey of the effects of aerobic dance on the lower extremity in aerobic instructors. *Journal of the American Podiatric Medical Association,* 91: 528-32.

Eickhoff-Shemek, J., and S. Selde. (2006). Evaluating group exercise leader performance: An easy and helpful tool. *ACSM Health and Fitness Journal* 10(1): 20-3.

Eller, D. (1996). News + views: Is aerobics dead? *Women's Sports and Fitness* January-February:19-20.

Eriksson, M., Hagberg, L., Lindholm, L., Malmgren-Olsson, E., Osterlind, J., Eliasson, M. (2010). Quality of life and cost-effectiveness of a 3-year trial of lifestyle intervention in primary health care. *Archives of Internal Medicine,* 170(16): 1470-79.

Flegal, K., B. Graubard, D. Williamson, and M. Gail. (2005). Excess deaths associated with underweight, overweight, and obesity. *JAMA* 293(15): 1861-7.

Fonda, J. (1981). *Jane Fonda's workout book.* New York: Simon & Schuster.

Francis, P. (1990). In step with science. *Fitness Management* 6(6): 37-38.

Francis, P., and L. Francis. (1988). *If it hurts, don't do it.* Rocklin, CA: Prima.

Garrick, J., Gillien, D., Whiteside, P. (1986). The epidemiology of aerobic dance injuries. *American Journal of Sports Medicine,* 14(1): 67-72.

Gladwell, M. (2005). *Blink: The power of thinking without thinking.* New York: Time Warner Book Group.

Gregor, P. (2006). Screening with meaning. *IDEA Fitness Journal* October:82-86.

Griffith, S. (2005). Integrate to elevate. *IDEA Fitness Journal* July-August: 39-44.

Hadeed, M., Juehl, K., Elliot, D., Sleigh, A. (2011). Exertional rhabdomyolysis after CrossFit exercise program. *Medicine & Science in Sports& Exercise*, 43(Suppl. 5): S152.

Hagan, M (2005). Group fitness takes center stage: 10 tips for creating a scheduling masterpiece. *IDEA Fitness Manager* March: 12-14.

Healthy People 2020. (2012). www.healthypeople.gov/2020/about/default.aspx

IDEA. (2007). Spanning 25 years: IDEA and fitness industry milestones 1982-2007. *IDEA Fitness Journal* July-August: 24-35.

Jakicic, J., and Otto, A. (2005). Physical activity considerations for the treatment and prevention of obesity. *American Journal Clinical Nutrition* 82(1): 2265-95.

Jazzercise. (2008). Jazzercise company info. www.jazzercise.com/companyinfo.htm.

Johnson, T. (2012) Health care costs and US competitiveness. Council on Foreign Relations. www.cfr.org/health-science-and-technology/health-care-costs-us-competitiveness/p13325

Jones, C., Christensen, C., Young, M. (2000). Weight training injury trends: A 20-year survey. *Physician & Sportsmedicine*, 28(7): 61-72.

Katzmarzyk, P., Church, T., Craig, C., Bouchard, C. (2009). Sitting time and mortality from all causes, cardiovascular disease, and cancer. *Medicine & Science in Sports and Exercise*, 41(5): 998-1005.

Kernodle, R. (1992). Space: The unexplored frontier of aerobic dance. *J Phys Educ Rec Dance* May-June:65-69.

Kerr, Z., Collings, C., Comstock, D. (2010). Epidemiology of weight training-related injuries presenting to United States emergency departments 1990-2007. *American Journal of Sports Medicine*, 38(4): 765-78.

Koszuta, L. (1986). Low-impact aerobics: Better than traditional aerobic dance? *Phys Sportsmed* 14(7): 156-61.

Lee, M., Mather, M. (2012). Population bulletin: U.S. labor force trends www.prb.org/pdf11/aging-in-america.pdf.

Lofshult, D. (2002). Group fitness trend watch 2002. *IDEA Health and Fitness Source* July-August: 69-76.

Malek, M., D. Nalbone, D. Berger, and J. Coburn. (2002). Importance of health science education for personal fitness trainers. *J Strength Cond Res* 16(1): 19-24.

Mutoh, Y., S. Sawai, Y. Takanashi, and L. Skurko. (1988). Aerobic dance injuries among instructors and students. *Phys Sportsmed* 16(12): 81-86.

National Business Group Health. (2011). Survey. http://businessgrouphealth.org/pdfs/2010%20NBGH%20Fidelity%20Employee%20Health%20Survey%20Report_FINAL_Jan2011.pdf

Nelson, M., W. Rejeski, S. Blair, P. Duncan, J. Judge, A. King, C. Macera, and C. Castenada-Sceppa. (2007). Physical activity and public health in older adults: Recommendation from the American College of Sports Medicine and the American Heart Association. *Medicine Science Sports Exercise*, 39(8): 1435-45.

Nogawa-Wasman, D. (2002). How to make group fitness profitable with fee-based programming. *IDEA Health and Fitness Source* May:29-35.

Pate, R., O'Neill, J., Lobelo, F. (2008). The evolving definition of "sedentary." *Exercise and Sport Sciences Reviews*, 36(4): 173-78.

Patel, A., Bernstein, L., Deka, A., Feigelson, H., Campbell, P., Gapstur, S., Colditz, G., Thun, M. (2010). Leisure time spent sitting in relation to total mortality in a prospective cohort of US adults. *American Journal of Epidemiology*, 172(4): 419-29.

Pronk, N., Martinson, B., Kessler, R., Beck, A., Simon, G., Wang. P. (2004). The association between work performance and physical activity, cardiorespiratory fitness, and obesity. *Journal of Occupational Environmental Medicine*, 46(1): 19-25.

Richie, D., S. Kelso, and P. Bellucci. (1985). Aerobic dance injuries: A retrospective study of instructors and participants. *Phys Sportsmed* 13(2): 130-40.

Santana, J. (2002). The four pillars of human movement. *IDEA Personal Trainer* February: 22-8. Schroeder, J. & Donlin, A. (2013). 2013 IDEA Fitness Programs and Equipment Trends Report, *IDEA Fitness Journal*, 10:6, 34-45.

Schuster, K. (1979). Aerobic dance: A step to fitness. *Phys Sportsmed* 7(8): 98-103.

Segar, M., Eccles, J., Richardson, C. (2012). Rebranding exercise: Closing the gap between values and behavior. *International Journal of Behavioral Nutrition and Physical Activity*, 8(94). doi:10.1186/1479-5868-8-94

Seidman, D. (2007). *How: Why how we do anything means everything.* Hoboken, NJ: Wiley & Sons.

Seligman, M. (2011). *Flourish.* New York, NY: Free Press.

Sipes, C., Ritchie, D. (2012). The significant 7: Principles of functional training for mature adults. *IDEA Fitness Journal*, Jan.

Sorenson, J., and B. Bruns. (1983). *Jacki Sorensen's aerobic lifestyle book.* New York: Poseidon Press.

Taylor, W. (2011). Prolonged sitting and the risk

of cardiovascular disease and mortality. *Current Cardiovascular Risk Reports*, 5: 350-57.

Tharrett, S., O'Rourke, F., Peterson, J. (2011*). Legends of fitness.* Monterey, CA: Healthy Learning.

Tharrett, S., Peterson, J. (2012) *Fitness management.* 3rd ed. Monterey, CA: Healthy Learning.

Thompson, W. (2012). Worldwide survey of fitness trends for 2013. *ACSM's Health and Fitness Journal*, 16(6): 8-17.

U.S. Census Bureau. (2012). International database. Table 094. Midyear population, by age and sex. www.census.gov/population/projections.

van der Ploeg, H., Chey, T., Korda, R., Banks, E., Bauman, A. (2012). Sitting time and all-cause mortality risk in 222,487 Australian adults. *Archives of Internal Medicine*, 172(6): 494-500.

Whaley, M. (2003). ACSM credentialing: The more towards formal education. *Health and Fitness Journal* July-August: 31-2.

Whitmer, R., Gunderson, E., Barrett-Connor, E. Quesenberry, C. & Yaffe, K. (2005). Obesity in middle age and future risk of dementia: a 27 year longitudinal population-based study. *British Medical Journal,* 330:1360.

Wolf, C. (2001). Moving the body. *IDEA Personal Trainer* June:23-31.

Chapter 2

Ahmed, C., Wiltonm, W., Pituch, K. (2002). Relations of strength training to body image among a sample of female university students. *Journal of Strength and Conditioning Research*, 16(4): 645-48.

Alan, K. (2003). Building socialization into choreography. *IDEA Fitness Edge*, Sept.: 1-5.

American College of Sports Medicine [ACSM]. (2014). *ACSM's guidelines for exercise testing and prescription.* 9th edition. Chapters 7 and 34. Baltimore, MD: Wolters Kluwer/Lippincott Williams & Wilkins.

Baicker, K., Cutler, D., Song, Z. (2010). Workplace wellness programs can generate savings. *Health Affairs*, 29(2): 1-8.

Bain, L., Wilson, T., Chaikind, E. (1989). Participant perceptions of exercise programs for overweight women. *Research Quarterly*, 60(2): 134-43.

Beals, K. (2003). Mirror, mirror on the wall, who is the most muscular one of all? *ACSM's Health and Fitness Journal*, Mar.-Apr.: 6-11.

Bednarski, K. (1993). Convincing male managers to target women customers. *Working Woman*, June: 23-28.

Begley, S. (2006). How to keep your aging brain fit: Aerobics. *Wall Street Journal*. Nov. 16: D1.

Blair, S. (2009). Physical inactivity, the biggest public health problem of the 21st century. *British Journal of Sports Medicine*, 43:1-2.

Bortz, W. (2003). Prevention: A solution to combat rising health care costs. *ACSM's Health and Fitness Journal*, Nov.-Dec.: 6-8

Bray, S., Gyurcsik, N., Culos-Reed, S., Dawson, K., Martin, K. (2001). An exploratory investigation of the relationship between proxy efficacy, self-efficacy and exercise attendance. *Journal of Health Psychology*, 6(4): 425-34.

Burke, S., Carron, A., Eys, M., Ntoumanis, N., & Estabrooks, P. (2006). Group versus individual approach? A meta-analysis of the effectiveness of interventions to promote physical activity. *Sport and Exercise Psychology Review*, 2(1): 19-35.

Capra, F. (1982). *The turning point*. New York: Bantam Books.

Carron, A., Hausenblas, H., Mack, D. (1996). Social influence and exercise: A meta-analysis. *Journal of Sports Exercise Psychology*, 18: 1-16.

Carron, A., Widmeyer, W., Brawley, L. (1988). Group cohesion and individual adherence to physical activity. *Journal of Sport Exercise Psychology*, 10: 127-38.

Center for Disease Control (CDC) (2008) www.cdc. gov/physicalactivity/everyone/guidelines/index. html.

Clapp, J., Little, K. (1994). The physiological response of instructors and participants to three aerobics regimens. *Medicine & Science in Sports & Exercise*, 26(8): 1041-46.

Claxton, C., Lacy, A. (1991). Pedagogy: The missing link in aerobic dance. *Journal of Physical Education, Recreation and Dance*, Aug.: 49-52.

Davis, C. (1994). The role of physical activity in the development and maintenance of eating disorders. *Psychological Medicine*, 24: 957-67.

de Vreede, P.M., Samson, M., VanMeeteren, N. (2005). Functional-task exercise vs. resistance strength exercise to improve daily tasks in older women: A randomized, controlled trial. *Journal of the American Geriatrics Society*, 53(1): 2-10.

Edmundson, A. (2007). *Globalized e-learning cultural challenges*. Hershey, PA: Information Science.

Eklund, R., Crawford, S. (1994). Social physique anxiety, reasons for exercise, and attitudes toward exercise settings. *Journal of Sports Exercise Psychology*, 16: 70-82.

Estabrooks, P. (2000). Sustaining exercise participation through group cohesion. *Exercise and Sports Sciences Review*, 28(2): 63-67.

Estabrooks, P., Carron, A. (1999). The influence of the group with elderly exercisers. *Small Group Research*, 30(4): 438-52.

Evans, E. (1993). Body image: Programming for a healthy perspective. *NIRSA Journal*, Fall: 46-51.

Evans, E., Connor, P. (1995). Body image of water aerobic instructors. Abstract. *Medicine & Science in Sports & Exercise*, 27(5): 852.

Evans, E., Kennedy, C. (1993). The body image problem in the fitness industry. *IDEA Today*, May: 50-56.

Floyd, A., Moyer, A. (2009). Group vs. individual exercise interventions for women with breast cancer: A meta-analysis. *Health Psychology Review*, 4(1), 22-41.

Fox, L., Rejeski, J., Gauvin, L. (2000). Effects of leadership style and group dynamics on enjoyment of physical activity. *American Journal of Health Promotion*, 15(5): 277-83.

Francis, L. (1991). Improving aerobic dance programs: The key role of colleges and universities. *Journal of Physical Education, Recreation and Dance*, 62(7): 59-62.

Francis, P. (2012). Is there a public health role for fitness professionals? *IDEA Fitness Journal*, Jan.: 53-59.

Franco, O., deLaet, C., Peters, A., Jonker, J., Mackenbach, J., Nusselder, W. (2005). Effects of physical activity on life expectancy with cardiovascular disease. *Archives of Internal Medicine*, 165: 2363-69.

Freeman, R. (1988). *Bodylove: Learning to like our looks and ourselves.* New York, NY: Harper-Collins.

Gaesser, G. (1999). Thinness and weight loss: Beneficial or detrimental to longevity? *Medicine & Science in Sports & Exercise*, 31(8): 1118-28.

Goleman, D. (1998). *Working with emotional intelligence.* New York: Bantam Books.

Goleman, D. (2006). *Social Intelligence: The new science of social intelligence.* New York, NY: Bantam Dell.

Grant, S., Todd, K., Aitchison, T., Kelly, P., Stoddart, D. (2004). The effects of a 12-week group exercise programme on physiological and psychological variables and function in overweight women. *Public Health*, 118(1): 31-42.

Heinzelmann, F., Bagley, P. (1970). Response to physical activity programs and their effects on health behavior. *Public Health*, 86: 905-11.

Hooker, S. (2003). The exercise/fitness professional's expanding role in promoting physical activity and the public's health. *ACSM's Health and Fitness Journal*, May-June: 7-11.

Howley, E., Bassett, D., Thompson, D. (2005). How to get them moving: Balancing weight with physical activity part II. *ACSM's Health and Fitness Journal*, Jan.-Feb.: 19-24.

Ibbetson, J. (1996). Body image and self-esteem: Factors that affect each and recommendations for fitness professionals. *NIRSA Journal*, Fall: 22-27.

Impett, E., Daubenmier, J., Hirschman, A. (2006). Minding the body: Yoga, embodiment, and well-being. *Sexuality Research and Social Policy*, 3(4): 39-48.

Jakicic, J.M., Marcus, B.H., Gallagher, K.I., Napolitano, M., Lang, W. (2003). Effect of exercise duration and intensity on weight loss in overweight, sedentary women. *Journal of the American Medical Association*, 290(10): 1323-30.

Kahlkoetter, J. (2002). Respect your body. *Triathlete* February:48-9.

Kandarian, M. (2006). Seven secrets for totally outrageous teaching. *IDEA Fitness Journal*, Sept.: 86-88.

Kennedy, C. (2004). Making a REAL Difference. *IDEA Health and Fitness Source*, Jan.: 40-44.

Kennedy, C., Legel, D. (1992). *Anatomy of an exercise class: An exercise educator's handbook.* Champaign, IL: Sagamore.

Krane, V., Shipley, S., Waldron, J., Michalenok, J. (2001). Relationships among body satisfaction, social physique anxiety, and eating behaviors in female athletes and exercisers. *Journal of Sports Behavior*, 24(3): 247-64.

Kravitz, L. (2007). The 25 most significant health benefits of physical activity and exercise. *IDEA Fitness Journal*, Oct.: 56-61.

Massie, J., Sheperd, R. (1971). Physiological and psychological effect of training: A comparison of individual and gymnasium programs, with a characterization of the exercise "drop-out." *Medicine & Science in Sports & Exercise*, 3: 110-17.

McGonigal, K. (2007). Facilitating fellowship. *IDEA Fitness Journal*, June: 73-79.

Miller, W. (1999). How effective are traditional dietary and exercise interventions for weight loss? *Medicine & Science in Sports & Exercise*, 31(8): 1129-34.

Mookadam, F., Arthur, H. (2004). Social support and its relationship to morbidity and mortality after acute myocardial infarction: Systematic overview. *Archives of Internal Medicine*, 164(14): 1514-18.

Muller-Riemenschneider, F., Reinhold, T., Willich, S. (2009). Cost-effectiveness of interventions promoting physical activity. *British Journal of Sports Medicine*, 43:70-76.

Murray, S., Touyz, S. (2012). Muscle dysmorphia: Towards a diagnostic consensus. *Australian and New Zealand Journal of Psychiatry*, 47(3): 206-7.

Nardini, M., Raglin, J., Kennedy, C. (1999). Body image, disordered eating, obligatory exercise and body composition among women fitness instructors. Abstract. *Medicine & Science in Sports & Exercise*, 31 (Suppl. 5): S297.

Olson, M., Williford, L., Brown, R., Pugh, S. (1996). Self-reports on the Eating Disorder Inventory by female aerobic instructors. *Perception in Motor Skills*, 82: 1051-58.

Ornish, D., (1998). *Love and survival*. New York: Harper-Collins.

Ostbye, T., Dement, J., Krause, K. (2007). Obesity and workers compensation: Results from the Duke Health and Safety Surveillance System. *Archives of Internal Medicine*, 167: 766-74.

Pate, R. R., Pratt, M., Blair, S.N., Haskell, W.L., Macera, C.A., Bouchard, C., Bushner, D., Ettinger, W., Health, G.W., King, A.C. (1995). Physical activity and public health: A recommendation from the Centers for Disease Control and Prevention and the American College of Sports Medicine. *Journal of the American Medical Association*, 273(5): 402-7.

Popowych, K. (2005). A studio society: Creating a positive program experience by fostering and developing participant relationships. *IDEA Fitness Journal*, Nov.-Dec.: 72-73.

Seidman, D. (2007). *How: Why how we do anything means everything*. Hoboken, NJ: Wiley and Sons.

Seligman, M. (2011). *Flourish*. New York, NY: Free Press.

Silberstein, L., Striegel-Moore, R., Rodin, J. (1987). *Feeling fat: A woman's shame*. Hillsdale, NJ: Erlbaum.

Spink, K., Carron, A. (1992). Group cohesion and adherence in exercise classes. *Journal of Sports Exercise Psychology*, 14: 78-86.

Spink, K., Carron, A. (1993). The effects of team building on the adherence patterns of female exercise participants. *Journal of Sports Exercise Psychology*, 15: 39-49.

Spink, K. Carron, A. (1994). Group cohesion effects in exercise classes. *Small Group Research*, 25(1): 26-42.

Stephens, T., Craig, S. (1990). *The well-being of Canadians: Highlights of the 1988 Campbell's Survey*. Ottawa: Canadian Fitness and Lifestyle Research Institute.

Uchino, B. (2006). Social support and health: A review of physiological processes potentially underlying links to disease outcomes. *Journal of Behavioral Medicine*, 29(4): 377-87.

Wallace, A. (2002). True thighs. *More*, Sept.: 90-95.

Weir, T. (2004). "New PE" objective: Get kids in shape. *USA Today*. www.usatoday.com/sports/2004-12-15-phys-ed-cover_x.htm

Westcott, W. (1991). Role-model instructors. *Fitness Management*, Mar.: 48-50.

Yager, Z., Jennifer, A. (2005). The role of teachers and educators in the prevention of eating disorders and child obesity: What are the issues? *Eating Disorders*, 13(3): 261-78.

Chapter 3

American College of Sports Medicine. 1978. The recommended quantity and quality of exercise for developing and maintaining fitness in healthy adults. *Medicine and Science in Sports and Exercise*, 10: vii-x.

American College of Sports Medicine. 2014. *ACSM's Guidelines for Exercise Testing and Prescription, 9th ed*. Baltimore, MD: Wolters Kluwer/ Lippincott Williams & Wilkins.

Cinque, C. (1989). Back pain prescription: Out of bed and into the gym. *Physician and Sportsmedicine*, 17(9): 185-8.

Devereaux, M. (2009). Low back pain. *Medical Clinics of North America*, 93(2): 477-501.

Frymoyer, J.W., Cats-Baril, W.L. (1991). An overview of the incidences and costs of low back pain. *Orthopedic Clinics of North America*, 22: 263.

Garber, CE, Blissmer, B., Deschenes, M.R., Franklin, B.A., Lamonte, M.J., Lee, I.M., Nieman, D.C., Swain, D.P. (2011). American College of Sports Medicine Position Stand. Quantity and quality of exercise for developing and maintaining cardiorespiratory, musculoskeletal, and neuromotor fitness in apparently healthy adults: guidance for prescribing exercise. *Medicine and Science in Sports and Exercise*, Jul;43(7): 1334-59.

Kellett, K., Kellett, D., Nordholm, L. (1991). Effects of an exercise program on sick leave due to back pain. *Physical Therapy*, 71: 283-93.

Kennedy, C. (1997). Exercise analysis. *IDEA Today*, January: 70-73.

Kennedy, C. (2003). Functional exercise progression. *IDEA Personal Trainer*, February: 36-43.

Kennedy, C. (2004). Making a real difference. *IDEA Health and Fitness Source*, January: 40-44.

Yoke, M., Kennedy, C. (2004). *Functional exercise progressions*. Monterey, CA; Healthy Learning.

Chapter 4

American Council on Exercise (2000). Group Exercise Instructor Manual. San Diego: American Council on Exercise.

Atkinson, G., Wilson, D., Eubank, M. (2004). Effects of music on work-rate distribution during a cycle time trial. *International Journal of Sports Medicine*, 62, 413-19.

Bain, L., Wilson, T., Chaikind, E. (1989). Participant perceptions of exercise programs for overweight women. *Research Quarterly*, 60(2): 134-43.

Biscontini, L. (2010). Music management: effectively (and legally) unleash the power of music. *ACE Certified News*, Sept.

Choi, P., Van Horn, J., Picker, D., Roberts, H. (1993) Mood changes in women after an aerobics class: A preliminary study. *Health Care Women International*, 14(2): 167-77.

Clapp, J., Little, K. (1994). The physiological response of instructors and participants to three aerobics regimens. *Medicine & Science in Sports & Exercise*, 26(8): 1041-46.

Dwyer, J. (1995). Effect of perceived choice of music on exercise intrinsic motivation. *Health Values*, 19(2): 18-26.

Estivill, M. (1995). Therapeutic aspects of aerobic dance participation. *Health Care Women International*, 16(4): 341-50. Faulkner, S., Faulkner, C. (1996). *NLP: The new technology of achievement*. New York, NY: Harper-Collins.

Harmon, N.M., Kravitz, L. (2007). The effects of music on exercise. *IDEA Fitness Journal*, Sept.: 72-77.

IDEA. (2002). Opinion statement. Recommendations for music volume in fitness settings *IDEA Fitness Edge*, 2003(4).

Karageorghis, C.I., Priest, D.L., Terry, P.C., Chatzisarantis, N., Lane, A.M. (2006). Redesign and initial validation of an instrument to assess the motivational qualities of music in exercise: The Brunel Music Rating Inventory-2. *Journal of Sports Sciences*, 24(8); 899-909.

Long, J., Williford, H., Olson, M., Wolfe, V. (1998). Voice problems and risk factors among aerobics instructors. *Journal of Voice*, 12(2): 197-207.

Monroe, M. (1999). And the beat goes on. *IDEA Health and Fitness Source*, October: 31-37.

National Institutes of Health [NIH]. 2012. Throat disorders. Bethesda, MD: National Library of Medicine. nlm.nih.gov/medlineplus/throatdisorders.html

Otto, R.M., Parker, C., Smith, T., Wygand, J., Perez, H. (1986). The energy cost of low impact and high impact aerobic exercise. Abstract. *Medicine & Science in Sports & Exercise*, 18: S523.

Otto, R.M., Yoke, M., Wygand, J., Larsen, P. (1988). The metabolic cost of multidirectional low impact and high impact aerobic dance. Abstract. *Medicine & Science in Sports & Exercise*, 20(2): S525.

Parker, S., Hurley, B., Hanlon, D., Vaccaro, P. (1989). Failure of target heart rate to accurately monitor intensity during aerobic dance. *Medicine & Science in Sports & Exercise*, 21 (2): 230-34.

Tendy, S.M. (2010). How fast is that music? *IDEA Fitness Journal*, Apr: 64-66.

Webb, T. (1989). Aerobic Q signs. *IDEA Today*, 10:30-31.

Williford, H.N., Blessing, D., Olson, M., Smith, F. (1989). Is low-impact aerobic dance an effective cardiovascular workout? *Physician & Sportsmedicine*, 17(3): 95-109.

Williford, H.N., Scharff-Olson, M., Blessing, D.L. (1989). The physiological effects of aerobic dance: A review. *Sports Medicine*, 8(6): 335-45.

Wininger, S. (2002). Instructors' and classroom characteristics associated with exercise enjoyment by females. *Perceptual Motor Skills*, 94(2): 395-800.

Yamashita, S., Iwai, K., Akimoto, T., Sugawara, J., Kono, I. (2006). Effects of music during exercise on RPE, heart rate and the autonomic nervous system. *Journal of Sports Medicine and Physical Fitness*, 46, 425-30.

Yoke, M., Otto, R., Larsen, P., Kamimukai, C., Wygand, J. (1989). The metabolic cost of instructors' low impact and high impact aerobic dance sequences. In *IDEA 1989 research symposium manual*. San Diego, CA: IDEA.

Yoke, M., Otto, R., Wygand, J., Kamimukai, C. (1988). The metabolic cost of two differing low impact aerobic dance exercise modes. Abstract. *Medicine & Science in Sports & Exercise*, 20(2): S527.

Chapter 5

Burke, S.M., Carron, A.V., Eys, M.A., Estabrooks, P.A. (2006). Group versus individual approach? A meta-analysis of the effectiveness of interventions to promote physical activity. *Sport and Exercise Psychology Review*, 1: 19-35.

DuBois, R., Hagen, R. (2007). *Success Perfect*. Monterey, CA: Coaches Choice.

Epstein, J.A., Harackiewicz, J.M. (1992). Winning is not enough: The effects of competition and achievement orientation on intrinsic interest. *Personality and Social Psychology Bulletin*, 18: 128-38.

Garcia, S.M., Avishalom, T. (2009). The N-effect: More competitors, less competition. *Psychological Science*, 20: 871-77.

Gavin, J. (2007). Transformational coaching. *IDEA Fitness Journal*, June.

IDEA. (2013). 2013 IDEA fitness programs and equipment trends report. *IDEA Fitness Journal*, June: 34- 45.

Knowles, M.S., Holton, E.F., Swanson, R.A. (2011). *The adult learner*. 7th ed. Burlington, MA: Elsevier.

Martens, R. (2012). *Successful Coaching*. 4th ed. Champaign, IL: Human Kinetics.

Veach, T.L., May, J.R. (2005). Teamwork: For the good of the whole. In S. Murphy (ed). *The Sport Psych Handbook* (pgs. 171-89). Champaign, Il: Human Kinetics.

Yoke, M., Kennedy, C. (2004). *Functional exercise progressions*. Monterey, CA, Healthy Learning.

Chapter 6

Alter, M.J. (2004). *The science of flexibility*. 3rd ed. Champaign, IL: Human Kinetics.

American College of Sports Medicine [ACSM]. (2014). *ACSM's guidelines for exercise testing and prescription*. 9th ed. Chapter 7. Baltimore, MD: Wolters Kluwer/Lippincott Williams & Wilkins;

Anderson, B., Anderson, J. (2010). *Stretching: 30th anniversary ed*. Bolinas, CA: Shelter Publications.

Anderson, P. (2000). The active range warm-up: Getting hotter with time. *IDEA Fitness Edge*, Apr.: 6-10.

Appel, A. (2007). The right rehearsal. *IDEA Fitness Journal*, Jan. 94.

Astrand, P., Rodahl, K. (1977). *Textbook of work physiology*. New York, NY: McGraw Hill.

Bacurau, R., Monteiro, G., Ugrinowitsch, C., Tricoli, V., Cabral, L., Aoki, M. (2009). Acute effect of a ballistic and a static stretching exercise bout on flexibility and maximal strength. *Journal of Strength and Conditioning Research*, 23: 304-8.

Blahnik, J., Anderson, P. (1996). Wake up your warm up! *IDEA Today,* June: 46-53.

Cramer, J., Housh, T., Weir, J., Johnson, G., Coburn, J., Beck, T. (2005). The acute effects of static stretching on peak torque, mean power output, electromyography, and mechanomyography. *European Journal of Applied Physiology*, 93: 530-39.

Fowles, J., Sale, D., MacDougall, J. (2000). Reduced strength after passive stretch of the human plantar flexors. *Journal of Applied Physiology* 89: 1179-88.

Garber, C., Blissmer, B., Deschenes, M., Franklin, B., Lamonte, M., Lee, I., Niemann, D., Swain, D. (2011). American College of Sports Medicine position stand. Quantity and quality of exercise for developing and maintaining cardiorespiratory, musculoskeletal, and neuromotor fitness in apparently healthy adults: Guidance for prescribing exercise. *Medicine & Science in Sports & Exercise*, 43(7): 1334-59.

Girouard, C., Hurley, B. (1995). Does strength training inhibit gains in range of motion from flexibility training in older adults? *Medicine & Science in Sports & Exercise,* 27(10): 1444-49.

Herbert, R., deNoronha, M., Kamper, S. (2011). Stretching to prevent or reduce muscle soreness after exercise. Review. *Cochrance Library*, issue 7. www.thecochranelibrary.com

Howley, E., Thompson, D. (2012). *Fitness professionals handbook*. 6th ed. Champaign, IL: Human Kinetics.

Kenney, W.L., Wilmore, J.H., D.L. Costill. (2011). *Physiology of sports and exercise.* Champaign, IL: Human Kinetics.

Kubo, K., Kanehisa, H., Fukunaga, T. (2001). Is passive stiffness in human muscles related to the elasticity of tendon structures? *European Journal of Applied Physiology* 85: 226-32.

Kubo, K., Kanehisa, H., Fukunaga, T. (2002). Effect of stretching training on the viscoelastic properties of human tendon structures in vivo. *Journal of Applied Physiology* 92: 595-601.

Lally, D. (1994). Stretching and injury in distance runners. *Medicine & Science in Sports & Exercise* 26(5): S84.

McArdle, W.D., Katch, F.I., Katch, V.I. (2009). *Exercise physiology: Energy, nutrition, and human performance*. 7th ed. Philadelphia, PA: Lippincott Williams & Wilkins.

McHugh, M., Cosgrave, C. (2010). To stretch or not to stretch: The role of stretching in injury prevention and performance. *Scandinavian Journal of Medicine & Science in Sports*, 20(2): 169-81.

Meroni, R., Giuseppe, C. Lanzarini, C., Giancesare, M., Barindelli, G., Gessaga, V., Cesana, C., DeVito, G. (2010). Comparison of active stretching technique and static stretching technique in hamstring flexibility. *Clinical Journal of Sport Medicine*, 20(1): 8-14.

Neiman, D. (2010). *Exercise testing and prescription*. 7th ed. New York, NY: McGraw-Hill.

Nelson, A., Driscoll, N., Landin, D., Young, M., Schexnayder, I. (2005). Acute effects of passive muscle stretching on sprint performance. *Journal of Sports Science*, 23: 449-54.

Shrier, I. (1999). Stretching before exercise does not reduce the risk of local muscle injury: A critical review of the clinical and basic science literature. *Clinical Journal of Sports Medicine*, 9: 221-27.

Shrier, I., Gossal, K. (2000). Myths and truths of stretching. *Physician and Sportsmedicine*, 28(8): 57-63.

Taylor, D., Dalton, J., Seaber, A., Garrett, W. (1990). Viscoelastic properties of muscle-tendon units: The biomechanical effects of stretching. *American Journal of Sports Medicine*, 18: 300-9.

Thacker, S., Gilcrest, J., Stroup, D., Kimsey, C. (2004). The impact of stretching on sports injury risk: A systematic review of the literature. *Medicine & Science in Sports& Exercise*, 36(3): 371-88.

Van Mechelen, W., Hlobil, H., Kemper, C., Voorn, W., deJongh, H. (1993). Prevention of running injuries by warm-up, cool-down, and stretching exercises. *American Journal of Sports Medicine*, 21: 711-19.

Walter, J., Figoni, F., Andres, F. (1995). Effect of stretching intensity and duration on hamstring flexibility. Abstract. *Medicine & Science in Sports & Exercise*, 27(5): S240.

Witvrouw, E., Mahieu, N., Danneels, L., McNair, P. (2004). Stretching and injury prevention: An obscure relationship. *Sports Medicine*, 34(7): 443-49.

Chapter 7

American College of Sports Medicine [ACSM]. (2014). *ACSM's Guidelines for Exercise Testing and Prescription*. 9th ed. Baltimore, MD: Wolters Kluwer/Lippincott Williams & Wilkins.

American Council on Exercise. 2011. *Group exercise instructor manual*. 3rd edition, San Diego: American Council on Exercise.

American Heart Association and the American College of Sports Medicine. (2002). Automated external defibrillators in health/fitness facilities. *Circulation*, 112(24): 1-211.

Balady, F., Chaitman, B., Foster, C., Froelicher, E., Gordan, N., VanCamp, S. (2002). AHA/ACSM scientific statement. Automated external defibrillators in health/fitness facilities: Supplement to the AHA/ACSM recommendations for cardiovascular screening, staffing, and emergency policies at health/fitness facilities, *Circulation*, 105: 1147-50.

Bates, M. (2008). *ACSM's health and fitness facility standards and guidelines*. 2nd ed. Champaign, IL: Human Kinetics.

Borg, G. (1982). Psychophysical bases of perceived exertion. *Medicine & Science in Sports & Exercise*, 14: 377-81.

Dunbar, C., Robertson, R., Baun, R., Blandin, M., Metz, K., Burdett, R., Goss, R. (1992). The validity of regulating exercise intensity by ratings of perceived exertion. *Medicine & Science in Sports & Exercise*, 24(1): 94-99.

Foster, C., Porcari, J. (2010). *personal training manual*. American Council on Exercise, San Diego, CA. Chapter 7.

Frangolias, D., Rhodes, E. (1995). Maximal and ventilatory threshold responses to treadmill and water immersion running. *Medicine & Science in Sports & Exercise* 27(7): 1007-13.

Galati, T. (2010) ACE IFT model for cardiorespiratory training: Phases 1-4. *ACE Certified News*, Aug.

Gellish, R., Goslin, B., Olson, R., McDonald, A., Russi, G., Moudgil, V. (2007). Longitudinal modeling of the relationship between age and maximal heart rate. *Medicine & Science in Sports & Exercise*, 39: 822-29.

Goleman, D. (2006). *Social Intelligence*. New York, NY: Random House.

Grant, S., Corbett, K., Todd, K., Davies, C., Aitchison, T., Mutrie, N., Byrne, J., Henderson, E., Dargie, H. (2002). A comparison of physiological response and rating of perceived exertion in two modes of aerobic exercise in men and women over 50 years of age. *British Journal of Sports Medicine*, 36: 276-81.

Janot, J. (2005). Comparing intensity monitoring methods. *IDEA Fitness Journal*, Apr.: 38-41.

Klika, B. (2012). Buddy up to cool down, *IDEA Fitness Journal*, Feb. 9:2.

Miller, W., Wallace, J., Eggert, K. (1993). Predicting max HR and the HR-VO_2 relationship for exercise prescription in obesity. *Medicine & Science in Sports& Exercise*, 25: 1007-81.

Parker, S., Hurley, B., Hanlon, D., Vaccaro, P. (1989). Failure of target heart rate to accurately monitor intensity during aerobic dance. *Medicine & Science in Sports & Exercise*, 21(2): 230-34.

Riley, S. (2005). The Pros and Cons of Automated External Defibrillators. *IDEA Fitness Manager*, July, 17:4.

Roach, B., Croisant, P., Emmett, J. (1994). The appropriateness of heart rate and RPE measures of intensity during three variations of aerobic dance.

Abstract. *Medicine & Science in Sports & Exercise,* 26(Suppl. 5): 24.

Roberg, R., Landwehr, R. (2002). The surprising history of the "HRmax = 220 - age" equation. *Journal of Exercise Physiology-Online.* 5(2): 1-10.

Robertson, R., Goss, F., Auble, T., Cassinelli, D., Spina, R., Glickman, E., Galbreath, R., Silberman, R., Metz, K. (1990). Cross-modal exercise prescription at absolute and relative oxygen uptake using perceived exertion. *Medicine & Science in Sports & Exercise,* 22(5): 653-59.

Schroeder, J. & Donlin, A. (2013). 2013 IDEA Fitness Programs and Equipment Trends Report, *IDEA Fitness Journal,* 10:6, 34-45.

Shechtman, N. (2008). A wet wind-down. *IDEA Fitness Journal,* Oct. 5:10.

Tanaka, H., Monahan, D., Seals, D. (2001). Age-predicted maximal heart rate revisited. *Journal of the American College of Cardiology,* 37: 153-56.

Tharrett, S., Peterson, J. (2012). *Fitness management.* 3rd ed. Monterey, CA: Healthy Learning.

Whaley, M., Kaminsky, L., Dwyer, G. (1992). Predictions of over- and underachievement of age-predicted maximal heart rate. *Medicine & Science in Sports & Exercise,* 24: 1173-79.

Wolohan, J.T. (2008). Supervision: Fitness centers may have duty of care regarding AEDs. *Athletic Business,* May www.athleticbusiness.com/articles/article.aspx?articleid = 1758&zoneid = 33.

Chapter 8

Aerobics and Fitness Association of America [AFAA]. (2010). *Fitness: Theory & practice.* 5th ed. Sherman Oaks, CA: Aerobics and Fitness Association of America.

Alter, M. (2004). *Science of flexibility.* 3rd ed. Champaign, IL: Human Kinetics.

American College of Sports Medicine [ACSM]. (2002). Position stand. Progression models in resistance training for healthy adults. *Medicine & Science in Sports & Exercise* 34(2): 364-80.

American College of Sports Medicine [ACSM]. (2010). *ACSM's Guidelines for Exercise Testing and Prescription.* 8th ed. Baltimore, MD: Lippincott Williams & Wilkins.

American College of Sports Medicine. [ACSM] (2014). *ACSM's Guidelines for Exercise Testing and Prescription, 9th ed.* Baltimore, MD: Wolters Kluwer/Lippincott Williams & Wilkins.

Anderson, O. (2003). Squatting exercise: How safe is squatting? www.pponline.co.uk/encyc/0827.htm

Bandy, W.D., Irion, J.M. (1994). The effect of time of static stretch on the flexibility of the hamstring muscles. *Physical Therapy,* 74: 845-52.

Beckham, S.G. and Earnest, C.P. (2000). Metabolic cost of free weight circuit weight training. *Journal of Sports Medicine and Physical Fitness,* 40: 118-25.

Blessing, D., Wilson, G., Puckett, J., Ford, H. (1987). The physiological effects of 8 weeks of aerobic dance with and without hand-held weights. *American Journal of Sports Medicine,* 15(5): 508-10.

Cosio-Lima, L.M., Jones, M.T., Paolone, V.J., Winter, C.R. (2001). The effects of a physioball training program on trunk and abdominal strength and static balance measures. Abstract. *Medicine & Science in Sports & Exercise,* 33(5): S1825.

Cressey, E.M., West, C.A., Tiberio, D.P., Kraemer, W.J. and Maresh, C.M. (2007). The effects of 10 weeks of lower-body unstable surface training on markers of athletic performance. *Journal of Strength and Conditioning Research,* 21(2): 561-67.

Feigenbaum, M.S., Pollock, M.L. (1999). Prescription of resistance training for health and disease. Medicine and Science in Sports and Exercise, Jan.31(1): 38-45.

Feland, J.B. (2000). The effect of stretch duration on hamstring flexibility in an elderly population. Abstract. *Medicine & Science in Sports & Exercise,* 32(5): S354.

Frymoyer, J.W., Cats-Baril, W.L. (1991). An overview of the incidences and costs of low back pain. *Orthopedic Clinics of North America* 22(2): 263-71.

Kravitz, L., Heyward, V.H., Stolarczyk, L.M., Wilmerding, V. (1997). Does step exercise with hand-weights enhance training effects? *Journal of Strength and Conditioning Research,* 11(3): 194-99.

Kreighbaum, E., Barthels, K. (1996). The deep squat. In *Biomechanics: A qualitative approach for studying human movement.* 4th ed. (pgs. 203-4). Boston: Allyn and Bacon.

Marshall, P.W., Murphy, B.A. (2006). Increased deltoid and abdominal muscle activity during Swiss ball bench press. *Journal of Strength and Conditioning Research,* 20(4): 745-50.

Miller, J.M., Rossi, M.D., Schurr, H., Brown, L.E., Whitehurst, M. (2001) Force production in healthy males during a horizontal press that uses elastics for resistance. Abstract. *Medicine & Science in Sports & Exercise,* 33(5): S139.

Myers, T. (2008). *Anatomy trains: Myofascial meridians for manual and movement therapists.* 2nd ed. UK: Elsevier.

National Strength and Conditioning Association. (2005). Session review: The end of the single set versus multiple set discussion. *NSCA bulletin*, 26, 7

Nobrega, A.C.L., Paula, K.C., Carvalho, A.C.G. (2005) Interaction between resistance training and flexibility training in healthy young adults. *Journal of Strength and Conditioning Research*, 19(4): 842-46.

Otto, R.M., Carpinelli, R.N. (2006). A critical analysis of the single versus multiple set debate. *Journal of Exercise Physiology*-online, 9(1): 32-57.

Page, P., Ellenbecker, T. (2003). *The scientific and clinical application of elastic resistance*. Champaign, IL: Human Kinetics.

Pearson, D., Faigenbaum, A., Conley, M., Kraemer, W. (2000). National Strength and Conditioning Association. Basic guidelines for the resistance training of athletes. *Strength and Conditioning Journal*, 22(4): 14-27.

Rancour, J., Holmes, C.F., Cipriani, D.J. (2009). The effects of intermittent stretching following a 4-week static stretching protocol: A randomised trial. *Journal of Strength and Conditioning Research*, 23(8): 2217-22.

Rhea, M.R., Alvar, B.A., Ball, S.D., Burkett, L.N. (2002). Three sets of weight training superior to one set with equal intensity for eliciting strength. *Journal of Strength and Conditioning Research*, 16: 525-29.

Sorace, P., LaFontaine, T. (2005). Resistance training muscle power: Design programs that work! *ACSM Health and Fitness Journal*, 9(2): 6-12.

Stanforth, D., Stanforth, P.R., Hahn, S., Phillips, A. (1998). A 10 week training study comparing Resistaball and traditional trunk training. www.ingentaconnect.com/content/jmrp/jdms/1998/00000002/00000004/art00002

Stanforth, D., Stanforth, P.R., Velasquez, K.S. (1993). Aerobic requirement of bench stepping. *International Journal of Sports Medicine*, 14(3): 129-33.

Stanforth, P.R., Stanforth, D. (1996). The effect of adding external weight on the aerobic requirement of bench stepping. *Research Quarterly in Exercise and Sport*, 67: 469-72.

Stoppani, J. (2005). *Encyclopedia of muscle strength*. Champaign, IL: Human Kinetics.

Sullivan, M.G., Dejulia, J.J., Worrell, T.W. (1992). Effect of pelvic position and stretching method on hamstring muscle flexibility. *Medicine & Science in Sports & Exercise*, 24(12): 1383-89.

Thacker, S.B., Gilchrist, J., Stroup, D.F., Kemsey, C.D. Jr. (2004). The impact of stretching on sports injury risk: A systematic review of the literature. *Medicine & Science in Sports & Exercise*, 36 (3): 371-78.

Willardson, J.M. (2004). The effectiveness of resistance exercises performed on unstable equipment. *Journal of Strength and Conditioning Research*, 26(3): 70-74.

Wolfe, B.L, LeMura, B.M., Cole, P.J. (2004). Quantitative analysis of single versus multiple-set programs in resistance training. *Journal of Sports and Conditioning Research*, 18: 35-47.

Yoke, M. (2010). *Personal fitness training: Theory and practice*. Sherman Oaks, CA: Aerobics and Fitness Association of America.

Yoke, M., Kennedy, C. (2004). *Functional exercise progressions*. Monterey, CA: Healthy Learning.

Yoke, M., Otto, R., Wygand, J., Kamimukai, C. (1988). The metabolic cost of two differing low impact aerobic dance exercise modes. Abstract. *Medicine & Science in Sports & Exercise*, 20(2): S527.

Chapter 9

Aerobics and Fitness Association of America. (2010). *Fitness: Theory & practice*. 5th ed. Sherman Oaks, CA: Aerobics and Fitness Association of America.

American College of Sports Medicine (2014). *ACSM's Guidelines for Exercise Testing and Prescription, 9th ed*. Baltimore, MD: Wolters Kluwer, Lippincott Williams & Wilkins.

American Council on Exercise. (2010). *ACE personal trainer manual*. 4th ed. San Diego, CA: American Council on Exercise.

Anders, M. (2007). Function follows fitness. *ACE Fitness Matters*, July-Aug.: 7-10.

Archer, S. (2007). Fitness and wellness intertwine: A major industry arises. *IDEA Fitness Journal*, July-Aug.: 36-47.

Astrand, P. (1992). Why exercise? *Medicine & Science in Sports & Exercise*, 24(2): 153-62.

Bird, M., Hill, K.D., Ball, M., Hetherington, S., Williams, A.D. (2010). The long-term benefits of a multi-component exercise intervention to balance and mobility in healthy older adults: Relationship between physical functioning and physical activity in the lifestyle interventions and independence for elders pilot. *Archives of Gerontology and Geriatrics*, 58(10): 1918–24.

Chin, A.P.M.J., van Uffelen, J.G., Riphagen, I, van Mechelen, W. (2008). The functional effects of physical exercise training in frail older people: A systematic review. *Sports Medicine*, 38(9): 781-93.

Cook, G. (2010). *Movement: Functional movement systems*. Santa Cruz, FL: On Target.

deVreede, P., Samson, M., VanMeeteren, N. (2005). Functional-task exercise vs. resistance strength exercise to improve daily tasks in older women: A randomized, controlled trial. *Journal of the American Geriatrics Society* 53(1): 2-10.

Fiatarone, M.A., O'Neill, E., Ryan, N. (1994). A randomized controlled trial of exercise and nutrition for physical frailty in the oldest old. *New England Journal of Medicine*, 330(25): 1769-75.

Garber, C., Blissmer, B., Deschenes, M., Franklin, B., Lamonte, M., Lee, I., Nieman, D., Swain, D. (2011). American College of Sports Medicine position stand. Quantity and quality of exercise for developing and maintaining cardiorespiratory, musculoskeletal, and neuromotor fitness in apparently healthy adults: Guidance for prescribing exercise. *Medicine & Science in Sports & Exercise*, 43(7): 1334-59.

Gatts, S. (2008). Neural mechanisms underlying balance control in tai chi. *Medicine and Sports Science*, 52: 87-103.

Hewett, T.E., Myer, G.D., Ford, K.R. (2005). Reducing knee and anterior cruciate ligament injuries among female athletes: A systematic review of neuromuscular training interventions. *Journal of Knee Surgery*, 18(1): 82-88.

Hrysomallis, C. (2007). Relationship between balance ability, training and sports injury risk. *Sports Medicine*, 37(6): 547-56.

Jahnke, R., Larkey, L., Rogers, C., Etnier, J., Lin, F. (2010). A comprehensive review of health benefits of quigong and tai chi. *American Journal of Health Promotion*, 24(6): el-e25.

Karinkanta, S., Heinonen, A., Sievanen, H., et al. (2007). A multi-component exercise regimen to prevent functional decline and bone fragility in home-dwelling elderly women: Randomized, controlled trial. *Osteoporosis International*, 18(4): 453-62.

Kennedy-Armbruster, C. Sexauer, L., Wyatt, W., Shea, J. (2012). Effects of Navy SHAPE on fitness parameters, functional movement screening (FMS) and self-reported sitting time. *Medicine & Science in Sports & Exercise*, 44(Suppl. 5 #3102).

Liu-Ambrose, Khan, K.M., Eng, J.J., Lord, S.R., McKay, H.A. (2004). Balance confidence improves with resistance or agility training. *Gerontology*, 50(6): 373-82.

Morrison, S., Colberg, S.R., Mariano, M., Parson, H.K., Vinik, A.I. (2010). Balance training reduces falls risk in older adults with type 2 diabetes. *Diabetes Care*, 33(4): 74

Myers, T. (2009). *Anatomy trains: Myofascial meridians for manual and movement therapists.* 2nd ed. UK: Elsevier.

Nelson, M.E., Rejeski, W.J., Blair, S.N., et al. (2007). Physical activity and public health in older adults: Recommendation from the American College of Sports Medicine and the American Heart Association. *Medicine & Science in Sports & Exercise*, 39(8): 1435-45.

Rikli, R., Jones, C. (1999). Development and validation of a functional fitness test for community-residing older adults. *Journal of Aging and Physical Activity*, 7(2): 129-61.

Rose, D.J. (2010). *Fall proof! A comprehensive balance and mobility training program.* 2nd ed. Champaign, IL: Human Kinetics.

Santana, J.C. (2002). The four pillars of human movement. *IDEA Personal Trainer*, Feb.: 22-28.

Shumway-Cook, A., Woollacott, M. (2000). Attentional demands and postural control: The effect of sensory context. *Journal of Gerontology*, 55A: M10-M16.

Willardson, J.M., Fontana, F.E., Bressel, E. (2009). The effect of surface stability on core muscle activity for dynamic resistance exercises. *International Journal of Sports Physiology Performance*, 4: 97-109.

Wolfe, B.L., Lemura, L.M., Cole, P.J. (2004). Quantitative analysis of single vs. multiple-set programs in resistance training. *Journal of Strength and Conditioning Research*, 18(1): 35-47.

Chapter 10

Adams, K.J., Allen, N.B., Schumm, J.E., Swank, A.M. (1997). Oxygen cost of boxing exercise utilizing a heavy bag. Abstract. *Medicine & Science in Sports & Exercise*, 29(5): S1067.

Albano, C., Terbizan, D.J. (2001). Heart rate and RPE difference between aerobic dance and cardio-kickboxing. Abstract. *Medicine & Science in Sports & Exercise*, 33(5): S604.

Anning, J.H., Armstrong, C., Mylona, E., Norkus, S., Sterner, R., Andres, F. (1999). Physiological responses during cardiovascular kickboxing: A pilot study. Abstract. *Medicine & Science in Sports & Exercise*, 31(5): S403.

Bellinger, B., St. Clair, G.A., Oelofse, A., Lambert, M. (1997). Energy expenditure of a noncontact boxing training session compared with submaximal treadmill running. *Medicine & Science in Sports & Exercise*, 29(12): 1653-56.

Bissonnette, D., Guzman, N., McMillan, L., Catalano, S., Giroux, M., Greenlaw, K., Vivolo, S., Otto, R.M., Wygand, J. (1994). The energy requirements of karate aerobic exercise versus low impact aerobic dance. Abstract. *Medicine & Science in Sports & Exercise*, 26(5): S58.

Buschbacher, R.M., Shay, T. (1999). Martial arts. *Physical Medicine & Rehabilitation Clinics of North America*, 10(1): 35-47.

Davis, S.E., Romaine, L.J., Harrison, K. (2002). Incidence of injury in kickboxing. Abstract. *Medicine & Science in Sports & Exercise*, 34(5): S1438.

Ergun, A.T., Plato, P.A., Cisar, C.J. (2006). Cardiovascular and metabolic responses to noncontact kickboxing in females. *Medicine & Science in Sports & Exercise*, 38(5): S497.

Franzese, P., Taglione, T., Flynn, C., Wygand, J., Otto, R.M. (2000). The metabolic cost of specific Taebo exercise movements. Abstract. *Medicine & Science in Sports & Exercise*, 32(5): S150.

Frymoyer, J.W., Cats-Baril, W.L. (1991). An overview of the incidences and costs of low back pain. *Orthopedic Clinics of North America*, 22:263.

Greene, L., Kravitz, L, Wongsathikun, J., Kemerly, T. (1999). Metabolic effect of punching tempo. Abstract. *Medicine & Science in Sports & Exercise*, 31(5): S674.

Jackson, K., Edginton-Bigelow, K., Bowsheir, C., Weston, M., Grant, E. (2011). Feasibility and effects of a group kickboxing program for individuals with multiple sclerosis: A pilot report. *Journal of Bodywork and Movement Therapy*, 16(1): 7-13.

Kravitz, L., Greene, L., Wongsathikun, J. (2000). The physiological responses to kick-boxing exercise. Abstract. *Medicine & Science in Sports & Exercise*, 32(5): S148.

McKinney-Vialpando, K. (1999). *Cardio TKO: Aerobic kickboxing for the fitness professional*. 2nd ed. Idaho Falls, ID: Safax Fitness Training.

O'Driscoll, E., Steele, J., Perez, H.R., Yreys, S., Snowkroft, N., Locasio, F. (1999). The metabolic cost of two trials of boxing exercise utilizing a heavy bag. Abstract. *Medicine & Science in Sports & Exercise*, 31(5): S676.

Perez, H.R., O'Driscoll, E., Steele, J., Yreys, S., Snowkroft, N., Steizinger, C., Locasio, F. (1999). Physiological responses to two forms of boxing aerobics exercise. Abstract. *Medicine & Science in Sports & Exercise*, 31(5): S673.

Romaine, L.J., Davis, S.E., Casebolt, K., Harrison, K.A. (2003). Incidence of injury in kickboxing participation. *Journal of Sports and Conditioning Research*, 17(3): 580-586.

Scharff-Olsen, M., Williford, H.N., Duey, W.J., Walker, S., Crumpton, S., Sanders, J. (2000). The energy cost of martial arts aerobic exercise. Abstract. *Medicine & Science in Sports & Exercise*, 32(5): S149.

Wingfield, L.D., Dowling, E.A., Branch, J.D., Colberg, S.R., Swain, D.P. (2006). Differences in VO2 between kickboxing and treadmill exercise at similar heart rates. *Medicine & Science in Sports & Exercise*, 38(5): S497.

Chapter 11

Aerobics and Fitness Association of America. (2010). *Fitness: Theory & Practice*. 5th ed. Sherman Oaks, CA: Aerobics and Fitness Association of America.

Arslan, F. (2011). The effects of an 8-week step-aerobic dance exercise programme on body composition parameters in middle-aged, sedentary, obese women. *International Sports Medicine Journal*, 12(4): 160-68.

Bemben, M.G., Clary, S.R., Barnes, C., Bemben, D.A., Knehans, A.W. (2006). Effects of ballates, step aerobics, and walking on balance in women aged 50-75 years. *Medicine & Science in Sports & Exercise*, 38(5): S445.

Calarco, L., Otto, R., Wygand, J., Kramer, J., Yoke, M, D'Zamko, F. (1991). The metabolic cost of six common movement patterns of bench-step aerobic dance. Abstract. *Medicine & Science in Sports & Exercise*, 23(4): S839.

Clary, S., Barnes, C., Bemben, D., Knehans, A., Bemben, M. (2006). Effects of ballates, step aerobics, and walking on balance in women aged 50-75 years. *Journal of Sports Science and Medicine*, 5: 390-99.

Francis, P. (1990). In step with science. *Fitness Management*, 6(6): 37-38.

Francis, P.R., Francis, L., Miller, G., Tichenor, K., Rich, B. (1994). *Introduction to Step Reebok*. San Diego, CA: San Diego University.

Francis, P.R., Poliner, J., Buono, M.J., Francis, L.L. (1992). Effects of choreography, step height, fatigue and gender on metabolic cost of step training. Abstract. *Medicine & Science in Sports & Exercise*, 24(5): S69.

Greenlaw, K., McMillan, S., Catalano, S., Vivolo, S., Giroux, M., Wygand, J., Otto, R.M. (1995). The energy cost of traditional versus power bench step exercise at heights of 4, 6, and 8 inches. Abstract. *Medicine & Science in Sports & Exercise*, 33(5): S123.

Hale, B.S., Raglin, J.S. (2002). State anxiety responses to acute resistance training and step aerobic exercise across eight weeks of training. *Journal of Sports Medicine and Physical Fitness*, 42(1): 108-12.

Hallage, T., Krause, M.P., Haile, L., Miculis, C.P., Nagle, E.F., Reis, R.S., da Silva, S.G. (2010). The effects of 12 weeks of step aerobics training on functional fitness in elderly women. *Journal of Strength and Conditioning Research*, 24(8): 2261-66.

Hallage, T., Krause, M.P., Miculis, C.P., da Silva, S.G. (2009). Effect of 12 weeks of step aerobics training on VO2 max of older adult women. Abstract. *Medicine & Science in Sports & Exercise*, 41(5): S2517.

IDEA. (2011). 2011 IDEA Fitness programs and equipment trends report. *IDEA Fitness Manager*, July-Aug.: 1-7.

Johnson, B.F., Johnston, K.D., Winnier, S.A. (1993). Bench-step aerobic ground forces for two steps of variable bench heights. Abstract. *Medicine & Science in Sports & Exercise*, 25(5): S1100.

Kin Isler, A., Kosar, S.N., Korkusuz, F. (2001). Effects of step aerobics and aerobic dancing on serum lipids and lipoproteins. *Journal of Sports Medicine and Physical Fitness*, 41(3): 380-85.

Kraemer, W.J., Keuning, M., Ratamess, N.A., Volek, J.S., McCormick, M., Bush, J.A., Nindl, B.C., Gordon, S.W., Mazzetti, S.A., Newton, R.U., Gomez, A.L., Wickham, R.B., Rubin, M.R., Hakkinen, K. (2001). Resistance training combined with bench step aerobics enhances women's health profile. *Medicine & Science in Sports & Exercise*, 33(2): 259-69.

Kravitz, L, Heyward, V.H., Stolarczyk, L.M., Wilmerding, M.V. (1995). Effects of step training with and without handweights on physiological and lipid profiles of women. Abstract. *Medicine & Science in Sports & Exercise*, 27(5): S1012.

Kravitz, L., Heyward, V., Stolarczyk, L., Wilmerding, V. (1997). Does step exercise with handweights enhance training effects? *Journal of Strength and Conditioning Research*, 11(3): 194-99.

Lloyd, L.K. (2011). Cardiovascular responses to aerobic bench stepping performed with and without choreographed arm movements. Abstract. *Medicine & Science in Sports & Exercise*, 43(5): S1927.

Moses, R.D. (1993). Ground reaction forces in bench aerobics. Abstract 49. Paper presented at the 22nd Annual Meeting of the Southeast Regional Chapter of the American College of Sports Medicine, Greensboro, NC.

Mosher, P.E., Ferguson, M.A., Arnold, R.O. (2005). Lipid and lipoprotein changes in premenstrual women following step aerobics dance training. *International Journal of Sports Medicine*, 26: 669-74.

Olson, M., Williford, H., Blessing, D., Greathouse, R. (1991). The cardiovascular and metabolic effects of bench-stepping exercise in females. *Medicine & Science in Sports & Exercise*, 23(11): 1311-18.

Scharff-Olson, M., Williford, H.N., Blessing, D.L., Moses, R., Wang, T. (1997) Vertical impact forces during bench-step aerobics: Exercise rate and experience. *Perceptual and Motor Skills*, 84(1): 267-74.

Scharff-Olson, M., Williford, H.N., Duey, W.J., Barber, J., Baldwin, S. (1997). Physiological responses of males and females to bench step exercise at two different rates. Abstract. *Medicine & Science in Sports & Exercise*, 29(5): S160.

Stanforth, D., Stanforth, P.R., Velasquez, K.S. (1993). Aerobic requirement of bench stepping. *International Journal of Sports Medicine*, 14(3): 129-33.

Stanforth, D., Velasquez, K., Stanforth, P. (1991). The effect of bench height and rate of stepping on the metabolic cost of bench stepping. Abstract. *Medicine & Science in Sports & Exercise*, 23(4): S143.

Step Reebok. (1997). *1997 revised guidelines for Step Reebok*. Canton, MA: Reebok University Press.

Wang, N., Scharff-Olson, M., Williford, H.N. (1993). Energy cost and fuel utilization during step aerobics exercise. Abstract. *Medicine & Science in Sports & Exercise*, 25(5): S630.

Wen, H., Tsai, K., Maiw, S., Lee, C., Fang, C. (2007). The effects of step-aerobics and resistance training on BMD and immune functioning in postmenopausal women. *Medicine & Science in Sports & Exercise*, 39(5): S229.

Wilson, J.R., Putman, D.H., Beckham, S, Ricard, M.D. (2010). Bench height and step cadence effects in aerobic dance on force impact and metabolic cost. Abstract. *Medicine & Science in Sports & Exercise*, 42(5): S2775.

Woodby-Brown, S., Berg, K., Latin, R.W. (1993). Oxygen cost of aerobic dance bench stepping at three heights. *Journal of Strength and Conditioning Research*, 7(3): 163-67.

Workman, D., Kern, D., Earnest, C. (1993). Cardiorespiratory responses of isolated arm movements and hand weighting during bench stepping aerobic dance in women. Abstract. *Medicine & Science in Sports & Exercise*, 25(5): S466.

Chapter 12

Battista, R., Foster, C., Andrew, J., Wright, G., Alejandro, L., Porcari, J. (2008). Physiologic responses during indoor cycling. *Journal of Strength and Conditioning*, 22(4): 1236-41.

Boyer, B., Porcari, J., Foster, C. (2010). Krank it! *ACE Fitness Matters*, March/April: 6-9.

Caria, M., Tangianu, F., Concu, A., Crisafulli, A., Mameli, O. (2007). Quantification of Spinning bike performance during a standard 50-minute class. *Journal of Sports Sciences*, 25(4): 421-29.

Chapman, A., Vicenzino, B., Blanch, P., Hodges, P. (2004). Do muscle recruitment patterns differ between trained and novice cyclists? *Medicine & Science in Sports & Exercise*, 30(5): S954.

Chinsky, A., DeFrancisco, J., Flanagan, K., Otto, R.M., Wygand, J. (1998). A comparison of two types of spin exercise classes. Abstract. *Medicine & Science in Sports & Exercise*, 30(5): S954.

Flanagan, K., DeFrancisco, J., Chinsky, A., Wygand, J., Otto, R.M. (1998). The metabolic and cardiovascular response to select positions and resistances during Spinning exercise. Abstract. *Medicine & Science in Sports & Exercise*, 30(5): S944.

Foss, O., Hallen, J. (2004). The most economical cadence increases with increasing workload. *European Journal of Applied Physiology*, 92: 443-51.

Francis, P.R., Witucki, A.S., Buono, M.J. (1999). Physiological response to a typical studio cycling session. *ACSM's Health and Fitness Journal*, 3(1): 30-36.

Gollwitzer, P., Sheeran, P. (2006). Implementation intentions and goal achievement: A meta-analysis of effects and processes. *Advances in Experimental Social Psychology*, 38: 69-119.

Hotting, K., Reich, B., Holzschneider, K., Kauschke, K., Schmidt, T., Reer, R., Braumann, K., Roder, B. (2012). Differential cognitive effects of cycling versus stretching/coordination training in middle-aged adults. *Health Psychology*, 31(2): 145-55.

John, D.H., Schuler, P. (1999). Accuracy of using RPE to monitor intensity of group indoor stationary cycling. Abstract. *Medicine & Science in Sports & Exercise*, 31(5): S643.

Lopez-Minarro, P., Rodriguez, J. (2010). Heart rate and overall ratings of perceived exertion during Spinning cycle indoor session in novice adults. *Science and Sports*, 25(5): 238-44.

Lucia, A., San Juan, A., Montilla, M., Canete, S., Santalla, A., Earnest, C., Perez, M. (2004). In professional road cyclists, low pedaling cadences are less efficient. *Medicine & Science in Sports & Exercise*, 36: 1048-54.

McArdle, W.D., Katch, F.I., Katch, V.L. (2009). *Exercise physiology: Energy, nutrition, and human performance*. 7th ed. Philadelphia: Lippincott, Williams & Wilkins.

Mora-Rodriguez, R., Aguado-Jimenez, R. (2004). Performance at high pedaling cadences in well-trained cyclists. *Medicine & Science in Sports & Exercise*, 38(5): 953-57.

Olson, J., Binns, A., Bliss, J., Swyden, A., Gray, M., DiBrezzo, R. (2012). Impact of instructor cues on changes in cycling form during a spin class. *Medicine & Science in Sports & Exercise*, 44(Suppl. 5 #2195).

Schroeder, J. & Donlin, A. (2013). 2013 IDEA Fitness Programs and Equipment Trends Report, *IDEA Fitness Journal*, 10:6, 34-45.

Thompson, W. (2012). Worldwide survey of fitness trends for 2013. *ACSM's Health and Fitness Journal*, 16(6): 8-17.

Williford, H.N., Scharff-Olson, M., Bradford, A., Walker, S., Crumpton, S. (1999). Maximum cycle ergometry and group cycle exercise: A comparison of physiological responses. Abstract. *Medicine & Science in Sports & Exercise*, 31(5): S423.

Chapter 13

American College of Sports Medicine [ACSM]. (2014). *ACSM's guidelines for exercise testing and prescription*. 9th ed. Baltimore: Lippincott Williams & Wilkins.

Baldwin. (2007). Add Water to the Mix. *IDEA Fitness Journal*, Mar.33-35.

Bartels, M., Bourne, G., Dwyer, J. (2010). High-intensity exercise for patients in cardiac rehabilitation after myocardial infarction. *Physical Medicine and Rehabilitation*, 2(2): 151-55.

Behm, D., Drinkwater, E., Willardson, J., Cowley, P. (2010). Canadian Society for Exercise Physiology position stand. The use of instability to train the core in athletic and nonathletic conditioning. *Applied Physiology, Nutrition, and Metabolism*, 35(1): 109-12.

Burgomaster, K.A., Howarth, K.R., Phillips, S.M., Rakobowchuk, M., Macdonald, M.J., McGee, S.L., Gibala, M.J. (2008). Similar metabolic adaptations during exercise after low volume sprint interval and traditional endurance training in humans. *Journal of Physiology*, 586(1): 151-60.

Cayot, T., Schick, E.R., Gochiocco, M.K., Wambold, S., Stacy, M.R., Scheuermann, B.W. (2011). Electromyographic analysis of suspension elbow flexion curls and standard elbow flexion curls. *Medicine & Science in Sports & Exercise*, 43(5): S1695.

Cook, Gray. (2010). *Movement: Functional movement systems*. Santa Cruz, CA: Target.

Crews, L. (2008). Sample class: Athletic Boot Camp. *IDEA Fitness Journal*, Feb.85-86.

Crews, L. (2009). Sample class: Zoomer Boot Camp. *IDEA Fitness Journal*, Mar.11.

Fernando, M., Borreani, S., Alves, J., Colado, J.C., Gramage, D., Martin, J. (2012). Lumbopelvic muscular activation during push-ups performed under different unstable surfaces. *Medicine & Science in Sports & Exercise*, 44(5): S1861.

Francis, P. (2012, Jan.). Is there a public health role for fitness professionals? *IDEA Fitness Journal*, Jan.: 53-59.

Gotchalk, L., Berger, R., Kraemer, W. (2004). Cardiovascular responses to a high-volume continuous circuit resistance training protocol. *Journal of Strength and Conditioning Research*, 18(4): 760-64.

Helgerud, J., Hoydal, K., Wang, E., Karlsen, T., Berg, P., Bjerkaas, M., Simonsen, T., Kibele, A., Behm, D. (2009). Seven weeks of instability and traditional resistance training effects on strength, balance and functional performance. *Journal of Strength and Conditioning Research*, 23(9): 2443-50.

McLain, S. (2005). Boot camp Ohio style. *IDEA Fitness Journal*, May: 31-33.

McMillan, S. (2005). Sample class: Sport step. *IDEA Fitness Journal*, Nov.-Dec.: 79-80.

Scheett, T., Aartun, J., Thomas, D., Herrin, J., Dudgeon, W. (2010). Physiological markers as a gauge of intensity for suspension training exercise. *Medicine & Science in Sports and Exercise*, 42(5): S2636.

Schroeder, J. & Donlin, A. (2013). 2013 IDEA Fitness Programs and Equipment Trends Report, *IDEA Fitness Journal*, 10:6, 34-45.

Slordahl, S.A., Madslien, V.O., Stoylen, A., Kjos, A., Helgerud, J., Wisloff, U. (2004). Atrioventricular plane displacement in untrained and trained females. *Medicine & Science in Sports and Exercise*, 37(9), 1871-75.

Sparks, R., Behm, D. (2010). Training adaptations associated with an 8-week instability resistance training program with recreationally active individuals. *Journal of Strength & Conditioning Research*, 24(7): 1931-41. doi:10.1519/JSC.0b013e3181df7fe4

Tharrett, S. (2012). *Fitness Management*. 3rd ed. Monterey, CA: Healthy Learning.

Thompson, C., Cobb, K., Blackwell, J. (2007). Functional training improves club head speed and functional fitness in older golfers. *Journal of Strength and Conditioning Research*, 21(1): 131-37.

Vogel, A. (2006). How to create a profitable boot camp program. *ACE Certified News*, Dec.-Jan.: 11-13.

Wisloff, U., Stoylan, A., Loennechen, J., Bruvold, M., Rognmo, O., Haram, P., Tjonna, A., Helgerud, J., Slordahl, S., Lee, S., Videm, V., Bye, A., Smith, G., Najjar, S., Ellingsen, O., Skjaerpe, R. (2007). Superior cardiovascular effect of aerobic interval training versus moderate continuous training in heart failure patients. *Circulation*, 115: 3086-94.

Zuhl, M., Kravitz, L. (2012). HIIT vs. continuous endurance training: Battle of the aerobic titans. *IDEA Fitness Journal*, Feb.

Chapter 14

Aquatic Exercise Association. (2010). *Aquatic fitness professional manual*. 6th ed. Nokomis, FL: Aquatic Exercise Association.

Archer, S. (2007). Fitness and wellness intertwine: A major industry arises. *IDEA Fitness Journal*, July-Aug.: 36-47.

Bates, A., Hanson, N. (1996). *Aquatic exercise therapy*. Philadelphia, PA: Saunders.

Batterham, S., Heywood, S., Keating, J. (2011). Systematic review and meta-analysis comparing land and aquatic exercise for people with hip and knee arthritis on functional, mobility and other health outcomes. *BMC Musculoskeletal Disorders*, 12: 123.

Benelli, P., Ditroilo, M., & DeVito, G. (2004). Physiological response to fitness activities: A comparison between land-based and water aerobics. *Journal of Strength & Conditioning Research,* 18(4): 719-22.

Bocalini, D., Serra, A., Murad, N., Levy, R. (2008). Water-versus land-based exercise effects on physical fitness in older women. *Geriatrics & Gerontology International*, 8(4): 265-71.

Bravo, G., Gauthier, P., Roy, P.M., Payette, H., Gaulin, P. (1997). A weight bearing, water-based exercise program for orthopedic women: Its impact on bone, functional fitness, and well-being. *Archives of Physical Medicine and Rehabilitation*, 78(12): 1375-80.

Brown, S., Chitwood, L., Beason, K., McLemore, D. (1997). Male and female physiologic responses to treadmill and deep water running at matched running cadences. *Journal of Strength and Conditioning Research*, 11(2): 107-14.

Bushman, B., Flynn, M., Andres, F., Lambert, C., Taylor, M., Braunl, W. (1997). Effect of 4 weeks of deep water run training on running performance. *Medicine & Science in Sports & Exercise*, 29(5): 694-99.

Byrnes, W. (1985). Muscle soreness following resistance exercise with and without eccentric actions. *Research Quarterly in Exercise and Sport*, 56: 283.

Craig, A.B., Dvorak, A.M. (1968). Thermal regulation of man exercising during water immersion. *Journal of Applied Physiology*, 25: 23-35.

D'Acquisto, L., D'Acquisto, D., Renne, D. (2001). Metabolic and cardiovascular responses in older women during shallow water exercise. *Journal of Strength and Conditioning Research*, 15(1): 12-19.

Davidson, K., McNaughton, L. (2000). Deep water running training and road running training improve VO2 max in untrained women. *Journal of Strength and Conditioning Research*, 14(2): 191-95.

DeMaere, J.M., Ruby, B.C. (1997). Effects of deep water and treadmill running on oxygen uptake and energy expenditure in seasonally trained cross country runners. *Journal of Sports Medicine and Physical Fitness*, 37(3): 175-81.

Evans, E., Cureton, K. (1998). Metabolic, circulatory and perceptual responses to bench stepping in water. *Journal of Strength and Conditioning Research*, 12(2): 95-100.

Eyestone, E., Fellingham, G., George, J., Fisher, G. (1993). Effect of water running and cycling on maximum oxygen consumption and 2-mile run performance. *American Journal of Sports Medicine*, 21(1): 41-44.

Frangolias, D., Rhodes, E. (1995). Maximal and ventilatory threshold responses to treadmill and water immersion running. *Medicine & Science in Sports & Exercise*, 27(7): 1007-13.

Frangolias, D., Rhodes, E., Taunton, J. (1996). The effects of familiarity with deep water running on maximal oxygen consumption. *Journal of Strength and Conditioning Research*, 10(4): 215-19.

Frangolias, D., Rhodes, E., Taunton, J., Belcastro, A., Coutts, K. (2000). Metabolic responses to prolonged work during treadmill and water immersion running. *Journal of Science and Medicine in Sport*, 3(4): 476-92.

Gangaway, J. (2010). Older adults: The need for exercise and the benefits of aquatics. *Topics in Geriatric Rehabilitation*, 26(2): 82-92.

Gehring, M., Keller, B., Brehm, B. (1997). Water running with and without a flotation vest in competitive and recreational runners. *Medicine & Science in Sports & Exercise*, 29(10): 1374-78.

Gulick, D. (2010). Effects of aquatic intervention on the cardiopulmonary system in the geriatric population. *Topics in Geriatric Rehabilitation*, 26(2): 93-103.

Hoeger, W., Warner, J., Fahleson, G. (1995). Physiologic responses to self-paced water aerobics and treadmill running. Abstract. *Medicine & Science in Sports & Exercise*, 27(5): 83.

Jentoft, E., Kvalvik, A., Mengshoel, A. (2001). Effects of pool-based and land-based aerobic exercise on women with fibromyalgia/chronic widespread muscle pain. *Arthritis Care and Research*, 45(1): 42-47.

Kennedy, C., Sanders, M. (1995). Strength training gets wet. *IDEA Today*, May: 25-30.

Killgore, G. (2009). Deep-water running: A practical review of the literature with an emphasis on biomechanics. *Physician and Sports Medicine*, 40(1): 116-26. doi:10.3810/psm.2012.02.1958

Kravitz, L. (1994). Getting Creative with Resistance Training. *IDEA Fitness Journal, May: 46-55.*

Loupias, J., Golding, L. (2004). Deep water conditioning: A conditioning alternative. *ACSM's Health and Fitness Journal*, Sept.-Oct.: 5-8.

Mayo, J. (2000). Practical guidelines for the use of deep water running. *Journal of Strength and Conditioning Research*, 22(1): 26-29.

Michaud, T., Brennan, D., Wilder, R., Sherman, N. (1995). Aquarunning and gains in cardiorespiratory fitness. *Journal of Strength and Conditioning Research*, 9(2): 78-84.

Michaud, T., Rodriguez-Zayas, J., Andres, F., Flynn, M., Lambert, C. (1995). Comparative exercise responses of deep-water and treadmill running. *Journal of Strength and Conditioning Research*, 9(2): 104-49.

Nagle, E., Robertson, R., Jakicic, J., Otto, A., Ranalli, J., Chiapetta, L. (2007). Effects of aquatic exercise and walking in sedentary obese women undergoing a behavioral weight-loss intervention. *IJARE* 1: 43-56.

Norton, C., Hoobler, K., Welding, A., Jensen, G.M. (1997). Effectiveness of aquatic exercise in the treatment of women with osteoarthritis. *Journal of Physical Therapy*, 5(3): 8-15.

Quinn, T., Sedory, D., Fisher, B. (1994). Physiological effects of deep water running following a land-based training program. *Research Quarterly in Exercise and Sport*, 65: 386-89.

Raffaelli, M., Lanza, M., Zanolla, L., Zamparo, P. (2010). Exercise intensity of head-out water-based activities (water fitness). *European Journal of Applied Physiology*, 109(5): 829-38.

Rica, R., Carneiro, R., Serra, A., Rodriguez, D., Pontese, F., Bocalini, D. (2012). Effects of water-based exercise in obese older women: Impact of short-term follow-up study on anthropometric, functional fitness and quality of life parameters. *Geriatrics & Gerontology International* 2013, 13(1): 209-14. doi:10.1111/j.1447-0594.2012.00889

Rodriguez, D., Silva, V., Prestes, J., Rica, R., Serra, A., Bocalini, D., Pontes, F. (2011). Hypotensive response after water-walking and land-walking exercise sessions in healthy trained and untrained women. *International Journal of General Medicine*, 4: 549-54.

Rotstein, A., Harush, M., Vaisman, N. (2008). The effect of a water exercise program on bone density of postmenopausal women. *Journal of Sports Medicine and Physical Fitness*, 48(3): 352-59.

Sanders, M. (2010). H2O solutions for active aging. *IDEA Fitness Journal*, Feb.46-53.

Sanders, M., Lawson, D. (2006). Use water's accommodating properties to help clients recovering from knee injuries return to sports. *IDEA Fitness Journal*, Sept.: 40-47.

Sato, D., Kaneda, K., Wakabayashi, H., Nomura, T. (2009). Comparison of 2-year effects of once and twice weekly water exercise on activities of daily living ability of community dwelling frail elderly. *Archives of Gerontology and Geriatrics*, 49(1): 123-28.

Simmons, V., Hansen, P. (1996). Effectiveness of water exercise on postural mobility in the well elderly: An experimental study on balance enhancement. *Journal of Gerontological Medicine and Science*, 51A(5): M233-38.

Suomi, R., Koceja, D.M. (2000). Postural sway characteristics in women with lower extremity arthritis before and after an aquatic exercise intervention. *Archives of Physical Medicine and Rehabilitation*, 8(6): 780-85.

Svedenhag, J., Seger, J. (1992). Running on land and in water: Comparative exercise physiology. *Medicine & Science in Sports & Exercise*, 24: 1155-60.

Takashima, N., Rogers, M., Watanabe, E., Brechue, W., Okada, A., Yamada, T., Islam, M., Hayano, J. (2002). Water-based exercise improves health-related aspects of fitness in older women. *Medicine & Science in Sports & Exercise*, 33(3): 544-51.

Templeton, M.S., Booth, D.L., O'Kelly, W.D. (1996). Effects of aquatic therapy on joint flexibility and functional ability in subjects with rheumatic disease. *Journal of Orthopedic Sports and Physical Therapy*, 23(6): 376-81.

Tsourlou, T., Benik. A., Dipla, K., Zafeiridis, A., Kellis, S. (2006). The effects of a twenty-four week aquatic training program on muscular strength performance in healthy elderly women. *Journal of Strength and Conditioning Research*, 20(4): 811-18.

U.S. Census Bureau. (2010). www.census.gov/prod/2010pubs/p25-1138.pdf

Vogel, A. (2006). What's hot in H2O? *IDEA Fitness Journal*, July-Aug.: 53-59.

Weltman, A. (1995). *The blood lactate response to exercise*. Champaign, IL: Human Kinetics.

Wilbur, R., Moffatt, R., Scott, B., Lee, D., Cucuzzo, N. (1996). Influence of water run training on the maintenance of aerobic performance. *Medicine & Science in Sports & Exercise*, 28(8): 1056-62.

World Health Organization. (2010). *Global health and aging*. www.who.int/ageing/publications/global_health.pdf

Chapter 15

Arpita. (1990). Physiological and psychological effects of hatha yoga: A review. *Journal of the International Association of Yoga Therapists*, 1(I & II): 1-28.

Bijlani, R.L., Vempati, R.P., Yadav, R.K., Ray, R.B., Gupta, V., Sharma, R., Mehta, N., Mahapatra, S.C. (2005). A brief but comprehensive lifestyle education program based on yoga reduces risk factors for cardiovascular disease and diabetes mellitus. *Journal of Alternative and Complementary Medicine*, 11(2): 267-74.

Boehde, D., Porcari, J. (2006). Does yoga really do the body good? *ACE Fitness Matters*, Sept.-Oct.: 7-9.

Carroll, J., Blansit, A., Otto, R.M., Wygand, J.W. (2003). The metabolic requirements of Vinyasa yoga. *Medicine & Science in Sports & Exercise*, 35(5): S155.

Cooper, S., Oberne, J., Newton, S., Harrison, V., Coon, J., Lewis, S., Tattersfield, A. (2003). Effect of two breathing exercises (Buteyko and pranayama) in asthma, a randomized controlled trial. *Thorax*, 58: 674-79.

Faulds, R. (2006). *Kripalu yoga: A guide to practice on and off the mat*. New York: Bantam Dell.

Galantino, M.L., Bzdewka, T.M., Eissler-Russo, J.L., Holbrook, M.L., Mogck, E.P. Geigle, P., Farrar, J.T. (2004). The impact of modified hatha yoga on chronic low back pain: A pilot study. *Alternative Therapy, Health, and Medicine*, 10:56-59.

Hawks, S.R., Hull, M.L., Thalman, R.L., Richins, P.M. (1995). Review of spiritual health: Definition, role, and intervention strategies in health promotion. *American Journal of Health Promotion*, 9(5): 371-78.

IDEA. (2013). 2013 IDEA fitness programs and equipment trends report. *IDEA Fitness Journal*, June: 34-45.

Jacobs, B.P., Mehling, W., Avins, A.L., Goldberg, H.A., Acree, M., Lasater, J.H., Cole, R.J., Riley, D.S., Mauer, S. (2004). Feasibility of conducting a clinical trial on hatha yoga for chronic low back pain: Methodological lesson. 10:80-83.

Javnbakht, M., Hejazi Kenari, R., Ghasemi, M. (2009). Effects of yoga on depression and anxiety of women. *Complementary Therapies in Clinical Practice*, 15(2): 102-4.

Kennedy, J.E., Abbott, R.A., Rosenberg, B.S. (2002). Changes in spirituality and well-being in a retreat program for cardiac patients. *Alternative Therapy, Health, and Medicine*, 8(4): 64-73.

Khalsa, S.B. (2004). Yoga as a therapeutic intervention: A bibliometric analysis of published research studies. *Indian Journal of Physiology and Pharmacology*, 48(3): 269-85.

Khalsa, S.B., Hickey-Schultz, L., Cohen, D., Steiner, N., Cope, S. (2012). Evaluation of the mental health benefits of yoga in a secondary school: A preliminary randomized controlled trial. *Journal of Behavioral Health Services and Research*, 39(1): 80-90.

Kim, S., Singh, H., Smith, J., Chrisman, C., Bemben, M., Bemben, D. (2011). Effects of an 8-month yoga intervention on bone markers and muscle strength in premenopausal women. Abstract. *Medicine & Science in Sports & Exercise*, 43(5): S865.

Kristal, A., Littman, A., Benitez, D., White, E. (2005). Yoga practice is associated with attenuated weight gain in healthy middle-aged men and women. *Alternative Therapy, Health, and Medicine*, 11(4): 28-33.

Lamb, T. (2004). Psychophysiological effects of yoga. International Association of Yoga Therapists. www.iayt.org

Mustian, K.M., Sprod, L., Peppone, L., Janelsins, M., Wharton, M., Webb, J., Esparaz, B., Kirschner, J., Morrow, G. (2011). Yoga significantly improves fatigue and circadian rhythm: A randomized, controlled trial among 410 cancer survivors. Abstract. *Medicine & Science in Sports & Exercise*, 43(5): S2750.

Ornish, D. (1998). *Love and Survival*. New York: Harper Collins.

Ornish, D., Brown, S.E., Scherwitz, L.W., Billings, J.H., Armstrong, W.T., Ports, T.A., McLanahan, S.M., Kirkeeide, R., Brand, R., Gould, K. (1990). Can lifestyle changes reverse coronary heart disease? The lifestyle heart trial. *Lancet*, 336: 129-33.

Rana, B.B., Pant, P.R., Pant, K.D., Balkrishna, A., Paygan, S. (2011). Effect of bhastrika pranayama and exercise on lung function capacity of athletes: A pilot study. Abstract. *Medicine & Science in Sports & Exercise*, 43(5): S2192.

Ross, A., Thomas, S. (2010). The health benefits of yoga and exercise: A review of comparison studies. *Journal of Alternative and Complementary Medicine*, 16(1): 3-12.

Schmid, A.A., Miller, K.K., Van Puymbroeck, M., Dierks, T.A., Altenburger, P., Schalk, N., Williams, L.S., DeBaun, E., Damush, T. (2012). Physical improvements after yoga for people with chronic stroke. Abstract. *Medicine & Science in Sports & Exercise*, 44(5): S1654.

Sherman, K.J., Cherkin, D.C., Erro, J., Miglioretti, D.L., Deyo, R.A. (2005). Comparing yoga, exercise, and a self-care book for chronic low-back pain: A randomized controlled trial. *Annals of Internal Medicine*, 143(12): 849-56.

Tran, M.D., Holly, R.G., Lashbrook, J., Amsterdam, E.A. (2001). Effects of yoga practice on the health-related aspects of physical fitness. *Preventive Cardiology*, 4(4): 165-70.

Vizcaino, M., King, G.A. (2012). Effect of yoga on anxiety, psychological stress, and cortisol of type 2 diabetes mellitus patients. *Medicine & Science in Sports & Exercise*, 44(5): S2034.

Wang, M.Y., Yu, S.Y., Haines, M., Hashish, R., Samarawickrame, S. Greendale, G., Salem, G. (2012). Can yoga improve balance performance in older adults? Abstract. *Medicine & Science in Sports & Exercise*, 44(5): S1675.

Williams, K.A., Petronis, J., Smith, D., Goodrich, D., Wu, J., Ravi, N., Doyle, R., Juckett, G., Kolar, M., Gross, R. (2005). Effect of Iyengar yoga therapy for chronic low back pain. *Pain*, 115: 107-17.

Williams, K., Steinberg, L, Petronis, J. (2003). Therapeutic application of Iyengar yoga for healing chronic low back pain. *International Journal of Yoga Therapy*, 13: 55-67.

Yoke, M., Kennedy, C. (2004) *Functional exercise progressions*. Monterey, CA: Healthy Learning.

Chapter 16

Amorim, T., Sousa, F., Machado, L., Santos, J.A. (2011). Effects of Pilates training on muscular strength and balance in ballet dancers. *Portuguese Journal of Sports Sciences*, 11(2): 147-50.

Anderson, B.D., Spector, A. (2000). Introduction to Pilates-based rehabilitation. *Orthopaedic Physical Therapy Clinics of North America*, 9(3): 395-410.

Bernardo, L.M. (2007). The effectiveness of Pilates training in healthy adults: An appraisal of the research literature. *Journal of Bodywork and Movement Therapies*, 11: 106-10.

Cholewicki, J., Panjabi, M.M., Khachatryan, A. (1997). Stabilizing function of trunk flexor-extensor muscles around a neutral spine posture. *Spine*, 22(19): 2207-12.

Herrington, L., Davies, R. (2005). The influence of Pilates training on the ability to contract the transverse abdominis muscle in asymtomatic individuals.

Journal of Bodywork and Movement Therapies, 9(1): 52-57.

Hodges, P.C., Richardson, C., Jull, G. (1996) Evaluation of the relationship between laboratory and clinical tests of transverse abdominis function. *Physiotherapy Research International*, 1(4): 269.

IDEA. (2011). 2013 IDEA fitness programs and equipment trends Report. *IDEA Fitness Journal*, June: 34-45.

Johnson, E.G., Larsen, A., Ozawa, H., Wilson, C.A., Kennedy, K.L. (2007). The effects of Pilates-based exercise on dynamic balance in healthy adults. *Journal of Bodywork and Movement Therapies*, 11(3): 238-42.

Kloubec, J.A. (2010). Pilates for the improvement of muscle endurance, flexibility, balance, and posture. *Journal of Strength and Conditioning Research*, 24(3): 661-67.

Lim, E.C.W., Poh, R.L.C., Low, A.Y., Wong, W.P. (2011). Effects of Pilates-based exercises on pain and disability in individuals with persistent, non-specific low back pain: A systematic review with meta-analysis. *Journal of Orthopaedic and Sports Physical Therapy*, 41(2): 70-80.

McGill, S. (2007). *Low back disorders, 2nd ed.* Champaign, IL: Human Kinetics.

Norris, C.M. (2000) *Back stability*. Champaign, IL: Human Kinetics.

Olson, M., Smith, C.M. (2005). Pilates exercise: Lessons from the lab: A new research study examines the effectiveness and safety of selected Pilates mat exercises. *IDEA Fitness Journal*, Nov.-Dec.: 38-43.

Olson, M., Williford, H., Martin, R., Ellis, M., Woolen, E., Esco, M. (2004). The energy cost of a basic, intermediate, and advanced Pilates mat workout. *Medicine & Science in Sports & Exercise*, 36(6): S357.

Otto, R., Yoke, M., McLaughlin, K., Morrill, J., Viola, A., Lail, A., Lagomarsine, M., Wygand, J. (2004). The effect of 12 weeks of Pilates training versus resistance training on trained females. Abstract. *Medicine & Science in Sports & Exercise*, 36(5): S356-57.

Pilates, J.H. (1945). *Pilates' return to life through contrology*. Available from Balanced Body: 800-PILATES.

Pilates Method Alliance. (2006). *PMA position statement: On Pilates*. Miami, FL: Pilates Method Alliance.

Rogers, K.V., Gibson, A.L. (2005). Effects of an 8-week mat Pilates training program on body composition, flexibility, and muscular endurance. (Unpublished master's thesis). Department of Sport and Exercise Science, Barry University, Miami Shores, FL.

Schroeder, J.M. Crussemeyer, J.A., Newton, S.J. (2002). Flexibility and heart rate response to an acute Pilates reformer session. *Medicine & Science in Sports & Exercise*, 34(5): S258.

Segal, N.A., Hein, J., Basford, J.R. (2004). The effects of Pilates training on flexibility and body composition: An observational study. *Archives of Physical and Medical Rehabilitation*, 85(12): 1977-81.

Shedden, M., Kravitz, L. (2006). Pilates exercise: A research-based review. *Journal of Dance Medicine & Science*, 10: 111-16.

Yoke, M., Kennedy, C. (2004). *Functional exercise progressions*. Monterey, CA: Healthy Learning.

Chapter 17

Aerobics and Fitness Association of America (AFAA) (2010), *Exercise Standards and Guidelines Reference Manual*, AFAA, Sherman Oaks, CA.

Anders, M. (2006). Budokon: Beyond fusion. *ACE Fitness Matters* May-June:6-9.

Asp, K. (2006). Group training, stroller-based exercise programs. *ACE Certified News*, Dec.-Jan.: 6-8.

Chodzko-Zajko, W., Beattie, L., Chow, R., Firman, J., Jahnke, R., Park, C., Rosengren, K., Sheppard, L., Yang, Y. (2006). Qi gong and tai chi: Promoting practices that promote healthy aging. *Journal on Active Aging*, Sept.-Oct.: 50-56.

Church, T., Thomas, D., Tudor-Locke, C., Katzmarzyk, P., Earnest, C., Rodarte, R., Martin, C. Blair, S., Bouchard, C. (2011). Trends over the 5 decades in U.S. occupation-related physical activity and their associations with obesity. *PLoS ONE*, 6(5): e19657. doi:10.1371/journal.pone.0019657

Davies, A. (2006). Baby steps. *IDEA Fitness Journal*, Nov.-Dec.: 86-88.

Gerard, J. (2006). Shake, lead and other new ways to get fit. *ACE Fitness Matters*, July-Aug.: 6-8.

Hoffman-Smith, K., Ma, A., Cheng-Tsung, Y., DeGuire, N., Smith, J. (2009). The effect of tai chi in reducing anxiety in an ambulatory population. *Journal of Complementary & Integrative Medicine*, 6(1): 1553-3840.

Holmes, M., Chen, W., Feskanich, D., Kroecke, C., Colditz, G. (2005). Physical activity and survival after breast cancer diagnosis. *Journal of the American Medical Association*, 293(20): 2479-86.

Holthusen, J., Porcari, J., Foster, C., Doberstein, S., Anders, M. (2011). ACE-sponsored research:

Hooping—effective workout or child's play? *ACE Certified News*, Jan.

Hooker, S. (2003). The exercise professional's expanding role in promoting physical activity and the public's health. *ACSM's Health and Fitness Journal*, May-June: 7-11.

IDEA Health and Fitness Association. (2011). *IDEA code of ethics: Group fitness instructors*, April: 8:4.

Kahn, J. (2008). What's shaking. *Boston Globe*, Jan.8.

Keller, J. (2008). Group energy. *IDEA Fitness Journal*, Jan.: 87.

Lan, C., Lai, J., Chen, S., Wong., M. (1998). 12-month tai chi training in the elderly: Its effect on health fitness. *Medicine & Science in Sports & Exercise*, 39(3): 345-51.

Lane, C. 2000. *Christy Lane's complete book of line dancing.* 2nd ed. Champaign, IL: Human Kinetics.

Li, F., Harmer, P., McAuley, E., Chaumeton, N., Eckstrom, E., Wilson, N. (2005). Tai chi and fall reductions in older adults: A randomized controlled trial. *Journal of Gerontology, Medicine, and Science*, 60A: 66-74.

Ludwig, J., A. VanGelder, J.W. Wygand, and R.M. Otto. (1994). The metabolic cost of fixed slideboard exercise at two different board lengths. Abstract. *Med Sci Sports Exerc* 26(5): S55.

Luettgen, M., Foster, C., Doberstein, S., Mikat, R., Porcari, J. (2012). Letter to the editor. *Journal of Sports Science and Medicine*, 11: 357-58.

McGlone, C., L. Kravitz, and J. Janot. (2002). Rebounding: A low-impact exercise alternative. *ACSM Health and Fitness Journal* 6(2): 11-5.

Melanson, E.L., Freedson, P.S., Webb, R., Jungbluth, S., Kozlowski, N. (1996). Exercise responses to running and in-line skating at self-selected paces. *Medicine & Science in Sports & Exercise*, 28(2): 247-50.

Nichols, J.F., C.L. Sherman, and E. Abbott. 2000. Treading is new and hot. *ACSM Health and Fitness Journal* 4(2): 12-7.

Otto, R.M., Maniguet, E., Peters, A., Boutagy, N., Gabbard, A., Wygand, J.W., Yoke M. (2011). The energy cost of Zumba exercise. Abstract. *Medicine & Science in Sports & Exercise*, 43(5): S1923.

Perez, B., Robinson, P., Herlong, K. (2011). *Instructor training manual: Zumba fitness.* Hollywood, FL: Zumba Fitness.

Pillarella, D. 1997. Ready, set, row! *IDEA Today* 15(8): 36-43.

Porcari, J.P. (1999). Pump up your walk. *ACSM's Health and Fitness Journal*, 3(1): 25-29.

Rosas, D., Rosas, C. (2006). NIA: The body's way. *IDEA Fitness Journal*, 3(2): 89-91.

Sallis, J., Cervero, R., Ascher, W., Henderson, K., Kraft, M., Kerr, J. (2006). An ecological approach to creating active living communities. *Annual Review of Public Health*, 27: 297-322.

Scheett, T., Aartun, J., Thomas, D., Herrin, J., Dudgeon, W. (2010). Physiological markers as a gauge of intensity for suspension training exercise. *Medicine & Science in Sports & Exercise*, 42(5): S2636.

Tharrett, S., Peterson, J. (2012). *Fitness Management.* 3rd edition. Monterey, CA: Healthy Learning.

Thompson, W. (2012). Worldwide survey of fitness trends for 2013. *ACSM's Health and Fitness Journal*, 16(6): 8-17.

van der Ploeg, H, Chey, T, Korda, R., Banks, E., Bauman, A. (2012). Sitting time and all-cause mortality risk in 222,487 Australian adults. *Archives of Internal Medicine*, 172(6): 494-500.

Wahbeh, H., Elsas, S., Oken, B. (2008). Mind–body interventions. *Neurology*, 70(24): 2321-28.

Walach, H., Ferrari, M., Sauer, S., Kohls, N. (2012). Mind-body practices in integrative medicine. *Religions*, 3(1), 50-81.

Wang, C., Schmid, C., Rones, R., Kalish, R., Yinh, J., Goldenberg, D., Lee, Y., McAlindon, T. (2010). A randomized trial of tai chi for fibromyalgia. *New England Journal of Medicine*, 363:743-54.

Webb, M. (2006). Group training series: Reebok core board. *ACE Certified News* February-March:6-8.

Webb, M. 2005. Group training series: BOSU. *ACE Certified News* October-November:6-8.

Williams, A. (2012). Group fitness must haves. *IDEA Fitness Journal*, 9(7): 70-77.

Williford, H.N., N. Wang, M. Scharff-Olson, D.L. Blessing, and J. Buzbee. (1993). Energy expenditure of slideboard exercise training. Abstract. *Med Sci Sports Exerc* 25(5): S621.

Wolever, R., Bobinet, K., McCabe, K. MacKenzie, E. (2012). Effective and viable mind-body stress reduction in the workplace: A randomized control trial. *Journal of Occupational Health Psychology*, 17(2): 246-58.

Young, D., L. Appel, S. Jee, and E. Miller. (1999). The effects of aerobic exercise and t'ai chi on blood pressure in older people: Results of a randomized trial. *J Am Geriatr Soc* 47(3): 277-84.

Zumba Fitness. (2011). Instructor training manual. www.zumba.com/en-US/training/type.

Index

Page numbers ending in an *f* or a *t* indicate a figure or table, respectively.

About the Authors

Carol Kennedy-Armbruster, PhD, is a senior lecturer in the school of public health in the department of kinesiology at Indiana University at Bloomington. During her more than 30 years of teaching and training fitness leaders, she has served on the American Council on Exercise (ACE) and the American College of Sports Medicine (ACSM) credentialing committees, and she chaired the IDEA Water Fitness Committee. Her research interests are translational research for physical activity and functional movement experiences for an over-40 population.

Certified through ACE as a group fitness instructor, ACSM as a health fitness instructor, and FMS as a functional movement specialist, Kennedy-Armbruster is a regular presenter at fitness conferences. At Indiana University, she managed the recreational sport fitness and wellness program that included more than 100 group exercise sessions per week before moving to the department of kinesiology to assist with the creation of the health fitness specialist undergraduate major.

Kennedy-Armbruster earned her bachelor's degree in leisure studies from the University of Illinois and her master's degree in exercise and sport science from Colorado State University. She completed her PhD in human performance at Indiana University while working with a military over-40 population. She has created and taught methods of group leadership classes at three major universities and continues to engage in and lead group movement experiences.

Kennedy-Armbruster and her family reside in Greenwood, Indiana. She enjoys outdoor activities, biking, tennis, reading, traveling, and spending time with her family and friends.

Mary M. Yoke, MA, MM, has more than 30 years of experience teaching and training group exercise leaders. In addition to leading group exercise classes on a regular basis, she is a lecturer in the school of public health in the department of kinesiology at Indiana University at Bloomington, where she teaches several undergraduate courses in exercise leadership. She is an adjunct board member and master trainer for the Aerobics and Fitness Association of America (AFAA) and served on the American College of Sports Medicine (ACSM) credentialing committee for six years. She is an associate editor for ACSM's Health & Fitness journal.

Yoke has led seminars for fitness professionals in Europe, Asia, Africa, and South America. She gives numerous presentations throughout the United States to both fitness professionals and the general public and is a regular presenter at fitness conferences. She is the author of three other books on fitness as well as three videos.

Yoke has obtained 22 certifications from organizations such as the ACSM, AFAA, American Council on Exercise (ACE), National Academy of Sports Medicine (NASM), and Stott Pilates. She received her master's degree in exercise physiology from Adelphi University, where she has coauthored several research studies on group exercise. Yoke also holds a bachelor's and master's degree in music. She is a former opera singer and an accomplished classical pianist. Yoke enjoys hiking, biking, reading, cooking, and traveling.

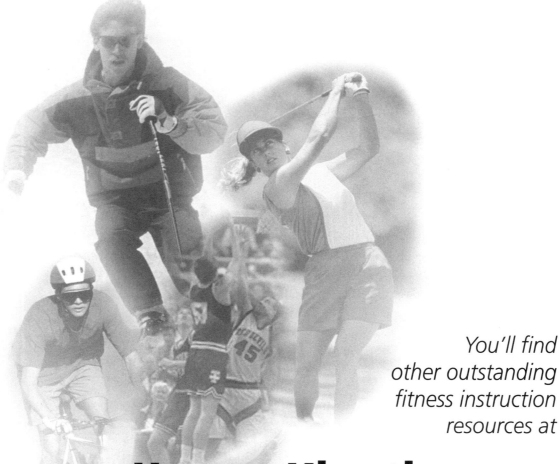

*You'll find
other outstanding
fitness instruction
resources at*

www.HumanKinetics.com

In the U.S. call

1-800-747-4457

Australia...08 8372 0999
Canada 1-800-465-7301
Europe...+44 (0) 113 255 5665
New Zealand...0800 222 062

HUMAN KINETICS
The Information Leader in Physical Activity & Health
P.O. Box 5076 • Champaign, IL 61825-5076 USA